ADVANCES IN

Pediatrics®

VOLUME 48

ADVANCES IN

Pediatrics®

VOLUMES 1 THROUGH 44 (OUT OF PRINT)

VOLUME 45

VOLUME 46

Testing for Cancer Susceptibility Genes in Children, *by Renata Laxova*

Effects of Fitness Training on Endocrine Systems in Children and Adolescents, *by David B. Allen*

Genetic Errors of Sexual Differentiation, *by Allen W. Root*

Advances in the Recognition and Treatment of Endocrine Complications in Children With Chronic Illness, *by Philip Scott Zeitler, Sharon Travers, and Michael S. Kappy*

Leptin: Molecular Biology, Physiology, and Relevance to Pediatric Practice, *by Frank B. Diamond, Jr and Duane C. Eichler*

Newer Pediatric Pathogens, *by Sheldon L. Kaplan*

Viral Hepatitis: Expanding the Alphabet, *by Jay A. Hochman and William F. Balistreri*

Parvovirus Infections in Children and Adults, *by James D. Cherry*

Syndromes Associated With Immunodeficiency, *by Jeffrey E. Ming, E. Richard Stiehm, and John M. Graham*

Protective Nutrients and Bacterial Colonization in the Immature Human Gut, *by Dingwei Dai and W. Allan Walker*

Umbilical Cord Blood Banking, *by Bertram H. Lubin, Marianna Eraklis, and Gina Apicelli*

Hydrops Fetalis: Lysosomal Storage Disorders *In Extremis, by Deborah L. Stone and Ellen Sidransky*

Overgrowth Syndromes: An Update, *by M. Michael Cohen, Jr*

Recent Advances in Canavan Disease, *by Reuben Matalon and Kimberlee MichalsMatalon*

Advances in Pediatric Pharmacology, Toxicology, and Therapeutics, *by Cheston M. Berlin, Jr*

VOLUME 47

Inborn Errors of Cholesterol Biosynthesis, *by Richard I. Kelley*

Atherogenesis in Children: Implications for the Prevention of Atherosclerosis, *by Robert E. Olson*

Improving the Health of Patients With Cystic Fibrosis Through Newborn Screening, *by Philip M. Farrell and the Wisconsin Cystic Fibrosis Neonatal Screening Study Group*

Cyclic Vomiting Syndrome: Evolution in Our Understanding of a Brain-Gut Disorder *by B U. K. Li and Jane P. Balint*

Childhood Migraine, *by William R. Turk*

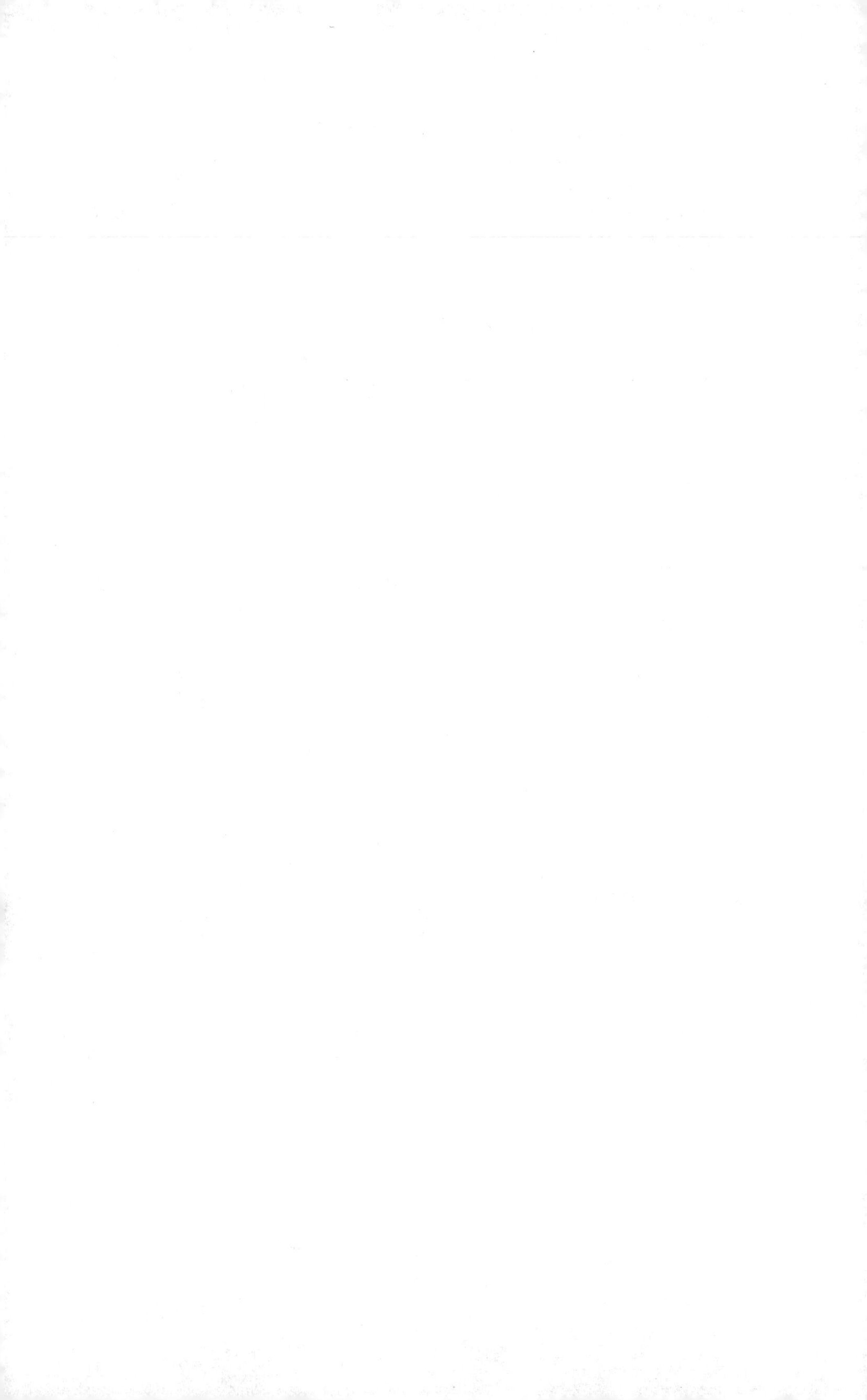

ADVANCES IN

Pediatrics®

VOLUME 48

Editor-in-Chief
Lewis A. Barness, MD
Professor, Department of Pediatrics, University of South Florida College of Medicine, Tampa

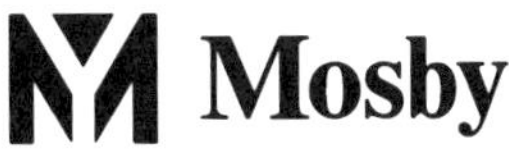

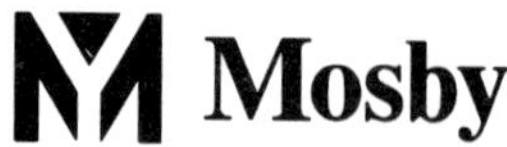

Publisher: Cynthia Baudendistel
Managing Editor: Colleen Cook
Manager, Literature Services and Continuity Editing: Idelle Winer
Production Editor: Amanda Maguire
Project Supervisor, Production: Joy Moore
Composition Specialist: Betty Dockins
Illustrations and Permissions Coordinator: Chidi C. Ukabam

Printed in the United States of America
Printing/binding by The Maple-Vail Book Manufacturing Group

Editorial Office:
Mosby, Inc.
11830 Westline Industrial Drive
St. Louis, Missouri 63146

International Standard Serial Number: 0065-3101
International Standard Book Number: 0-323-01526-3

Associate Editors

Darryl C. DeVivo, MD
Sidney Carter Professor of Neurology, Professor of Pediatrics, Columbia University College of Physicians and Surgeons; Director, Colleen Giblin Research Laboratories, Attending Neurologist and Pediatrician, Neurological Institute and Babies Hospital, Presbyterian Hospital, New York

Michael M. Kaback, MD
Professor, Departments of Pediatrics and Reproductive Medicine, University of California, San Diego School of Medicine; Chief, Division of Medical Genetics, Department of Pediatrics, University of California, San Diego

Grant Morrow III, MD
Professor, Department of Pediatrics, The Ohio State University College of Medicine; Medical Director, Children's Research Institute, Columbus

Abraham M. Rudolph, MD
Professor of Pediatrics Emeritus, Senior Staff, Cardiovascular Research Institute, University of California, San Francisco

Walter W. Tunnessen, Jr, MD
Senior Vice President, American Board of Pediatrics; Clinical Professor of Pediatrics, University of North Carolina School of Medicine, Chapel Hill

Contributors

Agatino Battaglia, MD
Adjunct Professor of Child Neuropsychiatry, Attending Neurologist and Pediatrician, Division of Child Neurology and Psychiatry, University of Pisa, Italy; Head, Center for the Study of Congenital Malformation Syndromes of Neuropsychiatric Interest, Stella Maris Clinical Research Institute, Pisa, Italy

Cheston M. Berlin, Jr, MD
University Professor of Pediatrics, and Professor of Pharmacology, The Pennsylvania State University College of Medicine, M.S. Hershey Medical Center, Hershey, Pa

Carol D. Berkowitz, MD
Professor of Clinical Pediatrics, University of California Los Angeles School of Medicine; Executive Vice Chair, Department of Pediatrics, Harbor-University of California Los Angeles Medical Center, Torrance

Mary E. Blue, PhD
Associate Professor of Neurology and Neuroscience, the Neuroscience Laboratory, Kennedy Krieger Institute and Johns Hopkins University School of Medicine, Baltimore, Md

Jane C. Burns, MD
Chief, Division of Allergy and Immunology, Professor, Department of Pediatrics, University of California San Diego School of Medicine, La Jolla

John C. Carey, MD
Professor of Pediatrics, University of Utah; Attending Clinical Geneticist, Division of Medical Genetics, Department of Pediatrics, University of Utah Health Sciences Center, Salt Lake City

Ka Wah Chan, MBBS, FRCPC
Professor of Pediatrics, The University of Texas M.D. Anderson Cancer Center, Houston

Frank B. Diamond, Jr, MD
Professor of Pediatrics, University of South Florida College of Medicine, Tampa

Cara B. Ebbeling, PhD
Instructor in Pediatrics, Harvard Medical School; Research Associate, Division of Endocrinology, Children's Hospital, Boston, Mass

Beverly S. Emanuel, PhD
Professor of Pediatrics, University of Pennsylvania School of Medicine; Charles E.M. Upham Professor of Pediatrics, Chief, Division of Human Genetics and Molecular Biology, The Children's Hospital of Philadelphia, Philadelphia

Maria Gieron-Korthals, MD
Professor, Departments of Pediatrics and Neurology, University of South Florida, Tampa; Program Director, Pediatric Neurology, Tampa General Hospital, Tampa

Karen Harum, MD
Instructor of Pediatrics, Division of Neurology and Developmental Medicine, the Neuroscience Laboratory, Kennedy Krieger Institute and Johns Hopkins University School of Medicine, Baltimore, Md

Julien I.E. Hoffman, MD, FRCP
Professor of Pediatrics (Emeritus), Attending Pediatric Cardiologist, Moffitt-Long Hospitals, University of California Medical Center, San Francisco

Michael V. Johnston, MD
Professor of Neurology and Pediatrics, Division of Neurology and Developmental Medicine, the Neuroscience Laboratory, Kennedy Krieger Institute and Johns Hopkins University School of Medicine, Baltimore, Md

Atilano G. Lacson, MD, FRCPC
Clinical Associate Professor, Departments of Pathology and Pediatrics, University of South Florida, Tampa; Staff Pathologist, All Children's Hospital, St Petersburg, Fla

Peter Lee, MD
Fellow, Division of Pediatric Gastroenterology and Nutrition, Children's Hospital Medical Center, Cincinnati, OH

Alexander K. C. Leung, MBBS, FRCPC, FRCP (UK & Irel), FRCPCH, FAAP
Clinical Associate Professor of Pediatrics, The University of Calgary; Pediatric Consultant, Alberta Children's Hospital, Calgary, Alberta, Canada

David S. Ludwig, MD, PhD
Assistant Professor in Pediatrics, Harvard Medical School; Director, Obesity Program, Division of Endocrinology, Children's Hospital, Boston, Mass

Marilyn J. Manco-Johnson, MD
Professor of Pediatrics, University of Colorado Health Sciences Center; Director, Mountain States Regional Hemophilia and Thrombosis Center, Aurora, Colo

Donna McDonald-McGinn, MS
Associate Director, Division of Clinical Genetics, The Children's Hospital of Philadelphia, Philadelphia, Pa

O. Thomas Mueller, PhD
Associate Professor of Pediatrics, University of South Florida; Director, Molecular Genetics Laboratory, All Children's Hospital, St Petersburg, Fla

Akira Nishimura, MD, PhD
Postdoctoral Fellow, Division of Neurology and Developmental Medicine, the Neuroscience Laboratory, Kennedy Krieger Institute and Johns Hopkins University School of Medicine, Baltimore, Md; Assistant Professor, Kyoto Prefectural University, Kyoto, Japan

Rachelle Nuss, MD
Associate Professor of Pediatrics, University of Colorado School of Medicine; Associate Director, Mountain States Regional Hemophilia and Thrombosis Center, University of Colorado Health Sciences Center, Aurora

James Pekar, PhD
Assistant Professor of Radiology, F.M. Kirby Center for Functional Brain Imaging, Kennedy Krieger Institute and Johns Hopkins University School of Medicine, Baltimore, Md

Wm. Lane M. Robson, MD, FRCP(C), FRCP (Glasg) FAACP
Chief of Pediatrics, Memorial Hospital of Rhode Island; Professor of Pediatrics, Brown University, Providence

Colin D. Rudolph, MD, PhD
Professor of Pediatrics, Medical College of Wisconsin, Chief, Pediatric Gastroenterology and Nutrition, Children's Hospital of Wisconsin, Milwaukee, Wis

Sulagna C. Saitta, MD, PhD
Assistant Professor of Pediatrics, The University of Pennsylvania School of Medicine; Attending Physician, The Children's Hospital of Philadelphia, Philadelphia, Pa

Janet E. Stockard-Pope, MS, CCC-A
Instructor, Department of Pediatrics, University of South Florida, Tampa

Tracy J. Wright, PhD
Postdoctoral Research Associate, Genomics Group, Life Sciences Division, Los Alamos National Laboratory, Los Alamos, NM, and Department of Human Genetics, University of Utah, Salt Lake City

Elaine H. Zackai, MD
Professor of Pediatrics, University of Pennsylvania School of Medicine; Director of Clinical Genetics, The Children's Hospital of Philadelphia, Philadelphia, Pa

Preface

Determining the meaning of the genome is an exciting achievement, but looking at the shape of a person's head to determine character, as practitioners of the 19th century art of phrenology claimed to do, is an even more astounding feat. In a fascinating article in this volume, Johnston, Nishimura, Harum, Pekar, and Blue describe why bumps on the head are still significant today. Sculpting the developing brain should be the start of further exciting studies.

First recorded in 1965, DiGeorge syndrome has since been cited in more than 400,000 instances and is associated with the most common chromosomal deletion in humans. Emanuel, McDonald-McGinn, Saitta, and Zackai thoroughly describe the phenotypic variations of this syndrome.

Until recently, Wolf-Hirschhorn syndrome was genetically and clinically confused. In their article, Battaglia, Carey, and Wright clarify many of its features. Proper recognition may lead to a better than expected outcome.

Prolonged QT interval has emerged as one of the most frightening cardiac threats. This channelopathy has been recognized as a cause of sudden death and perhaps sudden infant death. Hoffman discusses its manifestations, treatment, pathophysiology, and genetics.

Burns' discussion of the origin of Kawasaki disease reads like a novel; this is followed with new data on possible etiologies and treatment of the disease.

Much has been written on the epidemic of obesity in children worldwide. Ebbeling and Ludwig indicate that relatively simple dietary modifications may result in effective prevention and possible treatment.

The relationship of fetal growth to adult diseases has resulted in sophisticated studies of fetal growth. Diamond summarizes the late effects of fetal growth and then expands on the important factors influencing growth of the fetus and suggests the possibility of modification.

Lacson, Gieron-Korthals, and Mueller describe the peripheral neuropathies in the very young. Early recognition of these may be lifesaving to parents when definitive prognosis is provided.

Stockard-Pope shocks us with the statistic that "the prevalence of hearing impairment in infancy exceeds that of all other handicapping conditions for which mandated neonatal screening programs exist."(!!!) She stimulates us with the fascinating story of the development of hearing and its significance for other aspects of development.

Lee and Rudolph collate information on treatment of gastroesophageal reflux, its complications, and most impressively, its pathogenesis. They provide tips on indications for concern on this common phenomenon.

One must be fortified to read Berkowitz' description of fatal child neglect. The numbers are overwhelming.

A major expansion has occurred in observations of thrombophilia in infants and children. Experts in the field, Manco-Johnson and Nuss summarize known causes and treatment and approaches to diagnosis and prevention.

Recognition and prevention of iron-deficiency anemia give Alexander Leung and Ka Wah Chan an opportunity to summarize the new tests for earlier diagnosis.

Strange as it seems, Robson explores the genetics of enuresis and follows with exposition of effective treatment and thoughtful consideration.

Berlin has again beautifully reviewed the important drugs that have appeared or newly used in the last few years. This year, he especially emphasizes the proper use of many of these drugs.

We are anticipating with excitement the advances for the next volume.

Lewis A. Barness, MD

Contents

CHAPTER 1

Sculpting the Developing Brain

Michael V. Johnston, MD
Professor of Neurology and Pediatrics, Division of Neurology and Developmental Medicine, the Neuroscience Laboratory, Kennedy Krieger Institute and Johns Hopkins University School of Medicine, Baltimore, Md

Akira Nishimura, MD, PhD
Postdoctoral Fellow, Division of Neurology and Developmental Medicine, the Neuroscience Laboratory, Kennedy Krieger Institute and Johns Hopkins University School of Medicine, Baltimore, Md; Assistant Professor, Kyoto Prefectural University, Kyoto, Japan

Karen Harum, MD
Instructor of Pediatrics, Division of Neurology and Developmental Medicine, the Neuroscience Laboratory, Kennedy Krieger Institute and Johns Hopkins University School of Medicine, Baltimore, Md

James Pekar, PhD
Assistant Professor of Radiology, F.M. Kirby Center for Functional Brain Imaging, Kennedy Krieger Institute and Johns Hopkins University School of Medicine, Baltimore, Md

Mary E. Blue, PhD
Assistant Professor of Neurology and Neuroscience, the Neuroscience Laboratory, Kennedy Krieger Institute and Johns Hopkins University School of Medicine, Baltimore, Md

ABSTRACT

The developing brain experiences major construction during fetal life and for at least the first decade of childhood. Many more neurons and synaptic connections are produced than are needed for later function, and the mature brain is what remains after these excess building materials are "sculpted" away. This process is thought to be the basis for the developing brain's plasticity, or the capacity to adapt its behavior and circuitry to stimulation from the external environment. Plastic reorganization of the brain is now being studied in children and adults with new noninvasive tools such as functional brain magnetic resonance imaging. This exploratory tool and other new clinical methods demonstrate how the brain's functional "maps" undergo major reorganization in response to early environmental changes. The neurobiology of brain reorganization during development is also being studied with use of new insights into the molecular mechanisms for activity-dependent neuronal plasticity. Clinical disorders such as lead poisoning, metabolic and epileptic encephalopathies, and psychosocial deprivation may arise from disrupted brain plasticity. Several mental retardation syndromes and cognitive disorders recently recognized as being secondary to genetic disruption of intracellular signaling cascades may also disrupt this process. Understanding how the brain's circuitry is sculpted during development provides an important perspective for thinking about neurodevelopmental disorders.

Cognitive and motor development of infants and children reflects a brain that is under construction.[1] Although this process has often been considered to resemble a stepwise incremental process similar to construction of a building, recent neurobiologic evidence suggests that it is more like the sculpting of a statue. During fetal and postnatal development, more neurons and synaptic connections between neurons are produced than are needed to construct a mature brain.[2] Through the processes of programmed cell death and activity-dependent synaptic plasticity, these excess building materials (neurons and synaptic connections) are sculpted away or "pruned" to form the mature nervous system. For example, it is estimated that the cerebral cortex of a 2-year-old child contains nearly twice as many synapses as the adult.[3] This implies that during childhood, half of these synapses must be eliminated while the other half are preserved. This sculpting process may be heavily influenced by the child's experiences, parental influences, schooling, and other environmental influences as well as genetic programs.[4]

The major end product of all this scultping in the brain is a series of interwoven functional "brain maps."[5] Much of the brain, and especially the cerebral cortex, is organized by function into relatively discrete topographic "maps" that resemble the organization of different continents or countries on a globe. A major difference in topography between the brain and the globe is that cortical surface of the mature human brain is organized in sulci and gyri.

These maps include networks of neurons, often distributed among several regions, that are activated to serve special functions such as decoding or expressing language, perceiving sensory input from the fingers during typing or playing the piano, listening to music, or executing motor acts like hitting a baseball. Spatially organized maps in the brain help us find our way to work in the morning or find our car in a parking garage, and they help children learn to distinguish parents from strangers and learn to read. Even abstract cognitive tasks are thought to be executed by neuronal circuits organized spatially in maps.[6] The sculpting that unfolds during brain development can be thought of as shaping and refining these maps in response to patterned electrical stimulation provided by the primary senses. This spatial, topographic organization of the brain has turned out to be fortunate for clinical researchers in the new area of functional brain imaging, which visualizes the regions of the brain that are activated during specific tasks.[7] The relatively stable organization of functional maps from 1 person to another allows changes in them to be studied with computerized functional imaging methods. On the other hand, all the information available about brain development tells us that each person's maps are likely to be slightly different from everyone else. In a sense, one's brain, especially the cerebral cortex, is a complex, sculpted map of the world one has experienced over the years. Understanding the neurobiologic processes that shape developing neuronal circuits provides an important perspective on normal development as well as on the diagnosis and therapy for neurodevelopmental disorders.

THE SYNAPTIC "POWER CURVE"

In addition to its much larger size and complexity, 1 of the major features that distinguishes the developing human brain from that of other species is its massive cerebral cortex.[8] It is responsible for much of the neurobehavioral repertoire that makes us human. The thin sheet of neurons and synaptic connections and supporting glia that forms the cortex is folded into gyri and sulci to allow it to fit within the confines of the human skull.[8] The massive wave of neurogenesis, programmed cell death, and migration that creates the cerebral cortex is mostly complete by the third trimester of gestation, and the postnatal spurt in brain growth reflects the elaboration of axons, dendrites, and synapses as well as myelination.[9-11] Careful counting of synapses in the developing human postmortem brain indicates that several cortical areas including the frontal and occipital cortex have nearly twice as many synapses from the ages of approximately 2 to 10 years than at birth or in adulthood (Fig 1).[3,12] A similar profile of overproduction of cortical synapses and neurotransmitter receptors has been reported during development in rhesus monkeys.[13,14]

Positron emission tomography (PET) with the tracer 2-deoxy-2[18F]fluoro-D-glucose (FDG) and markers for regional cerebral blood flow have developed over more than 4 decades into powerful

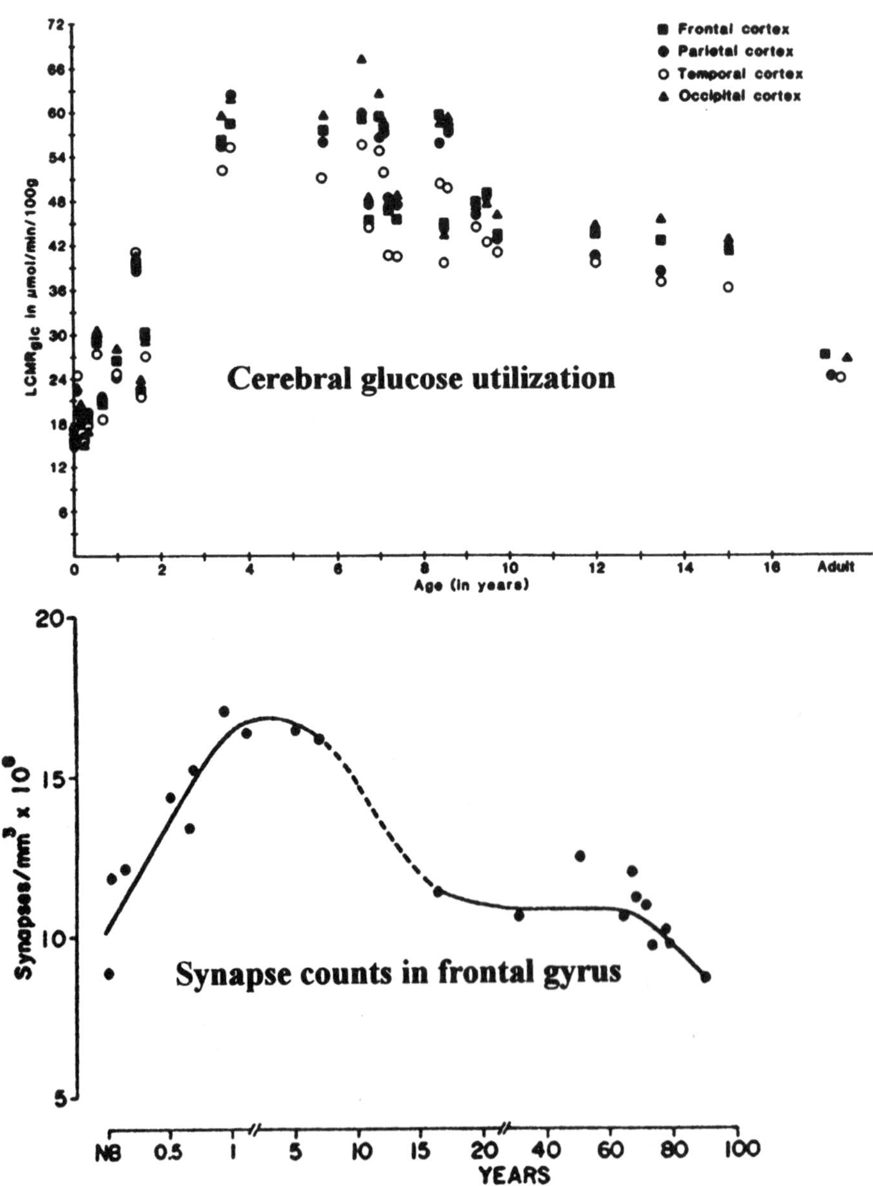

tools for quantitating functional brain activity.[15] Studies using these markers in the developing brain show a similar curve of enhanced uptake during 2 to 10 years of age, paralleling the estimates of synaptic number (Fig 1).[15,16] The similarity in curves is consistent with the hypothesis that glucose uptake in the brain primarily reflects the activity of synapses.[17] Several lines of evidence suggest that glucose consumption is highest in synapses rather than in neuronal cell bodies or in white matter.[18] Recent studies in animals with magnetic resonance MR spectroscopy indicate that glucose consumption in the brain is linked closely to the release and reuptake into glia of the excitatory amino acid neurotransmitter glutamate in synapses.[19] Therefore, both the synapse counting and PET results appear to reflect the overexpression and then pruning of cortical synapses during childhood. This developmental profile might be referred to as a synaptic "power curve" because its expression in humans may be responsible for a remarkable capacity to adapt to the environment and to recover from disruptions in brain development.

NEURONAL ACTIVITY PRUNES AND STABILIZES DEVELOPING SYNAPSE

Electrical activity is essential for the establishment and maintenance of neuronal synapses and is the major force that determines which connections will be eliminated or stabilized during brain development.[4] Although the broad overall patterns of regional synaptic proliferation and elimination are determined by genetic programs, circuits that serve specific functions are refined by local changes in neuronal activity and synaptic strength. One of the best

FIGURE 1.
Cerebral glucose metabolic rate and synaptic density are higher in young children than in the neonates or older children. Comparison of cortical glucose metabolic rate during development in children **(top)** with density of synapses in frontal cortex **(bottom)** determined in postmortem tissue. The 2 curves are very similar, consistent with the hypothesis that cerebral glucose metabolic rate reflects synaptic activity. *Abbreviation:* $LCMR_{glc}$, Local cerebral metabolic rate for glucose. (**Top figure**, based on positron emission tomography [PET] scanning for 2-deoxy-2[18F]fluoro-D-glucose [FDG]; reproduced with permission from Chugani HT: Metabolic imaging: A window on brain development and plasticity. *The Neuroscientist* 5:29-40, 1999, copyright © 1999 by Sage Publications, Inc. Reprinted by permission of Sage Publications, Inc. **Bottom figure,** reprinted from Huttenlocher PR: Synaptic density in human frontal cortex: Developmental changes and effects of aging. *Brain Res* 163:195-205, 1979, with permission from Elsevier Science.)

studied examples of plasticity lies in the developing visual system of cats, primates, and humans.[1,4,20] Visual information from both eyes is organized in visual cortex of each hemisphere in alternating "ocular dominance columns" or stripes seen in tangential sections to support binocular vision. Careful anatomical and electrophysiologic study of fetuses and postnatal animals indicates that axons carrying information from both eyes are initially mixed together but become segregated as electrical activity becomes established.[21] In the fetus, when external visual sensory information is not available, endogenous electrical activity appears to be generated by spontaneous waves of electricity in the immature retina.[22] Later, when visual sensory input is established, the ocular dominance columns are refined and if binocular visual input is normal, these ocular dominance columns occupy equal territory within visual cortex. However, if the vision of 1 eye is impaired by occlusion of the lids or blurred by strabismus during the critical period for visual plasticity, its projection territory is reduced while territory assigned to the opposite eye expands.[20]

It has been demonstrated experimentally many times that this reassignment of visual cortex, or ocular dominance shift, during development is related directly to the reduction in electrical activity in the occluded eye while the activity in the opposite eye is maintained.[4] The loss of visual cortex normally assigned to an eye that is occluded during childhood and its reassignment to axons serving the opposite one is correlated with the cortical blindness or amblyopia that occurs in children with congenital impairment of ocular function or strabismus.[4] The period during which pathologic occlusion can cause this reassignment and when correcting the problem and patching the opposite eye can correct it is referred to as the period of visual cortical plasticity. It is noteworthy that this period of maximal visual cortical plasticity extends over the first 10 years of life in children, the same interval over which maximal proliferation and pruning of synapses are occurring (Fig 2).[23] This indicates that under normal circumstances active axons from each eye seeking stable connections in the cortex can choose from a surplus of potential synapses until the end of this period. Under pathologic circumstances, this arrangement allows the difference in activity between the active eye and the silent eye to be amplified in terms of its impact on cortical organization because it is able to modulate the synaptic "power curve." Especially in primates, this developmental feature of cerebral cortex appears to be one of the factors responsible for exceptional ability to reorganize during critical periods.

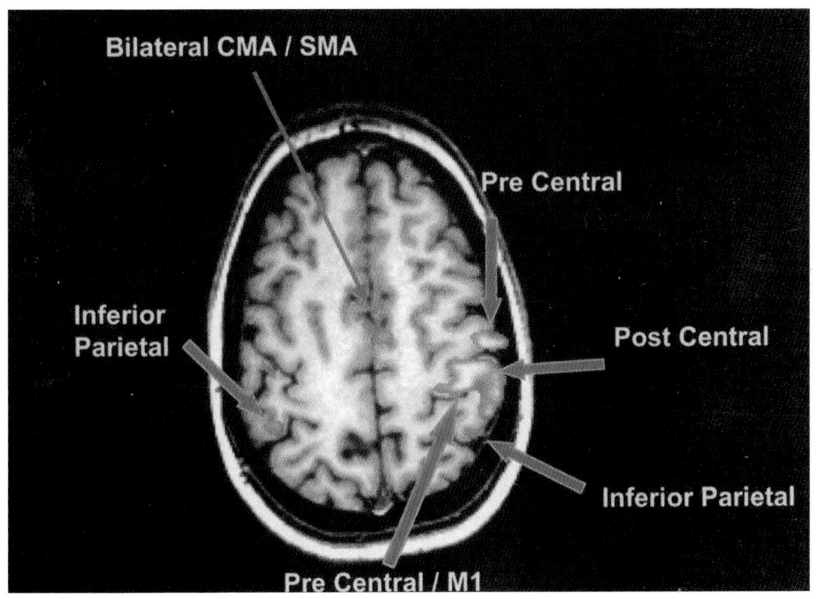

FIGURE 3.
Functional MRI (fMRI) of right-handed finger tapping. Blood oxygenation level–dependent (BOLD) fMRI was used to depict brain regions involved in one-handed finger tapping. Data were acquired by using a 1.5 Tesla MR scanner (Philips Medical Systems) during a 6-minute run, during which time the subject performed 3 cycles of alternating 1 minute of tapping the fingers of one hand at about 2 Hz with 1 minute of rest. Computer analysis of the resulting data yielded an "activation map" *(in color)* overlaid upon a high-resolution anatomical image *(in grayscale)* acquired separately during the scanning session. Activated regions depicted include precentral (motor) and postcentral (sensory) cortex, supplementary motor area (involved in motor planning), and bilateral inferior parietal areas (involved in self-monitoring). *Abbreviations: CMA, Central motor area; SMA, supplementary motor area.* (Data courtesy of A. Heemskerk, X. Golay, T. Brawner, P. van Zijl, and J. Pekar of the F.M. Kirby Research Center at Kennedy Krieger Institute, Baltimore, Md.)

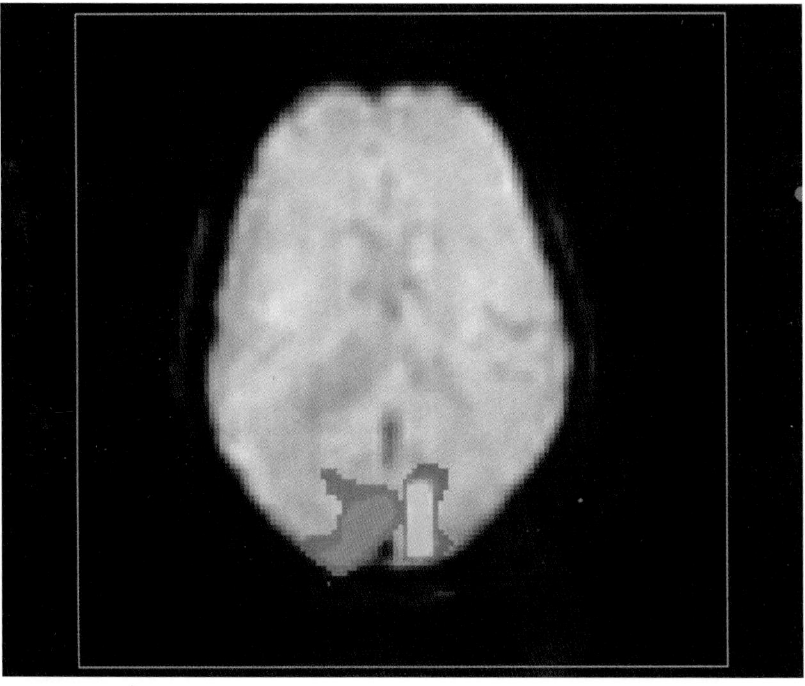

FIGURE 4.
Functional MRI (fMRI) of visual stimulus containing 2 independent components. Blood oxygenation level–dependent (BOLD) fMRI was used to reveal brain regions involved while observing a visual stimulus containing 2 independent components. Data were acquired using a 1.5 Tesla MR scanner (Philips Medical Systems) during a 4-minute run, during which time the subject viewed a visual stimulus, presented via a video projector upon a rear-projection screen. The visual stimulus consisted of 2 "patches" (in the left and right half of the subject's visual field) of a checkerboard pattern, flashing at 8 Hz; the 2 "patches" were slowly cycled on and off by using overlapping but independent timing. Analysis of the resulting data yielded 2 activation components, overlaid (in 2 different colors) upon a high-resolution anatomical image acquired separately during the scanning session. Results are consistent with the retinotopic mapping of the visual field onto primary visual cortex. (Data courtesy of V. Calhoun and J. Pekar; data acquired at the F.M. Kirby Research Center at Kennedy Krieger Institute, Baltimore, Md. See also Calhoun V, Pekar J: When and where are components independent? On the applicability of spatial- and temporal-ICA to functional MRI data. *Neuroimage* 11:682S, 2000.)

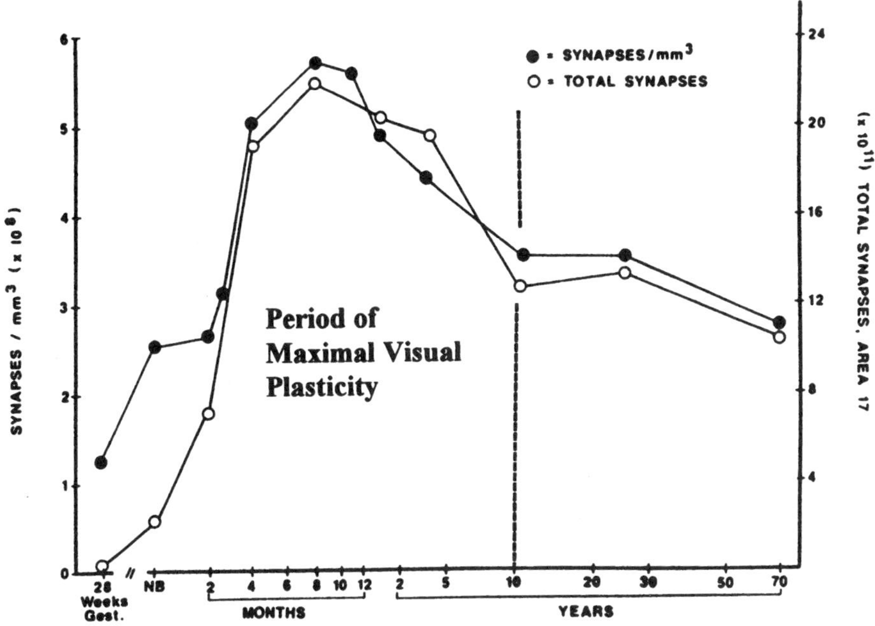

FIGURE 2.
Development of synapses in human visual cortex. (Reprinted from Huttenlocher PR: Morphometric study of human cerebral cortex development. *Neuropsychologia* 28:517-527, 1990, with permission from Elsevier Science.)

PLASTICITY MAY CONTRIBUTE TO RECOVERY OF CHILDREN FROM INSULTS SUCH AS HEMISPHERECTOMY

Several studies suggest that children recover more fully from neurologic injuries than adults.[15,24-26] It seems reasonable that the more favorable recovery may often be related to the robustness of the natural mechanisms in place to refine neuronal circuitry in response to environmental stimuli. This hypothesis is supported by studies of language acquisition in children exposed to deprivation or dominant hemisphere injury. After left hemispherectomy for intractable seizures, good speech recovery has been documented in children when the procedure was done from ages 9 to 14 years.[25,27] In contrast, much smaller areas of injury in the left hemisphere of adults produce permanent aphasia. It is possible that the good recovery in the epilepsy group may be related to stimulation of plastic reorganizational changes in the right hemisphere by earlier left hemisphere dysfunction related to the epileptic process. Preservation of ipsilateral corticospinal pathways subserving paraspinal musculature and body steering mechanisms has also been proposed as a mechanism for motor recovery after hemispherectomy in children.[28] Reactivation of ipsilateral motor pathways has also been suggested as a mechanism of recovery in adults with strokes, based on studies with PET.[29] Experimental models of hemispherectomy show large areas of neuronal sprouting and reinnervation of subcortical regions by the ipsilateral hemisphere left intact by the surgery.[24] These observations are consistent with the proposal that neuronal redundancy and a greater capacity for reorganization in the developing brain support better functional recovery.

Clinical experience suggests that certain rehabilitative therapies improve the speed and completeness of recovery from brain injuries, such as cerebral infarction and severe head injury. However, little objective information is available. Careful study of these interventions has sometimes yielded surprising results. For example, a rigorously reviewed report of a controlled trial of physical therapy on motor performance of infants with spastic diplegia suggested that there was little effect.[30] However, the infant cognitive stimulation therapy given to controls did seem to have a positive impact on motor ability. This may reflect the effects of "cross-modal" plasticity that has been reported in more recent studies.[31]

VISUALIZING SYNAPTIC PLASTICITY WITH FUNCTIONAL BRAIN IMAGING

Development of methods to measure functional brain activity, combined with protocols that activate discrete modalities such as vision, hearing, and finger movement, allows the brain to be mapped in living subjects.[5,7,15] The first practical high-resolution mapping method was PET with 2-deoxyglucose, but the field has expanded rapidly to include additional modalities, including functional magnetic resonance imaging (fMRI), magnetoencephalography (MEG), and transcranial magnetic stimulation (TMS). Each of these methods is being used to examine changes in spatial organization of cortical maps that might reflect plastic reorganization in the developing brain.

PET IMAGING

Two sets of experiments with PET imaging suggest changes that may reflect plastic reorganization of the developing brain after injury. Chugani and Jacob[32] examined the brains of children with hemispherectomy using FDG PET and found a low glucose metabolic rate in the basal ganglia and thalamus at 3 to 6 months, followed by a reappearance of activity in the caudate 1 to 2 years later. Since, as already discussed, glucose metabolic rate is tightly coupled to synaptic activity, this suggests that neural connections between other brain structures and the caudate have been reestablished. Potential candidates include the activation of unablated ipsilateral pathways from cerebral cortex to the basal ganglia or activation of latent, crossed corticostriatal pathways, which have been described in some species. Activation of primitive ipsilateral corticospinal pathways has been documented with TMS of the cortex in children with cerebral palsy related to hemisphere injury.[33]

Another example of cortical plasticity examined with PET was reported by Sadato et al[34,35] in Braille-reading individuals who had been blind from an early age. Brain activation was studied during Braille-reading and non–Braille-reading tactile discrimination tasks in the blind individuals by monitoring regional cerebral blood flow. During both tasks, the blind individuals activated the primary visual cortex and fusiform gyri, areas that are activated in sighted individuals by visual stimuli. Sighted individuals also activated the secondary somatosensory processing area when performing tactile discrimination tasks with the index fingers, whereas the Braille-reading blind individuals suppressed this area. These findings suggest that the tactile processing pathways to the secondary somatosensory processing area in sighted individuals have become rerouted in the Braille readers to the occipital regions normally reserved for visual shape discrimination. It appears that the brains of Braille readers have reassigned visual cortex silenced by early loss of its natural input to provide the higher level of tactile discrimination needed to read Braille. Studies in which the occipital cortex of these individuals was transiently inactivated with TMS showed that their tactile perception was distorted temporarily.[36] In a sense, the rewired brain has become able to "read" with the index finger.

MEG AND MUSICAL MAPS IN THE BRAIN

MEG is a technique that can be used to map regions of cortex that are stimulated by activation of sensory modalities, such as hearing or touching the skin.[37] The technique uses magnetic source imaging to detect the magnetic dipoles oriented at right angles to electricity generated by the firing neurons. In 1 set of experiments conducted by Elbert et al,[38] 9 musicians (6 violinists, 2 cellists, and 1 guitarist) who had played their instruments for 7 to 17 years were studied with MEG while the fingers of each hand were lightly touched with a standard technique. The results demonstrated that the cortical representation of the fingers on the left hand used to finger the stringed instruments was larger than the representation of the right hand and of the hands of age-matched control individuals who did not play. There was also a strong direct correlation between the expansion of the cortical somatosensory map assigned to the left-handed fingers and how early they began to play. The results are consistent with the hypothesis that early use of the fingers led to activity-dependent expansion of their cortical representations.

Another study showed complementary results in Braille readers who used 3 fingers together instead of 1 to read over a long period.[39] Using magnetic source imaging, the investigators found a substantial enlargement of the hand representation in the 3-finger Braille readers compared with single-finger Braille readers and sighted non-Braille readers. However, the cortical map of the 3-fingered Braille readers was disorganized compared with controls. The distortion of the finger map was correlated with their tendency to misidentify which finger was being touched during tactile sensory threshold determination. These findings suggested that use-dependent "smearing" of the cortical representation of the fingers had occurred in the 3-finger Braille readers associated with a reduction in the ability to discriminate 1 finger from another. This may have been adaptive for them, allowing them to process Braille with 3 fingers as if they were one.

In another series of experiments in musicians, Pantev et al[40] used MEG to map the cortical representation of piano tones compared with pure tones of the same frequency and loudness. These skilled musicians had played their instruments for more than 15 years and practiced for more than 20 hours per week. The cortical map of activation elicited by piano tones, but not for pure tones, was enlarged by 25% in the musicians compared with controls, and enlargement was correlated with the age at which they began to play. This suggests that the cortical tonotopic map for music undergoes activity-dependent functional reorganization during development of musical skill that is similar to changes in the somatosensory map. Although expansion of the somatosensory and tonotopic maps is correlated with length of practice in these musicians, it is unclear whether the larger map actually contributes to their musical skill. However, the results do indicate that all this practice has made their brains different from those of nonmusicians in a small way. It suggests that similar changes in cortical maps are likely to occur with many other types of early experience, such as exposure to different languages that feature special sounds.

FUNCTIONAL MRI

Functional MRI is emerging as the technique that promises to extend studies of brain plasticity into a wider range of pediatric conditions.[5,7] Because the technique does not use the radioactivity required for PET, the risk is far more acceptable for mapping the brains of normal children and those with relatively benign diseases. Software is also becoming available to allow fMRI studies to be performed on clinical MR scanners, making the technique more accessible than MEG.

Functional MRI uses the same basic principles as conventional MRI for protons, but the machine is set to measure the effects on protons of other molecules, such as hemoglobin, that have magnetic properties.[7] The iron-containing deoxygenated hemoglobin molecule can alter the rotating magnetic moment of the protons associated with water in the brain, referred to in MR as a "susceptibility effect." In the fMRI technique known as BOLD (blood oxygen level–dependent contrast), the MR acquisition protocol is modified to optimize these susceptibility effects to detect deoxygenated hemoglobin. When the brain is activated, a brisk regional increase in cerebral blood flow leads to a decrease in deoxyhemoglobin because more blood is provided than is actually needed to deliver oxygen to the tissue. If a BOLD image is acquired before and after brain activation, powerful computers can calculate the differences between them pixel by pixel to create a map that demonstrates only the pixels that are different. In the case of the BOLD protocol, these maps demonstrate regions in which regional cerebral blood flow has changed in response to the activation paradigm.

An example of functional activation of motor cortex visualized by the BOLD fMRI technique is shown in Fig 3. Although animal experiments indicate that there is a good correlation between these fMRI images and neuronal activation, the exact mechanisms involved are still debated. One likely hypothesis is that neuronal activation associated with release of excitatory neurotransmitters stimulates NMDA (N-methyl-D-aspartate)-type glutamate receptors, which in turn activate formation of the vasodilator neurotransmitter gas nitric oxide.[41] In general, there seems to be a good correlation between activation maps acquired by using the older techniques of PET regional cerebral blood flow and FDG uptake and the newer fMRI techniques using BOLD. A major limitation of fMRI is the relatively low "signal to noise" of 10% to 15% during acquisition of the BOLD signal. However, rapid advances in computer processing and engineering are expected to improve the technique.

Functional MRI Studies of Visual Processing in Infants and Children

Visually based behaviors are some of the first to develop in newborn infants, and as mentioned above, understanding the organization and plasticity of visual pathways in the brain has stimulated considerable clinical and research interest.[20,21,42] An example of the ability of fMRI to resolve distinct activation patterns in visual cortex is shown in Fig 4.

Functional MRI with the BOLD signal has been used to study the development of visual cortical activation in children from 1

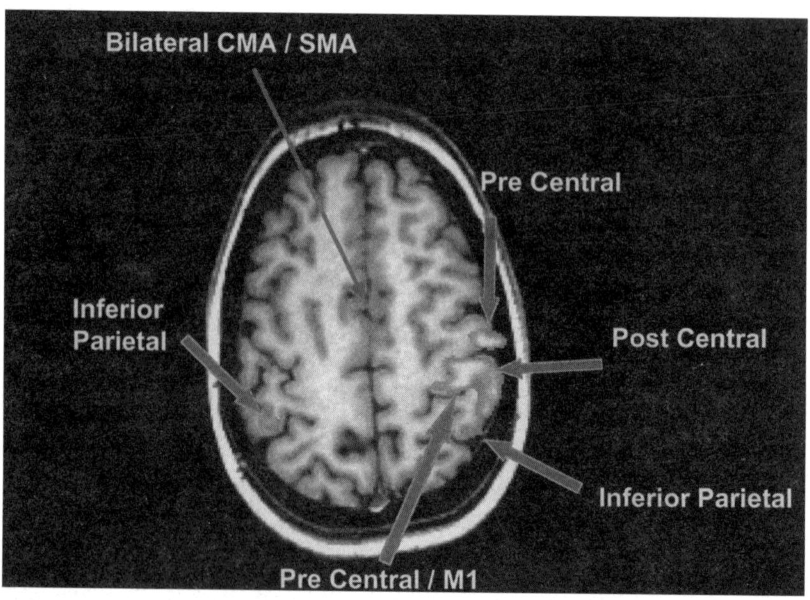

FIGURE 3.
(See color plate.) Functional MRI (fMRI) of right-handed finger tapping. Blood oxygenation level–dependent (BOLD) fMRI was used to depict brain regions involved in one-handed finger tapping. Data were acquired by using a 1.5 Tesla MR scanner (Philips Medical Systems) during a 6-minute run, during which time the subject performed 3 cycles of alternating 1 minute of tapping the fingers of one hand at about 2 Hz with 1 minute of rest. Computer analysis of the resulting data yielded an "activation map" *(in color)* overlaid upon a high-resolution anatomical image *(in grayscale)* acquired separately during the scanning session. Activated regions depicted include precentral (motor) and postcentral (sensory) cortex, supplementary motor area (involved in motor planning), and bilateral inferior parietal areas (involved in self-monitoring). *Abbreviations: CMA, Central motor area; SMA, supplementary motor area.* (Data courtesy of A. Heemskerk, X. Golay, T. Brawner, P. van Zijl, and J. Pekar of the F.M. Kirby Research Center at Kennedy Krieger Institute, Baltimore, Md.)

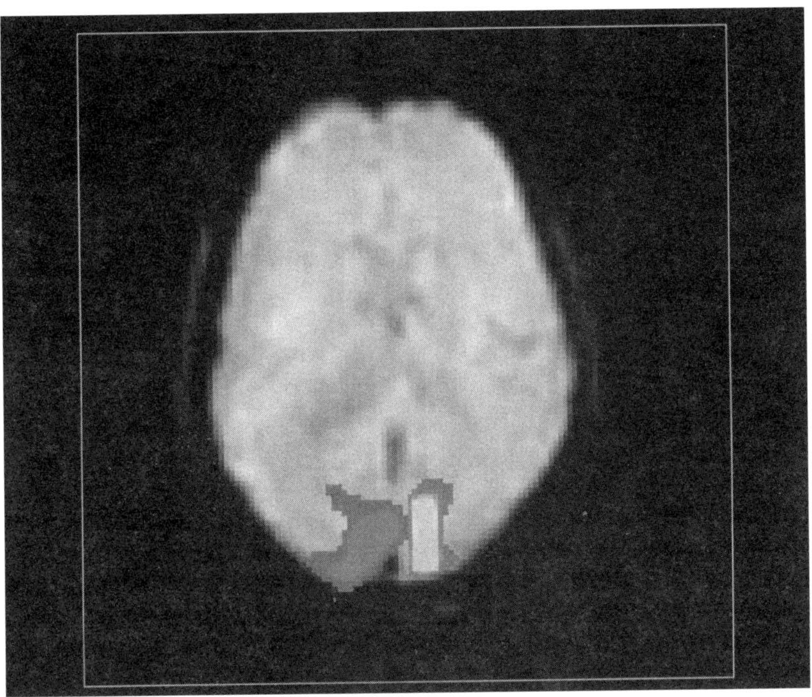

FIGURE 4.
(See color plate.) Functional MRI (fMRI) of visual stimulus containing 2 independent components. Blood oxygenation level–dependent (BOLD) fMRI was used to reveal brain regions involved while observing a visual stimulus containing 2 independent components. Data were acquired using a 1.5 Tesla MR scanner (Philips Medical Systems) during a 4-minute run, during which time the subject viewed a visual stimulus, presented via a video projector upon a rear-projection screen. The visual stimulus consisted of 2 "patches" (in the left and right half of the subject's visual field) of a checkerboard pattern, flashing at 8 Hz; the 2 "patches" were slowly cycled on and off by using overlapping but independent timing. Analysis of the resulting data yielded 2 activation components, overlaid (in 2 different colors) upon a high-resolution anatomical image acquired separately during the scanning session. Results are consistent with the retinotopic mapping of the visual field onto primary visual cortex. (Data courtesy of V. Calhoun and J. Pekar; data acquired at the F.M. Kirby Research Center at Kennedy Krieger Institute, Baltimore, Md. See also Calhoun V, Pekar J: When and where are components independent? On the applicability of spatial- and temporal-ICA to functional MRI data. *Neuroimage* 11:682S, 2000.)

day to 12 years of age by Martin et al.[43] They found that the primary visual cortical area does not respond functionally in the same manner as that of adults until 1.5 years of age. The site activated in the infants tended to be V2, the occipital cortical area located more anterior in the calcarine sulcus and more dorsal in the superior parietal lobule. In some infants, activation of V2 was also associated with activation of subcortical regions in the pulvinar of the thalamus and the quadrigeminal plate. These observations suggest that in young infants, a phylogenetically older subcortical visual pathway is being activated that bypasses the primary V1 visual cortex. Activation of V1 was far more frequent after the first year of life, correlating with behavioral and electrophysiologic studies of markedly improved vision and stereopsis later in infancy.

One interesting feature of the age-related activation patterns in these infants and children was that the early V2 cortical activation tended to be a negative BOLD signal, which became more progresively positive with age. Although the explanation for this is not entirely clear, 1 hypothesis is that this relative decrease in the ratio of deoxygenated to oxygenated hemoglobin is related to relatively higher consumption of oxygen by neuronal activity at this age. This would be consistent with the relatively higher synaptic density during the first year of life in humans compared with older children.[12] In fact, Yamada et al[44] recently showed that the BOLD signal in this region is positive before 8 weeks of age, the time at which rapid synaptic overproduction is just beginning. Another possible explanation which has been suggested is that vascular reactivity in response to neuronal activation is less robust at this age than in older children. These studies suggest that fMRI could be used to understand visual cortical plasticity in children and adults after injury, and possibly to develop ways to hasten functional recovery. Born et al[45] recently used this technique in young infants to try to predict later visual performance.

Functional MRI of Cortical Organization of Language in Deaf Individuals

Cortical reorganization has also been examined in individuals who are congenitally deaf.[46] Neville et al[46] measured activation of cerebral cortex activated during sentence reading in congenitally deaf individuals who learned American Sign Language (ASL) at an early age. Unlike normal controls, the deaf individuals did not activate classic left hemisphere language areas when reading

English sentences but did activate the left hemisphere when reading the same language conveyed by sign language. Both hearing and deaf individuals activated right hemisphere areas when processing ASL but not when processing English. This is consistent with previous reports that humans who sustained auditory deprivation since birth had enhanced ability to process discriminate motion.[46] The results suggest that the modality through which these individuals attained functional language at an early age (signing or oral English) heavily influenced the subsequent organization of their classic language areas.

In contrast to deaf signers, individuals who were not deaf but who learned ASL through contact with family members at an early age, displayed considerable individual differences during sentence processing for both English and ASL. Within the same experimental session, they displayed a strongly left-lateralized pattern of activation for reading English but activation of both left and right hemispheres for processing in ASL. These results are consistent with reports of a high degree of individual variability in cortical activation in bilingual speakers with normal hearing who learned their second language after 7 years of age.[46] They support the hypothesis that delayed or imperfect acquisition of a language leads to an anomalous pattern of brain organization for that language.

Reorganization of Motor Cortex

Very limited studies have been done with fMRI in children with early motor system injury. Chu et al[47] recently used this modality to demonstrate that somatosensory cortex associated with the hemiparetic hand in children after unilateral perinatal brain injury is reorganized.

NEUROBIOLOGY OF PLASTICITY

SYNAPTIC ACTIVITY IS MEDIATED BY NEUROTRANSMITTERS

Recognition that neuronal activity has a profound effect on establishment and refinement of developing synaptic connections has focused attention on the major transmitters that mediate these effects.[48] Synapses that use the excitatory neurotransmitter glutamate have received special attention because this amino acid mediates most of the excitatory neurotransmission in the brain.[49] This flexible dicarboxylic amino acid can assume several conformations to bind to several glutamate receptor subtypes including NMDA, AMPA (α-amino-3-hydroxy-5-methylisoxazoleproprionic acid), and metabotropic receptors. The NMDA receptor has been implicated in synaptic plasticity in visual cortex through experiments in which specific antagonists can block the ocular dominance shift in kittens at doses that do not disrupt neuronal activity.[50,51] NMDA receptors have also been implicated in synaptic pruning in the developing cerebellum and in segregation of optic stripes in the optic tectum of a 3-eyed tadpole model.[52-54] NMDA receptors are developmentally regulated so that they are more active and flux more calcium through their channels in the immature brain.[49,55]

NMDA receptors are also attractive candidates for mediators of activity-dependent refinement of developing brain circuitry because of their special physiologic characteristics as "coincidence detectors" (Fig 5).[56] To open the NMDA channel, the amino acids glutamate and glycine must occupy surface receptors, and simultaneously the membrane potential must be depolarized. This requires that the presynaptic release of neurotransmitter and the depolarization of the postsynaptic membrane of the adjacent neuron occur together. The most probable way for this to occur is for other excitatory axons on nearby synapses to be active at the same time. This type of patterned, concurrent activity in adjacent projections into visual cortex appears to be the most powerful for refining or reorganizing cortical columns in the developing brain. This principle of activity-dependent connectivity during development has been described by the phrase, "neurons that fire together, wire together."[1,4]

The involvement of NMDA receptors in the phenomenon of long-term potentiation (LTP) also provides a potential parallel to their involvement in developmental plasticity.[57] LTP is a form of activity-dependent synaptic strengthening that results when rapid receptor stimulation occurs along with membrane depolarization. It is easier to elicit LTP in the immature brain than in the adult brain, and the period of heightened LTP corresponds to the critical period for cortical plasticity in several rodent models.[58,59] LTP mediated by NMDA receptors is an attractive model for stabilization of synapses during development, as it is for increasing synaptic strength and memory storage in the mature brain.[60]

Several additional neurotransmitter actions have been implicated in stabilization and pruning of synapses in the developing brain involved in developmental neuronal plasticity. Long-term depression (LTD), an electrophysiologic phenomenon similar to LTP but acting in the opposite direction to depress synaptic strength, may be mediated by NMDA or other receptors.[61,62] Inhibitory neurotransmission may also be important for controlling plasticity. Inhi-

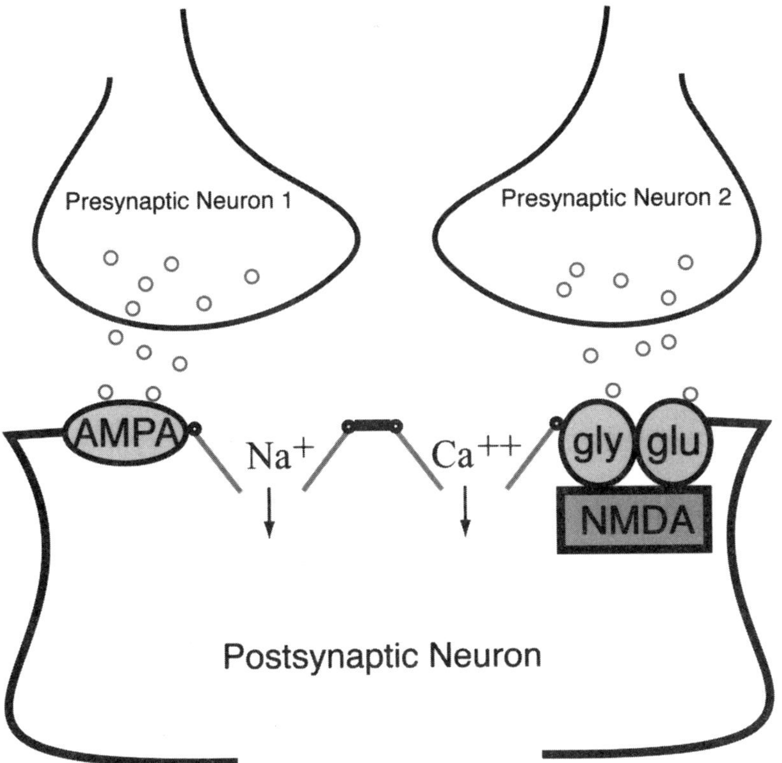

FIGURE 5.
Diagram of excitatory synapses with NMDA (N-methyl-D-aspartate) and AMPA (α-amino-3-hydroxy-5-methylisoxazoleproprionic acid) glutamate receptors side by side. Opening the NMDA receptor requires simultaneous activation of an AMPA receptor by an adjacent axon, which depolarizes the adjacent neuronal membrane. The arrangement makes it more likely that the NMDA receptor channel will open when there is coincident activity from a second neuron. This means the neurons firing together in a pattern are more likely to open the NMDA channel, which in turn can stimulate long-lasting synaptic plasticity. *Abbreviation: gly,* Glycine.

bition mediated by the inhibitory amino acid γ-aminobutyric acid (GABA) may modulate the ability of excitatory synapses to trigger LTP, and in 1 model has been shown to trigger the onset of the critical period for visual plasticity in mice.[63,64] These studies provide a link between excitatory and inhibitory mechanisms used in the mature brain and activity-dependent plasticity during development.

RETROGRADE OR TROPHIC SIGNALS RESPOND TO CHANGES IN ACTIVITY

When vision is impaired in 1 eye in developing cats or primates, regression of axons carrying impulses from the eye becomes apparent as the ocular dominance shifts in a few weeks, and microscopic reductions in the complexity of geniculocalcerine axonal arbors have been observed within a few days.[65] One possible explanation for this remodeling of presynaptic arbors is a change in the release of retrograde signals from target neurons. Signaling molecules such as neuronal growth factors and the neurotransmitter free-radical gas nitric oxide are known to be produced in neurons and are regulated by neuronal activity.[55,66,67] The neurotrophins brain-derived neurotrophic factor (BDNF), neurotrophin-3 (NT-3), and neurotrophin-4 (NT-4) have been implicated in this sculpting process because their receptors are expressed in developing cerebral cortex.[68]

The more rapidly acting gas nitric oxide is produced in neurons in response to stimulation of NMDA receptors, and it has been implicated in restricted refinement of developing neuronal connections in some models.[55]

INTRANEURONAL SIGNALING CASCADES IMPLICATED IN SYNAPTIC PLASTICITY

The neuronal receptors involved in activity-dependent plasticity produce changes in synaptic connectivity via intracellular protein phosphorylation cascades that regulate gene transcription (Fig 6).[69-74] Many of these cascades converge on phosphorylation of CREB (cyclic adenosine monophosphate [AMP] response element binding protein), a transcription factor that binds to a special nucleotide sequence near the promoter of numerous genes. Phosphorylation of CREB has been implicated in learning and memory in fruitflies, snails, and mice, making it a potentially important pathway for mediating activity-dependent changes in neuronal circuitry in the developing brain.[72] In cultured hippocampal neurons, CREB phosphorylation has been shown to play an important role in the plasticity of dendritic spines, a site for long-term plasticity in synaptic connections.[69] The mitogen-activated protein kinase (MAPK) cascade couples both protein kinase A and protein kinase C activity stimulated by a variety of neurotransmitter receptors to CREB phosphorylation.[71] Activation of MAPK is required for associative learning involving the hippocampus in mammals.[71] It seems likely that these intracellular signaling pathways mediate the effects of synaptic stimulation to shape neuronal circuits as well as learning and memory in the developing brain.

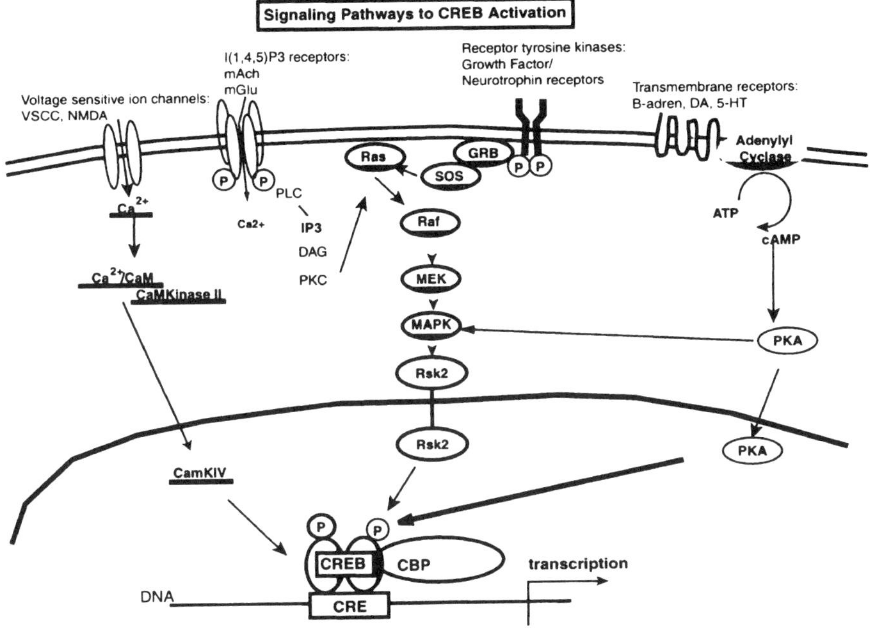

FIGURE 6.
Some intracellular cascades that are activated by neurotransmitter and trophic factor receptors. These cascades carry signals from the synapse to the nucleus, where transcription of genes leads to long-term synaptic plasticity. *Abbreviations: VSCC,* Voltage-sensitive calcium channels; *CaMKinase II,* calcium calmodulin-dependent protein kinase II; *mAch and mGlu,* metabotropic acetylcholine and glutamate receptors; *PLC,* phospholipase C; *IP3,* inositol triphosphase; *DAG,* diacylglycerol; *PKC,* protein kinase C; *Ras,* guanine nucleotide binding protein; *GRB, SOS,* adaptor proteins linking receptor tyrosine kinase receptors to Ras; *Raf,* serine/threonine protein kinase; *Mek,* protein kinase; *MAPK,* mitogen-activated protein kinase; *Rsk-2,* CREB kinase; *CREB,* cyclic AMP response element (CRE) binding protein; *CBP,* CREB binding protein; *B-adren,* β-adrenergic; *DA,* dopamine; *5-HT,* serotonin; *PKA,* protein kinase A. (Reproduced with permission from Harum KH, Alemi L, Johnston MV. Cognitive impairment in Coffin-Lowry syndrome correlates with reduced RSK 2 activation. *Neurology* 56:209-214, 2001.)

NEUROGENESIS: ANOTHER POTENTIAL PLASTICITY MECHANISM DURING POSTNATAL DEVELOPMENT

Although neurogenesis is markedly reduced in the postnatal brain, recent experiments suggest that it may persist in certain special areas such as the dentate gyrus of the hippocampus even in adulthood and may be stimulated by activity or injury.[75] Synaptic activity may stimulate neurogenesis in some situations. Exposure to an enriched environment and the opportunity to run in their cages stimulated neurogenesis in adult mice.[76] Adult rats who participated in an associative learning task also experienced a doubling of newborn neurons in the dentate gyrus.[77] Recently, it has been shown that injury can induce neurogenesis in adult mice in neocortical regions that do not normally demonstrate new neurons.[78] These studies suggest that neurogenesis could continue to play a role in brain plasticity in the developing brain long after the major waves of replication cease, especially after injury.

MODELS OF REORGANIZATION IN SOMATOSENSORY CORTEX

Evidence for reorganization of cortical maps in humans has stimulated research into basic mechanisms with animal models.[79,80] Several examples of morphological reorganization have been documented over the last decade, including a study by Pons et al[80] in adult macaque monkeys who had sensory denervation of the arm for several years. When these animals were examined electrophysiologically, it was found that the entire zone of cortex deprived of sensory input from the arm now responded to stimulation of the face.[80] In anatomical terms, this represents reorganization across 10 to 14 mm of cortex, a large distance to be accomplished by axonal sprouting alone. They initially suggested that some of this "rewiring" may occur at subcortical levels in the thalamus, brain stem, or spinal cord. Consistent with this hypothesis, Jain et al[81] showed that sprouting occurs in this model at the level of the trigeminal nucleus. However, work by Florence et al[82] indicates that growth of new intracortical connections does extend more than a centimeter.

Another study conducted in subhuman primates aimed to assess cortical plasticity in response to rehabilitative training of the arm similar to that provided to patients after strokes.[83] Nudo et al[83] found that small infarcts that damaged the motor cortex assigned to the hand and arm usually caused further loss of hand territory in adjacent, undamaged cortex. However, training the monkey to use the arm after the stroke caused the area assigned to the hand to expand into regions formerly assigned to the elbow and shoulder. These studies showed that the rehabilitative training could shape the reorganization of adjacent, intact cortex, which in turn might play a role in functional recovery.

Rodents have special features in their somatosensory cortex that make them attractive for plasticity studies. The so-called "whisker-to-barrel" pathway in mice and rats creates a somatosensory map across layer IV of the flat, ungyrated rodent cortex that can be visualized by using a simple cytochrome oxidase stain or special procedures for identifying neurotransmitter receptors or other cellular

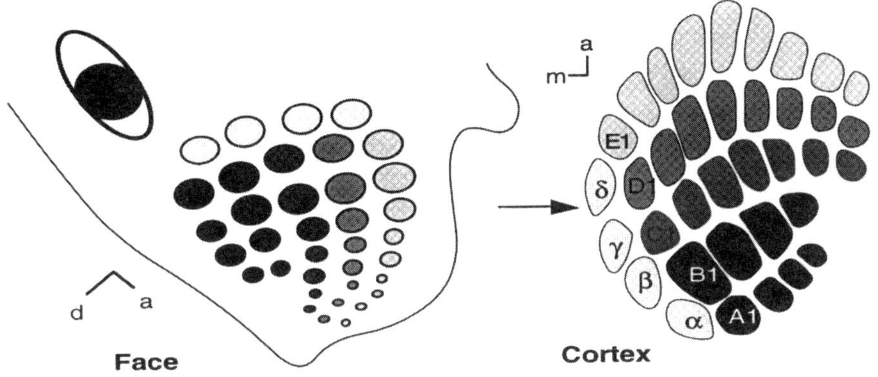

FIGURE 7.
The whisker-to-barrel system in somatosensory cortex of rodents. The diagram illustrates that the barrel pattern across the somatosensory cortex faithfully reproduces the pattern of whiskers on the rodent's snout. (Diagram provided by J. McCasland, PhD.)

markers (Fig 7).[84] The phrase "whisker-to-barrel" refers to the fact that each whisker on the rodent's snout sends sensory information to its own patch in layer IV of cortex referred to by neuroanatomists as "barrels" because of their appearance when cut crosswise to the surface.[84] This sensory pathway, transmitted by nerves in the snout up into the brain stem and thalamus and then into the cerebral cortex, creates an indispensable map of the rodent's world, which is filled with small dark passageways. This barrel-field map occupies a relatively large expanse of cortex in the rodent, similar to areas occupied by the hand and fingers in the human.

The whisker-to-barrel pathway is an excellent model system for understanding interactions between genetic programs and sensory stimulation from the outside world to create and sculpt developing cortical circuits.[79] During early barrel development, interactions between dendrites in cortical neurons and afferents projecting from the thalamus may determine which synaptic connections persist and which are eliminated.[85] Excitatory amino acid receptors appear to play an important role in this process, and the organization of the barrel patterns is reflected by a complex pattern of expression of different glutamate receptor subtypes.[86-89] Mice in which NMDA receptors have been genetically deleted in cerebral cortex do not form normal barrel patterns.[90] During postnatal development, barrels display periods in which serotonin receptors and G-protein linked metabotropic glutamate receptors are expressed in high densities and then pruned.[84,88] Although the details remain controversial, excitatory synapses in whisker sensory pathways play a major role in the refinement of these circuits during development.[91]

This rodent model of cortical development also holds promise for understanding ways to manipulate or enhance cortical plasticity. When whisker follicles are ablated within the first few days after birth, the barrels assigned to them shrink dramatically, while barrels in adjacent rows expand (Fig 8). These structural rearrangements are thought to occur through competition-type interactions, similar to those in the visual cortex described above.[92-94] The cortex associated with the lesioned whisker is inactive, whereas the expanded cortical regions are activated by the intact whiskers. A number of studies indicate a role for NMDA receptors and activity in the plastic response to whisker removal in rodents and functional cortical reorganization in higher animals.[95,96] NMDA-mediated synaptic plasticity involving LTP occurs at the same time in neonatal development when barrel patterning is susceptible to peripheral damage.[97,98] Plasticity from whisker ablation has also been shown to be blunted by administration of drugs that block NMDA receptors.[96] Recent work suggests that other neurotransmitters, such as acetylcholine, may have a potent effect to control plastic reorganization after whisker ablation.[99,100] A better knowledge of the molecular signals that control plasticity may have important clinical implications.

SYNAPTIC ACTIVITY REGULATES GENE EXPRESSION IN DEVELOPMENT

The neurobiologic model of synaptic plasticity that emerges from this experimental work indicates that patterned neuronal firing transmitted through synapses leads to postsynaptic changes in expression of genes such as growth factors, which in turn modify axonal and dendritic arbors (Fig 9). The model indicates that sensory experience, including the primary senses, nurturing, education, and stress, and other environmental factors, can influence brain circuitry during critical periods of development. The relative impact of natural genetic programs versus environmental influences is probably determined by numerous factors including age, genes, strength and duration of the environmental influence, and the intrinsic plasticity of the system. However, an important point is that activity at synapses is directly linked to changes in gene expression in the nucleus, making these terminals a focal point for understanding the influences of nature versus nurture in brain development.

CLINICAL PEDIATRIC DISORDERS INVOLVING DISRUPTED PLASTICITY

Plasticity in the developing brain is a double-edged sword: it endows the brain with great capacity to learn and adapt, but it also makes

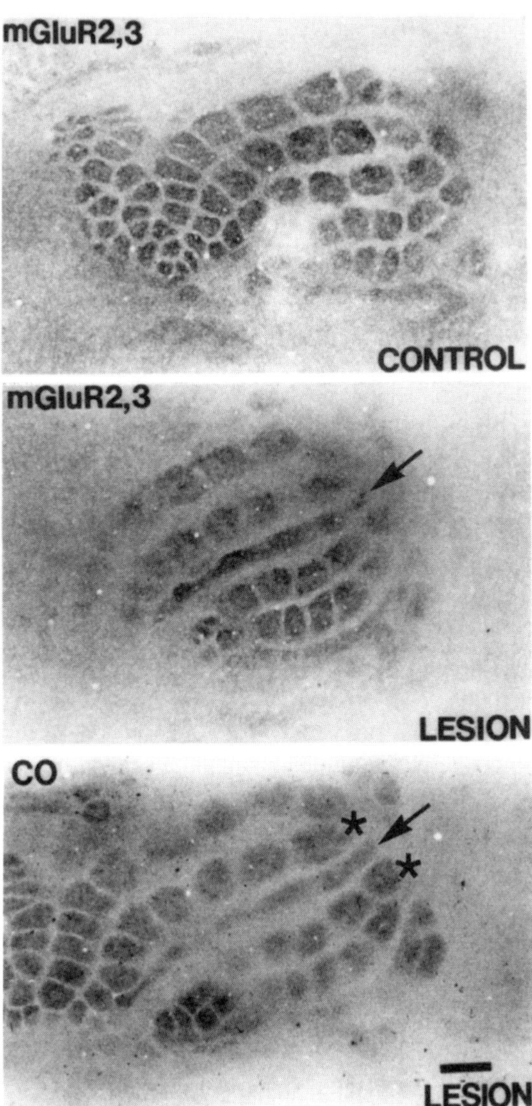

FIGURE 8.
Plasticity in the whisker-to-barrel pattern of somatosensory cortex after ablation of a row of whisker follicles in the neonatal period. The **top panel** shows the whiskers immunostained to show metabotropic glutamate receptors in a control animal. The **bottom 2 panels** show that the row indicated by the *arrow* has shrunk after neonatal ablation of corresponding whiskers. Staining for both metabotropic receptors *(mGluR2,3)* and cytochrome oxidase *(CO)* are shown. Barrels adjacent to the shrunken row have enlarged *(asterisks)* in comparison to normal barrels.

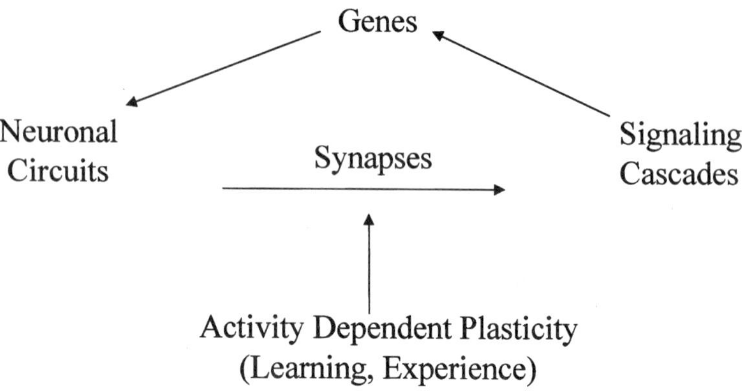

FIGURE 9.
Model showing how synaptic activity sculpts developing brain. Activity influences the developing brain by modifying synaptic function, stimulating intracellular signaling cascades, and modifying gene expression.

it vulnerable to a noxious environment or diseases that alter brain activity. Evidence suggests that certain toxins, such as lead and alcohol, may impair plasticity by altering activity-dependent neuronal activity. Metabolic disorders such as nonketotic hypergylcinemia and epileptic encephalopathies may have similar effects on the developing brain by altering the activation of excitatory amino acid receptors. In addition, a recently recognized group of genetic intracellular signaling disorders may impair the brain's ability to respond appropriately to neuronal synaptic activity, producing a variety of cognitive and mental retardation syndromes. The accumulating information about this mechanism for neurodevelopmental disorders discussed in the following sections may lead to better ways to intervene or prevent them.

LEAD POISONING MAY REDUCE INTELLIGENCE IN CHILDREN BY ALTERING NEURONAL PLASTICITY

Childhood lead poisoning continues as a major public health problem throughout the world, especially in poor urban children of the United States.[101] Lead is especially damaging to the developing brain, producing a dose-related decline in intelligence that is related to the blood level at 2 to 3 years of age.[102] Interestingly, lead's effect on the brain diminishes with age, producing much less effect in adults. Considerable experimental evidence suggests that lead has its major impact on developing neurons and their synapses, especially excitatory synapses that use glutamate as their neurotransmitter. At the low levels known to affect brain development and behavior in children, lead has stimulatory effects on 3 separate components of glutamate synapses: presynaptic release of glutamate, the NMDA receptor itself, and on protein kinase C, an enzyme that is downstream from glutamate receptors.[101-104] These effects have led to the hypothesis that low-level lead raises the background "noise" in excitatory synaptic neurotransmission in the developing brain.[101]

Experiments with the developing rodent barrel-field model described above showed that lead administered in the neonatal period impairs the development of the barrels in somatosensory cortex in a dose-dependent fashion.[105] In contrast, the total size of the cortex was unaffected, suggesting that lead had a selective effect on cortex innervated by thalamocortical axons carrying sensory information from the thalamus. Taken together with the electrophysiologic and biochemical evidence of the effect of lead on synapses, these observations suggest that lead may produce its permanent effect by disrupting the activity-dependent plasticity at developing synapses. This would be consistent with the fact that the toxin's maximal effect occurs in toddlers, at a time when cortical synaptogenesis is normally peaking.

OTHER TOXIC AND METABOLIC DISORDERS MAY ALTER PLASTICITY

Several other toxic and metabolic disorders of children may disrupt brain development by altering activity-dependent plasticity at developing synapses. For example, nonketotic hyperglycinemia, caused by a genetic defect in the glycine cleavage system, causes seizures and severe mental retardation in association with high levels of plasma glycine.[106] Glycine has 2 major actions as a neurotransmitter, one as an inhibitory transmitter in the brain stem, the other as a coagonist with glutamate at the NMDA receptor. In children with this disorder, reduction of glycine levels by administering sodium benzoate, and inhibiting glycine's effect with the NMDA receptor with dextromethorphan, can reduce seizures and improve outcome in some cases.[106] The major mechanism of glycine's toxic effect is likely to be through enhanced NMDA-mediated excitoxicity and disruption of activity-dependent plasticity in the immature brain.[49] The inherited metabolic disorder molybdenum cofactor deficiency also produces a severe encephalopathy with neuropathology that resembles glutamate-mediated excitotoxic injury.[49] This injury may be secondary to accumulation of the metabolite L-sulfocysteine, which can produce excitotoxic neuronal injury in experimental models.

Toxins that reduce activity-dependent neuronal plasticity by blocking glutamate receptors may also be responsible for serious neurodevelopmental disorders. Just as NMDA antagonists have been shown to block the experimental ocular dominance shift that occurs in the visual cortex of mammals, complete blockade of excitatory activity at these receptors earlier in development can cause neuronal death by apoptosis.[107] Developing neurons appear to require just the right amount of excitatory neurotransmission, and too much or too little can produce damage. This is probably a mechanism by which neurons that have not made effective neuronal contacts during development are eliminated.[107] Recent evidence suggests that at high concentrations, ethanol is a potent NMDA receptor antagonist, and experiments in rodents showed that fetal or early postnatal exposure can cause neuronal death by apoptosis. This evidence suggests that blockade of NMDA receptors by ethanol may be an important mechanism for the neurobehavioral abnormalities seen in fetal alcohol syndrome.[108]

EPILEPTIC ENCEPHALOPATHIES

The epileptic encephalopathies associated with Landau-Kleffner syndrome (LKS), infantile spasms, and Lennox-Gastaut syndrome are very likely to reflect, at least in part, the disruptive effects of abnormal electrical activity on brain development.[4,109-111] Some of these children are relatively normal before the onset of their epilepsy, and a severely abnormal electroencephalogram background is associated with loss of neurobehavioral skills, language skills, or both. Successful treatment, especially in the case of children with symptomatic infantile spasms who respond to corticotropin (ACTH) therapy, can lead to remarkably swift recovery.[110] In some cases of LKS, anticonvulsant treatment is associated with improvement in language.[111] The evidence described earlier that the developing brain depends to some extent on endogenously generated electrical rhythms suggests that the pathologic electrical patterns generated in these disorders could disrupt brain development even in the absence of underlying neuropathology.[4]

COGNITIVE DISORDERS ASSOCIATED WITH DEFECTS IN INTRACELLULAR SIGNALING

Research in genetics has demonstrated that the molecular lesions responsible for a number of poorly understood developmental cognitive disorders reside within signaling cascades involved in activity-dependent plasticity (Table 1). As a result, these lesions make it difficult for signals from the cell surface to be translated into the changes in gene expression within the nucleus. It is thought that these nuclear transcriptional effects are required for a long-term impact to be made on the developing brain, whether it be to encode a long-term memory, a change in synaptic strength, or a change in cortical map.

TABLE 1.
Cognitive Disorders Related to Molecular Defects in Intracellular Signaling

Disorder	Features	Defective Protein	Function
Neurofibromatosis type 1 (NF 1)	Learning disorder, neurofibromas, tumors	Neurofibromin	Ras/GTP Protein
Aarskog syndrome	Faciogenital dysplasia	Guanine nucleotide exchange factor	Activates rho GTPase Cdc42
X-linked MR	Seizures, ataxia	Oligophrenin-1	rho GTPase-activating protein (rhoGAP)
X-linked nonsyndromic MR	No dysmorphic features	PAK3 (p21- activated kinase 3	ser/threonine MAP kinase complexes with Ras-like proteins
Tuberous sclerosis-2	Seizures, tumors	Tuberin	GTPase- activating protein (GAP)
Coffin-Lowry syndrome	X-linked MR, dysmorphic	Rsk-2	CREB kinase
Complex X-linked MR	MR	Rsk-4	Similar to Rsk-2
Rubinstein-Taybi syndrome	MR, dysmorphic	CREB-binding protein	Transcriptional coactivator
X-linked α-thalassemia	MR, thalassemia	XH2 helicase	Unwinds DNA: transcription
Rett syndrome	X-linked, girls, encephalopathy	MeCP2	Transcriptional repressor, binds methyl-CpGs
Cretinism	MR, spasticity	Nuclear thyroid receptor	Transcriptional coactivator

Abbreviations: Ras, Guanine nucleotide binding protein; *GTP,* guanosine triphosphate; *MR,* mental retardation; *MAP,* mitogen-activated protein; *CREB,* cyclic AMP response element binding protein; *CPGs,* cytosine guanine containing nucleotides.

Several of these disorders, including neurofibromatosis type 1, the Aarskog syndrome, tuberous sclerosis type 2, and X-linked mental retardation associated with defects in oligophrenin 1 or PAK3 (p21-activated kinase 3), involve defects in pathways involving G proteins linked to membrane receptors.[112-115] Others involve defects in steps closer to the nucleus, including Coffin-Lowry syndrome, an X-linked disorder of the CREB phosphorylase Rsk-2; complex X-linked mental retardation associated with a defect in Rsk-4; and Rubinstein-Tabyi syndrome, caused by a defect in CREB-binding protein.[116-119] The X-linked α- thalassemia/retardation syndrome is secondary to a defect in a DNA helicase.[120] Rett syndrome, the X-linked neurobehavioral disorder that affects girls predominantly, has been associated with defects in the MeCP2 transcriptional repressor protein.[121]

These disorders probably disrupt brain development by restricting activity-dependent neuronal plasticity, and 2 of them, Rubinstein-Tabyi and Rett syndromes, are associated with morphological abnormalities in synaptic connections. Cretinism caused by thyroid hormone deficiency during a critical period in early brain development, also produces similar pathologic changes in the brain because it acts through a nuclear hormone receptor to facilitate transcription.[122] These signaling cascades are particularly important for "sculpting" developing dendrites.[123] Dendritic abnormalities are a relatively common feature of mental retardation syndromes, and they may point to unrecognized defects in these signaling pathways.[124,125] Similar molecular lesions have been associated with defects in learning and memory in lower animals.

Most of these disorders have dysmorphic features in somatic tissues as well as in brain function because the defective signaling pathways are ubiquitous in many cell types, although they may serve different functions. For example, neurofibromin, the defective protein in neurofibromatosis type 1, is a Ras/guanosine 5'-triphosphate protein that appears to play a role in cyclic AMP–dependent signaling in neurons and also serves in a tumor suppressor role in many tissues.[112] In Coffin-Lowry syndrome, patients have prominent facial, bony, and other somatic abnormalities along with cognitive defects. In cultured fibroblasts and lymphoblasts from a group of 5 boys with Coffin-Lowry syndrome and 2 female carriers, the functional ability of the Rsk-2 enzyme to phosphorylate a CREB analogue was found to be directly related to cognitive ability.[117] This is an area where more genetic lesions are likely to be discovered in the future, and these somatic abnormalities could provide clues to their identification.

CAN THERE BE TOO MUCH PLASTICITY?

Although neuronal plasticity is usually thought to be a good thing, enabling adaptability and flexibility as well as recovery from injury or accidental miswiring, some evidence indicates that it can sometime have unwanted consequences. This may be the case in phantom limb pain, a disorder that occurs commonly after amputation of an extremity.[126-128] Flor et al[126] used MEG to study adult patients who had arm amputations to determine the extent of the reorganization of their somatosensory cortex. They found that the area of cortex deprived of sensory input from the amputated arm is reassigned to a variable degree to the face and lip and that the degree of reorganization was directly related to the severity of phantom limb pain. They suggested that pain pathways previously connected to the amputated arm became permanently hyperactive during the course of cortical reorganization.

Similar studies have not been reported in children, but experiments in immature animals suggest that a similar maladaptive phenomenon could occur. Ruda et al[129] studied a rodent model of chronic hindpaw limb inflammation in neonates and found that as adults, they exhibited spinal neuronal circuits with increased inputs and heightened responses to stimulation. They also found an increase in the density of central terminals in the spinal cord originating from peripheral nerve fibers from the inflamed limb, suggesting that sprouting had occurred. These studies suggested the potential for dysfunctional plasticity in infants exposed to chronic pain.

Another clinical situation in which dysfunctional plasticity might contribute to disability is in patients with cerebral palsy. Dystonia, or sustained, twisting involuntary movements of the trunk or extremities, commonly appears to worsen some time after early injury to the basal ganglia in patients with extrapyramidal cerebral palsy.[130] Saint Hilaire et al[130] described a series of patients with dystonia attributed to perinatal asphyxia that was delayed until an average of 13 years after birth and continued to progress for as long as 3 decades. A similar phenomenon is often seen in children with progressive dystonia in a hemiparetic extremity from an early stroke or traumatic injury. Although these disorders have not been studied with functional imaging, it seems likely that they are related to maladaptive plastic reorganization of neuronal circuitry in cortical and basal ganglia motor pathways. Dystonia has been linked to abnormal reorganization of somatosensory cortex in adults with disorders such as writer's cramp or focal hand dystonia secondary to occupations such as piano playing.[131,132] Experimental injury to the basal ganglia in immature animals also produces abnormal reorganization of cholinergic neurons that may produce dysfunction.[133] Plastic reorganization of the hippocampus after early damage has also been associated with chronic epilepsy.[134] Therefore, some evidence indicates that too much as well as too little plasticity may cause neurodevelopmental disorders.

CONCLUSION

As more is learned about the neurobiology of the developing brain, many intuitive notions about nature versus nurture are confirmed. Experience does seem to play a large role in brain development, both positively and negatively, and we are learning exactly how this happens at the level of genes, molecules, and synapses. It has been suspected for some time that children do better after brain injuries than adults, and some of the potential reasons for this are now becoming more clear. The concept of the "synaptic power curve" is a relatively new but important one because it implies that for most of childhood, the brain is choosing which connections to eliminate, not growing new ones. An enlarging list of genetic and acquired disorders such as lead poisoning, epileptic encephalopathies, neurofibromatosis, and Coffin-Lowry syndrome may impair the brain by disrupting pathways that mediate activity-dependent plasticity. These pathways are also important for understanding the effects of early intervention enrichment programs and rehabilitative therapies.[135] Understanding how environment can sculpt the developing brain provides an important perspective on the causes and treatment of neurodevelopmental disabilities.

REFERENCES

1. Shatz CJ: The developing brain. *Sci Am* 267:60-67, 1992.
2. Cowan WM, Fawcett JW, O'Leary DD, et al: Regressive events in neurogenesis. *Science* 225:1258-1265, 1984.
3. Huttenlocher PR: Synaptic density in human frontal cortex: Developmental changes and effects of aging. *Brain Res* 163:195-205, 1979.
4. Penn AA, Shatz CJ: Brain waves and brain wiring: The role of endogenous and sensory-driven neural activity in development. *Pediatr Res* 45:447-458, 1999.
5. Toga AW, Mazziota JC, Frankowiak RSJ: *Brain Mapping: The Systems.* New York, Academic Press, 2000, p 659.
6. Courtney SM, Ungerleider LG, Keil K, et al: Transient and sustained activity in a distributed neural system for human working memory. *Nature* 386:608-611, 1997.

7. Cohen MS, Bookheimer SY: Localization of brain function using magnetic resonance imaging. *Trends Neurosci* 17:268-277, 1994.
8. Conel JL: *The Postnatal Development of the Human Cerebral Cortex*, 1st ed. Cambridge, Mass, Harvard University Press, 1939-1967.
9. Rabinowicz T, de Courten-Myers GM, Petetot JM, et al: Human cortex development: Estimates of neuronal numbers indicate major loss late during gestation. *J Neuropathol Exp Neurol* 55:320-328, 1996.
10. Sidman RL, Rakic P: Neuronal migration, with special reference to developing human brain: A review. *Brain Res* 62:1-35, 1973.
11. Yakovlev PI, Lecours AR: The myelogenetic cycles of regional maturation of the brain. *Regional Development of the Brain in Early Life.* Oxford, England, Blackwell, 1967.
12. Huttenlocher PR: Morphometric study of human cerebral cortex development. *Neuropsychologia* 28:517-527, 1990.
13. Rakic P, Bourgeois JP, Eckenhoff MF, et al: Concurrent overproduction of synapses in diverse regions of the primate cerebral cortex. *Science* 232:232-235, 1986.
14. Lidow MS, Goldman-Rakic PS, Rakic P: Synchronized overproduction of neurotransmitter receptors in diverse regions of the primate cerebral cortex. *Proc Natl Acad Sci U S A* 88:10218-10221, 1991.
15. Chugani HT: Metabolic imaging: A window on brain development and plasticity. *The Neuroscientist* 5:29-40, 1999.
16. Chugani HT, Phelps ME, Mazziotta JC: Positron emission tomography study of human brain functional development. *Ann Neurol* 22:487-497, 1987.
17. Magistretti PJ, Pellerin L, Rothman DL, et al: Energy on demand. *Science* 283:496-497, 1999.
18. Sokoloff L: Energetics of functional activation in neural tissues. *Neurochem Res* 24:321-329, 1999.
19. Sibson NR, Dhankhar A, Mason GF, et al: Stoichiometric coupling of brain glucose metabolism and glutamatergic neuronal activity. *Proc Natl Acad Sci U S A* 95:316-321, 1998.
20. Hubel DH, Wiesel TN: The period of susceptibility to the physiological effects of unilateral eye closure in kittens. *J Physiol* 206:419-436, 1970.
21. Crair MC, Gillespie DC, Stryker MP: The role of visual experience in the development of columns in cat visual cortex. *Science* 279:566-570, 1998.
22. Wong RO, Chernjavsky A, Smith SJ, et al: Early functional neural networks in the developing retina. *Nature* 374:716-718, 1995.
23. Vaegan, Taylor D: Critical period for deprivation amblyopia in children. *Trans Ophthalmol Soc U K* 99:432-439, 1979.
24. Villablanca JR, Hovda DA: Developmental neuroplasticity in a model of cerebral hemispherectomy and stroke. *Neuroscience* 95:625-637, 2000.
25. Boatman D, Freeman J, Vining E, et al: Language recovery after left hemispherectomy in children with late-onset seizures. *Ann Neurol* 46:579-586, 1999.

26. Johnston MV, Gerring JP: Head trauma and its sequelae. *Pediatr Ann* 21:362-368, 1992.
27. Vargha-Khadem F, Carr LJ, Isaacs E, et al: Onset of speech after left hemispherectomy in a nine-year-old boy. *Brain* 120:159-182, 1997.
28. Waxman SG: Nonpyramidal motor system and functional recovery after damage to the central nervous system. *J Neurol Rehabil* 2:1-6, 1988.
29. Chollet F, DiPiero V, Wise RJ, et al: The functional anatomy of motor recovery after stroke in humans: A study with positron emission tomography. *Ann Neurol* 29:63-71, 1991.
30. Palmer FB, Shapiro BK, Wachtel RC, et al: The effects of physical therapy on cerebral palsy. A controlled trial in infants with spastic diplegia. *N Engl J Med* 318:803-808, 1988.
31. Hamdy S, Rothwell JC, Aziz Q, et al: Long-term reorganization of human motor cortex driven by short-term sensory stimulation. *Nat Neurosci* 1:64-68, 1998.
32. Chugani HT, Jacob B: Metabolic recovery in caudate nucleus of children following cerebral hemispherectomy: Two case studies. *Ann Neurol* 36:794-797, 1995.
33. Maegaki Y, Maeoka Y, Ishii S, et al: Central motor reorganization in cerebral palsy patients with bilateral cerebral lesions. *Pediatr Res* 45:559-567, 1999.
34. Sadato N, Pascual-Leone A, Grafman J, et al: Activation of the primary visual cortex by Braille reading in blind subjects. *Nature* 380:526-528, 1996.
35. Sadato N, Pascual-Leone A, Grafman J, et al: Neural networks for Braille reading by the blind. *Brain* 121:1213-1229, 1998.
36. Cohen LG, Celnik P, Pascual-Leone A, et al: Functional relevance of cross-modal plasticity in blind humans. *Nature* 389:180-183, 1997.
37. Simos PG, Papanicolaou AC, Breier JI, et al: Insights into brain function and neural plasticity using magnetic source imaging. *J Clin Neurophysiol* 17:143-162, 2000.
38. Elbert T, Pantev C, Wienbruch C, et al: Increased cortical representation of the fingers of the left hand in string players. *Science* 270:305-307, 1995.
39. Sterr A, Muller MM, Elbert T, et al: Changed perceptions in Braille readers. *Nature* 391:134-135, 1998.
40. Pantev C, Oostenveld R, Engelien A, et al: Increased auditory cortical representation in musicians. *Nature* 392:811-814, 1998.
41. Heeger DJ, Huk AC, Geisler WS, et al: Spikes versus BOLD: What does neuroimaging tell us about neuronal activity? *Nat Neurosci* 3:631-633, 2000.
42. Dubowitz LM, Mushin J, De Vries L, et al: Visual function in the newborn infant: Is it cortically mediated? *Lancet* 1:1139-1141, 1986.
43. Martin E, Joeri P, Loenneker T, et al: Visual processing in infants and children studied using functional MRI. *Pediatr Res* 46:135-140, 1999.

44. Yamada H, Sadato N, Konishi Y, et al: A milestone for normal development of the infantile brain detected by functional MRI. *Neurology* 55:218-223, 2000.
45. Born AP, Miranda MJ, Rostrup E, et al: Functional magnetic resonance imaging of the normal and abnormal visual system in early life. *Neuropediatrics* 31:24-32, 2000.
46. Neville HJ, Corina DBD, Rauschecker J, et al: Cerebral organization for language in deaf and hearing subjects: Biological constraints and effects of experience. *Proc Natl Acad Sci (U S A)* 95:922-929, 1998.
47. Chu D, Huttenlocher PR, Levin DN, et al: Reorganization of the hand somatosensory cortex following perinatal unilateral brain injury. *Neuropediatrics* 31:63-69, 2000.
48. Katz LC, Shatz CJ: Synaptic activity and the construction of cortical circuits. *Science* 274:1133-1138, 1966.
49. McDonald JW, Johnston MV: Physiological and pathophysiological roles of excitatory amino acids during central nervous system development. *Brain Res Rev* 15:41-70, 1990.
50. Rauschecker JP, Hahn S: Ketamine-xylazine anaesthesia blocks consolidation of ocular dominance changes in kitten visual cortex. *Nature* 326:183-185, 1987.
51. Daw NW, Gordon B, Fox KD, et al: Injection of MK-801 affects ocular dominance shifts more than visual activity. *J Neurophysiol* 81:204-215, 1999.
52. Kakizawa S, Yamasaki M, Watanabe M, et al: Critical period for activity-dependent synapse elimination in developing cerebellum. *J Neurosci* 20:4954-4961, 2000.
53. Cline HT, Debski EA, Constantine-Paton M: N-methyl-D-aspartate receptor antagonist desegregates eye-specific stripes. *Proc Natl Acad Sci U S A* 84:4342-4345, 1987.
54. Rabacchi S, Bailly Y, Delhaye-Bouchaud N, et al: Involvement of the N-methyl D-aspartate (NMDA) receptor in synapse elimination during cerebellar development. *Science* 256:1823-1825, 1992.
55. Contestabile A: Roles of NMDA receptor activity and nitric oxide production in brain development. *Brain Res Brain Res Rev* 32:476-509, 2000.
56. Hebb DO: *The organization of behavior.* New York, Wiley, 1949.
57. Bliss TV, Collingridge GL: A synaptic model of memory: Long-term potentiation in the hippocampus. *Nature* 361:31-39, 1993.
58. Kirkwood A, Lee HK, Bear MF: Co-regulation of long-term potentiation and experience-dependent synaptic plasticity in visual cortex by age and experience. *Nature* 375:328-331, 1995.
59. Fox K, Daw NW: Do NMDA receptors have a critical function in visual cortical plasticity? *Trends Neurosci* 16:116-122, 1993.
60. Martin SJ, Grimwood PD, Morris RG: Synaptic plasticity and memory: An evaluation of the hypothesis. *Annu Rev Neurosci* 23:649-711, 2000.
61. Kirkwood A, Rioult MC, Bear MF: Experience-dependent modification of synaptic plasticity in visual cortex. *Nature* 381:526-528, 1996.

62. Rittenhouse CD, Shouval HZ, Paradiso MA, et al: Monocular deprivation induces homosynaptic long-term depression in visual cortex. *Nature* 397:347-350, 1999.
63. Hensch TK, Fagiolini M, Mataga N, et al: Local GABA circuit control of experience-dependent plasticity in developing visual cortex. *Science* 282:1504-1508, 1998.
64. Feldman DE: Inhibition and plasticity. *Nat Neurosci* 3:303-304, 2000.
65. Antonini A, Stryker MP: Rapid remodeling of axonal arbors in the visual cortex. *Science* 260:1819-1821, 1993.
66. Huang ZJ, Kirkwood A, Pizzorusso T, et al: BDNF regulates the maturation of inhibition and the critical period of plasticity in mouse visual cortex. *Cell* 98:739-755, 1999.
67. Hata Y, Stryker MP: Control of thalamocortical afferent rearrangement by postsynaptic activity in developing visual cortex. *Science* 265:1732-1735, 1994.
68. Lein ES, Hohn A, Shatz CJ: Dynamic regulation of BDNF and NT-3 expression during visual system development. *J Comp Neurol* 420:1-18, 2000.
69. Murphy DD, Segal M: Morphological plasticity of dendritic spines in central neurons is mediated by activation of cAMP response element binding protein. *Proc Natl Acad Sci U S A* 94:1482-1487, 1997.
70. Roberson ED, English JD, Adams JP, et al: The mitogen-activated protein kinase cascade couples PKA and PKC to cAMP response element binding protein phosphorylation in area CA1 of hippocampus. *J Neurosci* 19:4337-4348, 1999.
71. Atkins CM, Selcher JC, Petraitis JJ, et al: The MAPK cascade is required for mammalian associative learning. *Nat Neurosci* 1:602-609, 1998.
72. Kandel ER, Pittenger C: The past, the future and the biology of memory storage. *Philos Trans R Soc Lond B Biol Sci* 354:2027-2052, 1999.
73. Harum KH, Johnston MV: Developmental neurobiology: New concepts in learning, memory, and neuronal development. *MRDD Res Rev* 4:20-25, 1998.
74. Johnston MV, Harum KH: Recent progress in the neurology of learning: Memory molecules in the developing brain. *J Dev Behav Pediatr* 20:50-56, 1999.
75. Bjorklund A, Linduall O: Self-repair of the brain. *Nature* 405:892-895, 2000.
76. van Praag H, Kempermann G, Gage FH: Running increases cell proliferation and neurogenesis in the adult mouse dentate gyrus. *Nat Neurosci* 2:266-270, 1999.
77. Gould E, Beylin A, Tanapat P, et al: Learning enhances adult neurogenesis in the hippocampal formation. *Nat Neurosci* 2:260-265, 1999.
78. Magavi SS, Leavitt BR, Macklis JD: Induction of neurogenesis in the neocortex of adult mice. *Nature* 405:951-955, 2000.
79. Wall JT: Variable organization in cortical maps of the skin as an indication of the lifelong adaptive capacities of circuits in the mammalian brain. *Trends Neurosci* 11:549-557, 1988.

80. Pons TP, Garraghty PE, Ommaya AK, et al: Massive cortical reorganization after sensory deafferentation in adult macaques. *Science* 252:1857-1860, 1991.
81. Jain N, Florence SL, Qi HX, et al: Growth of new brainstem connections in adult monkeys with massive sensory loss. *Proc Natl Acad Sci U S A* 97:5546-5550, 2000.
82. Florence SL, Taub HB, Kaas JH: Large-scale sprouting of cortical connections after peripheral injury in adult macaque monkeys. *Science* 282:1117-1121, 1998.
83. Nudo RJ, Wise BM, SiFuentes F, et al: Neural substrates for the effects of rehabilitative training on motor recovery after ischemic infarct. *Science* 272:1791-1794, 1996.
84. Killackey HP, Rhoades RW, Bennett-Clarke CA: The formation of a cortical somatotopic map. *Trends Neurosci* 18:402- 407, 1995.
85. Agmon A, Yang LT, O'Dowd DK, et al: Organized growth of thalamocortical axons from the deep tier of terminations into layer IV of developing mouse barrel cortex. *J Neurosci* 13:5365-5382, 1993.
86. Blue ME, Johnston MV: The ontogeny of glutamate receptors in rat barrel field cortex. *Brain Res Dev Brain Res* 84:11-25, 1995.
87. Blue ME, Erzurumlu RS, Jhaveri S: A comparison of pattern formation by thalamocortical and serotonergic afferents in the rat barrel field cortex. *Cereb Cortex* 1:380-389, 1991.
88. Blue ME, Martin LJ, Brennan EM, et al: Ontogeny of non-NMDA glutamate receptors in rat barrel field cortex: I. Metabotropic receptors. *J Comp Neurol* 386:16-28, 1997.
89. Brennan EM, Martin LJ, Johnston MV, et al: Ontogeny of non-NMDA glutamate receptors in rat barrel field cortex: II. Alpha-AMPA and kainate receptors. *J Comp Neurol* 386:29-45, 1997.
90. Iwasato T, Datwani A, Wolf AM, et al: Cortex-restricted disruption of NMDAR1 impairs neuronal patterns in the barrel cortex. *Nature* 406:726-731, 2000.
91. Crair MC, Malenka RC: A critical period for long-term potentiation at thalamocortical synapses. *Nature* 375:325-328, 1995.
92. Jones EG: Cortical and subcortical contributions to activity-dependent plasticity in primate somatosensory cortex. *Annu Rev Neurosci* 23:1-37, 2000.
93. Fox K: A critical period for experience-dependent synaptic plasticity in rat barrel cortex. *J Neurosci* 12:1826-1838, 1992.
94. Fox K, Zahs K: Critical period control in sensory cortex. *Curr Opin Neurobiol* 4:112-119, 1994.
95. Kano M, Iino K: Functional reorganization of adult cat somatosensory cortex is dependent on NMDA receptors. *Neuroreport* 2:77-80, 1991.
96. Fox K, Schlaggar BL, Glazewski S, et al: Glutamate receptor blockade at cortical synapses disrupts development of thalamocortical and columnar organization in somatosensory cortex. *Proc Natl Acad Sci U S A* 93:5584-5589, 1996.

97. Fox K: The critical period for long-term potentiation in primary sensory cortex. *Neuron* 15:485-488, 1995.
98. Feldman DE, Nicoll RA, Malenka RC: Synaptic plasticity at thalamocortical synapses in developing rat somatosensory cortex: LTP, LTD, and silent synapses. *J Neurobiol* 41:92-101, 1999.
99. Hohmann CF, Berger-Sweeney J: Cholinergic regulation of cortical development and plasticity. New twists to an old story. *Perspect Dev Neurobiol* 5:401-425, 1998.
100. Kilgard MP, Merzenich MM: Cortical map reorganization enabled by nucleus basalis activity. *Science* 279:1714-1718, 1998.
101. Johnston MV, Goldstein GW: Selective vulnerability of the developing brain to lead. *Curr Opin Neurol* 11:689-693, 1998.
102. Needleman HL, Schell A, Bellinger D, et al: The long-term effects of exposure to low doses of lead in childhood. An 11-year follow-up report. *N Engl J Med* 322:83-88, 1990.
103. Guilarte TR, McGlothan JL: Hippocampal NMDA receptor mRNA undergoes subunit specific changes during developmental lead exposure. *Brain Res* 790:98-107, 1998.
104. Markovac J, Goldstein GW: Picomolar concentrations of lead stimulate brain protein kinase C. *Nature* 334:71-73, 1988.
105. Wilson MA, Johnston MV, Goldstein GW, et al: Neonatal lead exposure impairs development of rodent barrel field cortex. *Proc Natl Acad Sci U S A* 97:5540-5545, 2000.
106. Hamosh A, Johnston MV, Valle D: Nonketotic hyperglycinemia, in Scriver CR, Beaudet AL, Sly WS, et al (eds): *The Metabolic and Molecular Bases of Inherited Disease*, vol 1. New York, McGraw-Hill, 1995, pp 1337-1348.
107. Ikonomidou C, Bosch F, Miksa M, et al: Blockade of NMDA receptors and apoptotic neurodegeneration in the developing brain. *Science* 283:70-74, 1999.
108. Ikonomidou C, Bittigau P, Ishimaru MJ, et al: Ethanol-induced apoptotic neurodegeneration and fetal alcohol syndrome. *Science* 287:1056-1060, 2000.
109. Aicardi J: Infantile spasms and related syndromes, in Aicardi J (ed): *Epilesy in Children*. New York, Raven Press, 1986.
110. Lacy JR, Penny JK: *Infantile spasms,* New York, Raven Press, 1976, p 169.
111. Tuchman RF: Epileptiform disorders with cognitive symptoms, in Swaiman KF, Ashwol S (eds): *Pediatric Neurology*. St Louis, Mosby, 1999, pp 661-667.
112. Guo HF, Tong J, Hannan F, et al: A neurofibromatosis-1-regulated pathway is required for learning in *Drosophila*. *Nature* 403:895-898, 2000.
113. Pasteris NG, Buckler J, Cadle AB, et al: Genomic organization of the faciogenital dysplasia (FGD1; Aarskog syndrome) gene. *Genomics* 43:390-394, 1997.
114. Allen KM, Gleeson JG, Bagrodia S, et al: PAK3 mutation in nonsyndromic X-linked mental retardation. *Nat Genet* 20:25-30, 1998.

115. Nellist M, van Slegtenhorst MA, Goedbloed M, et al: Characterization of the cytosolic tuberin-hamartin complex. Tuberin is a cytosolic chaperone for hamartin. *J Biol Chem* 274:35647-35652, 1999.
116. Trivier E, De Cesare D, Jacquot S, et al: Mutations in the kinase Rsk-2 associated with Coffin-Lowry syndrome. *Nature* 384:567-570, 1996.
117. Harum KH, Alemi L, Johnston MV: Cognitive impairment in Coffin-Lowry syndrome correlates with reduced RSK-2 activation. *Neurology* 56:207-214, 2001.
118. Yntema HG, van den Helm B, Kissing J, et al: A novel ribosomal S6-kinase (RSK4; RPS6KA6) is commonly deleted in patients with complex X-linked mental retardation. *Genomics* 62:332-343, 1999.
119. Petrij F, Giles RH, Dauwerse HG, et al: Rubinstein-Taybi syndrome caused by mutations in the transcriptional co-activator CBP. *Nature* 376:348-351, 1995.
120. Picketts DJ, Higgs DR, Bachoo S, et al: ATRX encodes a novel member of the SNF2 family of proteins: Mutations point to a common mechanism underlying the ATR-X syndrome. *Hum Mol Genet* 5:1899-1907, 1996.
121. Amir RE, Van den Veyver IB, Wan M, et al: Rett syndrome is caused by mutations in X-linked MECP2, encoding methyl-CpG-binding protein 2. *Nat Genet* 23:185-188, 1999.
122. Love JD, Gooch JT, Nagy L, et al: Transcriptional repression by nuclear receptors: Mechanisms role in disease. *Biochem Soc Trans* 28:390-396, 2000.
123. Demyanenko GP, Tsai AY, Maness PF: Abnormalities in neuronal process extension, hippocampal development, and the ventricular system of L1 knockout mice. *J Neurosci* 19:4907-4920, 1999.
124. Armstrong DD, Dunn K, Antalffy B: Decreased dendritic branching in frontal, motor and limbic cortex in Rett syndrome compared with trisomy 21. *J Neuropathol Exp Neurol* 57:1013-1017, 1998.
125. Billuart P, Bienvenu T, Ronce N, et al: Oligophrenin-1 encodes a rhoGAP protein involved in X-linked mental retardation. *Nature* 392:923-926, 1998.
126. Flor H, Elbert T, Knecht S, et al: Phantom-limb pain as a perceptual correlate of cortical reorganization following arm amputation. *Nature* 375:482-484, 1995.
127. Harris AJ: Cortical origin of pathological pain. *Lancet* 354:1464-1466, 1999.
128. Roricht S, Meyer BU, Niehaus L, et al: Long-term reorganization of motor cortex outputs after arm amputation. *Neurology* 53:106-111, 1999.
129. Ruda MA, Ling QD, Hohmann AG, et al: Altered nociceptive neuronal circuits after neonatal peripheral inflammation. *Science* 289:628-631, 2000.
130. Saint Hilaire M-H, Burke RE, Bressman SB, et al: Delayed-onset dystonia due to perinatal or early childhood asphyxia. *Neurology* 41:216-222, 1991.
131. Bara-Jimenez W, Shelton P, Sanger TD, et al: Sensory discrimination

capabilities in patients with focal hand dystonia. *Ann Neurol* 47:377-380, 2000.

132. Bara-Jimenez W, Catalan MJ, Hallett M, et al: Abnormal somatosensory homunculus in dystonia of the hand. *Ann Neurol* 44:828-831, 1998.
133. Johnston MV, Hudson C: Effects of postnatal hypoxia-ischemia on cholinergic neurons in the developing rat forebrain: Choline acetyltransferase immunocytochemistry. *Brain Res* 431:41-50, 1987.
134. Lynch M, Sutula T: Recurrent excitatory connectivity in the dentate gyrus of kindled and kainic acid-treated rats. *J Neurophysiol* 83:693-704, 2000.
135. Ramey CT, Ramey SL: Prevention of intellectual disabilities: Early interventions to improve cognitive development. *Prev Med* 27:224-232, 1998.

CHAPTER 2

The 22q11.2 Deletion Syndrome

Beverly S. Emanuel, PhD
Professor of Pediatrics, University of Pennsylvania School of Medicine; Charles E.H. Upham Professor of Pediatrics, Chief, Division of Human Genetics and Molecular Biology, The Children's Hospital of Philadelphia, Philadelphia, Pa

Donna McDonald-McGinn, MS
Associate Director, Division of Clinical Genetics, The Children's Hospital of Philadephia, Philadelphia, Pa

Sulagna C. Saitta, MD, PhD
Assistant Professor of Pediatrics, The University of Pennsylvania School of Medicine; Attending Physician, The Children's Hospital of Philadelphia, Philadelphia, Pa

Elaine H. Zackai, MD
Professor of Pediatrics, University of Pennsylvania School of Medicine; Director of Clinical Genetics, The Children's Hospital of Philadelphia, Philadelphia, Pa

ABSTRACT

Estimates suggest that the 22q11.2 deletion occurs in approximately 1 in 4000 live births, making this disorder a significant health concern in the general population. The 22q11.2 deletion has been identified in the majority of patients with DiGeorge syndrome, velocardiofacial syndrome, and conotruncal anomaly face syndrome, suggesting that they are phenotypic variants of the same disorder. The findings associated with the 22q11.2 deletion are extensive and highly variable from patient to patient. In this chapter, we discuss the features of this disorder, with an emphasis on the clinical findings and an approach to the evaluation of these patients. In addition, we present the current understanding at the molecular level, of the genomic mechanisms and genes that are likely to play a central role in causing this frequent genetic condition.

The 22q11.2 deletion has been identified in most patients with the DiGeorge syndrome (DGS), velocardiofacial syndrome (VCFS), conotruncal anomaly face syndrome (CAFS), as well as some cases of autosomal dominant Opitz G/BBB syndrome and Cayler cardiofacial syndrome.[1-10] The list of findings associated with the 22q11.2 deletion is extensive and varies from patient to patient. Most children are initially seen by a cardiologist, most commonly for evaluation of conotruncal cardiac anomalies, or by a plastic surgeon for evaluation of a cleft palate, velopharyngeal incompetence (VPI) or both. Recent estimates indicate that the 22q11 deletion occurs in approximately 1 in 4000 live births.[11] Thus, this disorder is a significant health concern in the general population.

DGS, first described in 1965 by Dr Angelo DiGeorge,[12] is a development defect of the third and fourth pharyngeal pouches. DiGeorge himself credits Harington in 1829 for the first description of congenital absence of the thymus in an infant with seizures who, in all probability, also had congenital absence of the parathyroid glands. DGS is characterized by a conotruncal cardiac anomaly and aplasia or hypoplasia of the thymus and parathyroid glands. Most patients with diagnosed DGS are first seen as newborns or infants with significant cardiovascular malformations, including interrupted aortic arch type B, truncus arteriosus, or tetralogy of Fallot, along with T-cell abnormalities and hypocalcemia. In addition, patients with DGS may have mild facial dysmorphia including hypertelorism, prominent ears, a bulbous nasal tip, a small mouth, and micrognathia. Since the initial report by DiGeorge[12] in 1965, the spectrum of clinical features associated with DGS has been expanded to include anomalies such as cleft palate, cleft lip, renal agenesis, neural tube defects, and hypospadias.[7,13-16] Before the advances in medical and surgical management of children with complex congenital cardiac disease, DGS was associated with significant morbidity and mortality. Thus, developmental delay and learning disabilities were not initially recognized as common features of this disorder.

Although the etiology of DGS was thought to be heterogeneous,[17] recent cytogenetic and molecular studies have demonstrated that a chromosome 22q11.2 deletion is the cause of DGS in most cases.[1,3,18-20] The initial links between 22q11.2 and DGS came from reports of DGS patients with unbalanced translocations resulting in the loss of the short arm and proximal long arm of chromosome 22, and from patients with interstitial deletions of 22q11.2.[21-24] Subsequently, molecular studies demonstrated that approximately 90% of cytogenetically normal DGS patients have microdeletions of chromosome 22q11.21.[1,3,19]

In 1968, Strong[25] reported an association of cardiac abnormalities (right-sided aortic arch), learning disabilities, and a characteristic facial appearance in 4 members of 1 family. In 1978, Shprintzen et al[26] described an apparently autosomal dominant disorder combining cleft palate or VPI, cardiac anomalies (most notably ventricular septal defect [VSD] or tetralogy of Fallot), learning disabilities, and facial dysmorphia. He termed this combination of findings velocardiofacial syndrome. The presence of features common to DGS, such as neonatal hypocalcemia, conotruncal cardiac anomalies, and decreased lymphoid tissue in patients with diagnosed VCFS, suggested that these 2 disorders might share a common pathogenesis.[27] Cytogenetic studies with high-resolution banding techniques detected interstitial deletions of chromosome 22q11.2 in 20% of patients with VCFS. Molecular studies with chromosome 22 probes, identical to those used to detect patients with DGS, demonstrated that most individuals with VCFS also had the same submicroscopic deletion of 22q11.2.[2,3]

The phenotype associated with the 22q11.2 deletion is variable, and the observed differences between patients with a diagnosis of DGS or VCFS most likely represent an ascertainment bias. For example, most patients with DGS have been identified in the neonatal period with a major congenital heart defect, whereas many patients with VCFS have been diagnosed in a cleft palate or craniofacial center when speech and learning difficulties became evident, near school age. DGS and VCFS were previously described as 2 distinct disorders. However, in light of the significant phenotypic overlap, most clinicians consider deletion-positive DGS and VCFS patients to have variant manifestations of the same disorder, the 22q11.2 deletion syndrome.[28-31] In addition, a microdeletion of chromosome 22q11.2 has also been detected in patients with CAFS (conotruncal cardiac anomalies and dysmorphia),[4,5] autosomal dominant "Opitz" G/BBB syndrome (hypertelorism, laryngotracheoesophageal cleft, cleft palate, swallowing difficulty, genitourinary defects, mental retardation, and congenital heart defects),[7,9,10] and Cayler cardiofacial syndrome (asymmetric crying facies),[8] further enlarging the phenotypic scope of the deletion. In this chapter, we describe the structural and functional processes associated with the 22q11.2 deletion, by system, as well as the current status of the molecular analysis of the deletion.

GENERAL OBSERVATIONS

In the large series of patients reported by McDonald-McGinn et al,[32] males and females were equally likely to be affected (52% female, 48% male). Greater than three fourths of the patients were white (77%), which is thought to be the result of an ascertainment bias (see the section on dysmorphology). The majority of patients were ascertained through Clinical Genetics. However, many were diagnosed in Cardiology or Plastic Surgery and less often in Ear, Nose, and Throat, Neurology, Immunology, Endocrinology, and Child Development.[32]

STRUCTURAL AND FUNCTIONAL ANOMALIES ASSOCIATED WITH 22Q11.2 DELETION

CARDIAC

Congenital heart disease is the most common structural anomaly associated with the 22q11.2 deletion. In a series of 250 patients, McDonald-McGinn et al[32] reported heart disease in 75% of patients with the deletion. The cardiac manifestations of the syndrome vary widely, ranging from minor cardiac anomalies requiring no intervention to major defects requiring multiple surgical procedures or causing mortality. The most common defect reported was tetralogy of Fallot, followed by interrupted aortic arch type B, conoventricular septal defect, truncus arteriosus,

TABLE 1.
Distribution of Cardiac Defects in Patients With a 22q11.2 Deletion (N = 305)

Heart Defect	%
Tetralogy of Fallot	20
VSD	14
Interrupted aortic arch	12
Truncus arteriosus	6
Vascular ring	6
ASD/VSD	6
Atrial septal defect	3
Right aortic arch	2
Other	6
Normal	25
Total	100

Abbreviations: VSD, Ventricular septal defect; *ASD,* atrial septal defect.

TABLE 2.
22q11.2 Deletions in Patients With Conotruncal Cardiac Defects

	No. of Patients Studied	No. Deleted	% Deleted
Tetralogy of Fallot	131	20	15.3
Interrupted aortic arch	25	13	52.0
Truncus arteriosus	29	10	34.5
Perimembranous VSD	8	3	37.5
Total	193	46	23.8

Abbreviation: VSD, Ventricular septal defect.
(Data from Goldmuntz E, Driscoll DA, Budarf ML, et al: Microdeletions of chromosomal region 22q11 in patients with conotruncal cardiac defects. *J Med Genet* 30:807-812, 1993.)

and a vascular ring (Table 1). Less common abnormalities include transposition of the great arteries with a VSD and pulmonary atresia, coarctation of the aorta, hypoplastic left heart syndrome, and heterotaxy.[32,33] Children with severe cardiac defects most often present in the newborn period with cyanosis, a heart murmur, or symptoms of congestive heart failure. Patients with the 22q11.2 deletion diagnosed after the first year of life are unlikely to have a major cardiac anomaly, but a septal defect or arch anomaly such as a vascular ring might not have been diagnosed at an earlier age. Such anomalies may require intervention. Therefore, it is not unreasonable to suggest that a cardiac evaluation be performed in patients who have the deletion diagnosed at an older age.[34]

In 1 study, patients with congenital heart disease were tested based solely on their conotruncal cardiac lesion.[35] It was found that 52% of patients with interrupted aortic arch, 34.5% of patients with truncus arteriosus, 37.5% of patients with a conoventricular septal defect, and 15.3% of patients with tetralogy of Fallot tested positive for the 22q11.2 deletion (Table 2). The frequency of the 22q11.2 deletion did not vary in patients with tetralogy of Fallot based on the presence of pulmonary atresia as compared with pulmonary stenosis. However, in patients with tetralogy of Fallot and absent pulmonary valve syndrome, there was a suggestion of an increased incidence of the 22q11.2 deletion. This study strongly supports screening patients with these specific cardiac lesions to provide appropriate clinical management and recurrence risk counseling for the patients and their families.

PALATE

Similar to congenital heart disease, palatal anomalies are frequently associated with the 22q11.2 deletion (Table 3). In 1 large cohort,[32] 69% of patients with the deletion were found to manifest a palatal defect. In this group of patients, VPI was the most common palatal anomaly (29%), followed by submucosal cleft palate (15%), overt cleft palate (11%), bifid uvula (5%), and cleft lip or cleft lip and palate (1%). In this study, palatal evaluations were performed by a plastic surgeon and a speech pathologist using a standard history (which included inquiry regarding the presence of nasal regurgitation and frequent otitis media), physical examination, and speech evaluation. Patients underwent videofluoroscopy, nasendoscopy, or both, when indicated. Some patients demonstrated incomplete closure of the velopharyngeal mechanism during crying and swallowing but were too young to obtain an adequate speech sample, and therefore received a diagnosis of infantile VPI or occult submucosal cleft palate (8%). Other patients demonstrated no overt abnormality but were considered too young to provide an adequate speech sample (14%). Overall, only 17% of patients were completely cleared of palatal involvement.

This same study found that, as opposed to findings in the cardiac population, the testing of patients with an isolated cleft palate is unlikely to yield a diagnosis of the 22q11.2 deletion. This was confirmed by screening 50 patients with isolated cleft palate. None were found to have the 22q11.2 deletion. Therefore, it is unlikely that the 22q11.2 deletion is responsible for a significant proportion of patients with nonsyndromic cleft palate. In contrast, Kirschner[36] found that 37.5% of patients with VPI of unknown eti-

TABLE 3.
Cleft Palate Findings in Patients With a 22q11.2 Deletion (N = 234)

Defect	% of Total
Velopharyngeal incompetence	29
Submucosal cleft palate	15
Overt cleft palate	11
Bifid uvula	5
Cleft lip/palate	1
Suspected VPI/need follow-up	22
Normal	17

Abbreviation: VPI, Velopharyngeal incompetence.

ology were diagnosed with the 22q11.2 deletion. Therefore, deletion testing in patients with VPI of unknown origin may be warranted.

EAR, NOSE, AND THROAT

Ear, nose, and throat findings include overfolded helices, squared-off helices, cupped, microtic, and protuberant ears, preauricular pits, preauricular tags, and narrow canals. A prominent nasal root, bulbous nasal tip, hypoplastic alae nasae, and nasal dimple/bifid nasal tip were common. Laryngotracheal esophageal abnormalities, including stridor caused by a vascular ring, laryngomalacia, and laryngeal webs, were seen. Chronic otitis media and chronic sinusitis were also commonly seen, perhaps related to the high incidence of VPI and the presence of immune compromise.[32]

In a group of 49 patients from this series, 39% demonstrated hearing loss in 1 or both ears. Most had conductive hearing loss averaging 25 to 35 dB, whereas 1 patient demonstrated a reverse slope mixed hearing loss. Abnormal otoscopic evaluations in the affected ears revealed serous otitis media, retraction of the tympanic membrane, or perforation of the tympanic membrane. Three patients with normal otoscopic evaluation and tympanometry in the presence of permanent conductive or mixed hearing loss had either presumed or confirmed ossicular abnormality. Only 4 of the patients with hearing loss were found to have normal palatal function; 3 of those were the patients with presumed or confirmed ossicular abnormalities. Of the 61% of patients (30 patients) noted to have normal hearing sensitivity, 7 had bilateral pressure-equalization tubes, suggesting a history of middle ear dysfunction and prior conductive hearing loss. Because these problems are often linked to a patient's speech and palatal abnormalities, it is important to recognize and treat the otolaryngologic problems of children with the 22q11.2 deletion early in life.

FEEDING

Until recently, the significant feeding problems associated with the 22q11.2 deletion had not been appreciated. In the cohort reported by McDonald-McGinn et al,[32] 30% of patients with the 22q11.2 deletion had a history of feeding difficulties. Forty-five percent required gastrostomy tubes, and 50% required nasogastric tube feedings. Results of barium swallow studies in 23 patients indicated that the underlying problem in many patients was dysmotility in the pharyngoesophageal area that was independent of other structural abnormalities (cardiac defects and palatal anomalies). The major problems included nasopharyngeal reflux, prominence of the cricopharyngeal muscle, abnormal cricopharyngeal closure, and diverticulum. In addition, many patients had significant constipation. Successful management strategies include medication for gastrointestinal dysmotility, facilitation of bowel evacuation, treatment of gastroesophageal reflux with acid blockade and prokinetic agents, postural therapy, and spoon placement modifications.[37,38]

OCULAR

Ocular findings are frequently associated with the 22q11.2 deletion. The external findings include hooding of the upper lid (41%), ptosis (9%), hooding of the lower lid (6%), epicanthal folds (3%), and distichiasis (3%). Tortuous retinal vessels were present in 58% of cases, and posterior embryotoxon was seen in 69% of patients. No patients were found to have cataracts or colobomas.[32] Of note, posterior embryotoxon has been seen in 12% to 32% of control individuals, but the incidence in patients with the deletion is almost as high as the 89% seen in patients with Alagille syndrome.[39] In contrast, the incidence of astigmatism, myopia, and hyperopia were fairly comparable to that of the general population.

NEUROLOGIC

The 22q11.2 deletion has been associated with a variety of neurologic and psychological manifestations including hypotonia, developmental delay, and psychiatric abnormalities. Lynch[40] examined 47 consecutive patients with the 22q11.2 deletion and found the majority had neurologic abnormalities that were generally nonprogressive and highly variable. This finding suggests that diverse neurologic complications are a component of the 22q11.2 deletion, but no single manifestation is present in most patients. Findings in the series of patients described by McDonald-McGinn et al,[32] included seizures (with and without hypocalcemia), asymmetric crying facies, ataxia, cerebellar hypoplasia, enlarged Sylvian fissures, pituitary abnormalities, polymicrogyria, mega cisterna magna, and neural tube defects.[41,42]

The 22q11.2 deletion has also been associated with progressive central nervous system degeneration in adults who developed progressively worsening ataxia beginning at approximately 20 years of age.[40] Magnetic resonance imaging scans have been concordant with these findings.

SKELETAL

In the series by McDonald-McGinn et al,[32] chest radiographs were examined from 63 patients. Of these, 19% had vertebral anomalies including coronal clefts, hemivertebrae, and butterfly vertebrae. Rib anomalies, most commonly supernumerary ribs, were noted in 19%. Other anomalies such as hypoplastic scapulae were seen in 1.5%, and scoliosis has been reported, with a rate as high as 13%. A review for anomalies of the extremities was done on 108 patients; 6% had anomalies of the upper extremities, which included preaxial and postaxial polydactyly. Anomalies of the lower extremities, including postaxial polydactyly, club foot, overfolded toes, and 2,3 syndactyly, were noted in 15% of patients.[43]

The presence of butterfly vertebrae in the 22q11.2 deletion is particularly noteworthy in that it is a rare finding in the general population. In combination with tetralogy of Fallot, these findings could be mistakenly diagnosed as Alagille syndrome. This is especially significant in light of the high incidence of posterior embryotoxon in the 22q11.2 deletion patients. It is important to know that these skeletal findings are occasionally associated with the deletion so that one does not seek other diagnoses in the face of the patient's otherwise typical findings. Finally, the incidence of craniosynostosis is increased in patients with the 22q11.2 deletion.[44-46] Four patients had craniosynostosis: 3 bicoronal and 1 unicoronal. None were found to have a mutation in *FGFR1, 2, 3*, or *TWIST.* This association was also reported in 5 patients in the European collaborative study.[47]

RENAL

Previous reports have suggested that 10% to 37% of patients with the 22q11.2 deletion have renal or bladder abnormalities.[48] In a prospective study, 67 patients with no prior history of uropathy were evaluated with renal ultrasonography.[32] Of these patients, 37% were found to have renal abnormalities, which included calculi, single kidney, small kidneys, echogenic kidney, horseshoe kidney, bladder wall thickening, multicystic dysplastic kidney, duplicated collecting system, and renal tubular acidosis. The high incidence of renal abnormalities in this population is similar to that reported by others and supports screening patients by renal ultrasound for these abnormalities.[13]

ENDOCRINE

The major endocrine problems associated with the 22q11.2 deletion include hypoparathyroidism and growth disorders. Hypoparathyroidism can result in transient, persistent, or late-onset hypocalcemia, and patients can present with seizures, tetany, or be asymptomatic.[49] In the series by McDonald-McGinn et al,[32] 49% of 158 patients had confirmed hypocalcemia. Two patients (ages 8 and 12 years) who had hypocalcemia in infancy did not have the 22q11.2 deletion diagnosed until school age. Although they both required learning support, neither had any other medical problems.

The other associated endocrine problem is short stature. When a patient with 22q11.2 deletion has short stature or slow growth velocity, genetic short stature must be ruled out before growth hormone deficiency is investigated. Weinzimer et al[50] examined 95 patients between the ages of 1 and 15 years and found 41% to be below the 5th percentile in height. Of these, heights in 4 patients were significantly below the 5th percentile, and all were found to have low levels of growth factors, insulin-like growth factor-1 and insulin-like growth factor binding protein-3. The growth hormone response to pharmacologic stimulation was indicative of growth hormone deficiency in 3 of the 4 patients and normal in the fourth. Magnetic resonance imaging performed in the patients demonstrated a small pituitary gland in 2 of the 3. Two of the patients were treated with growth hormone and have demonstrated a dramatic improvement in height. One patient's height was –2.5 SD and after 2 years of therapy improved to –1.8 SD, with the growth velocity standard deviation score (SDS) changing from –1.6 to +0.7 SDS. The second patient's height was –3.2 SD and after 2 years of therapy improved to –1.6 SD, with the growth velocity SDS changing from –3.7 to +2.7.[50] Other hormonal disorders have been noted in children with the 22q11.2 deletion, including delayed puberty and hyperthyroidism.[49,51]

IMMUNE

In children with the 22q11.2 deletion, the extent of immunodeficiency is highly variable and does not correlate with any other phenotypic features. It is caused by impaired formation of thymic tissue and decreased production of T cells. There may also be secondary T-cell functional defects, humoral deficits, or both. In a series conducted by Sullivan et al,[52] 60 patients older than 6 months had immunologic evaluations including T-cell production and gross T-cell function. In patients older than 1 year, immunoglobulin production and function as well as more sensitive studies of T-cell function were also evaluated. Seventy-seven percent of patients were considered to be immunodeficient regardless of their clinical presentation. Sixty-seven percent had impaired T-cell production, 23% had humoral defects, 19% had impaired T-cell function, and 13% had IgA deficiency.[52,53] Nineteen infants had T-cell studies at birth and again at 1 year of age. Their findings were compared with those of deletion-negative controls. The results indicated that newborns with deletions have significantly fewer cells of thymic lineage compared with controls and that improvement in T-cell production is variable in deletion patients. Patients with the most significant deficiencies in T-cell production improved the most in the first year of life.[54]

T-cell disorders are often associated with autoimmune disease, specifically autoimmune hemolytic anemia, idiopathic thrombocytopenic purpura (ITP), autoimmune enteropathies, and arthritis. Sullivan (personal communication) reported the presence of juvenile rheumatoid arthritis (3 polyarticular, 2 pauciarticular) in 5 of 317 patients studied. Six patients had ITP, one of whom had chronic ITP. One patient with ITP had concomitant autoimmune hemolytic anemia, 1 patient had vitiligo, and 1 patient had rheumatic fever. This rate is much greater than the incidence seen in the general population for these disorders. Therefore, it appears that the frequency of autoimmune disease, in general, is higher in patients with the chromosome 22q11.2 deletion.[55]

In addition, Graves disease is associated with the 22q11.2 deletion. Recently, Kawame et al[51] described 4 patients with Graves disease and the 22q11.2 deletion. This association is not believed to be a coincidence and suggests that Graves disease is an uncommon but component manifestation of the 22q11.2 deletion. Therefore, evaluation of thyroid hormone levels is indicated when features suggestive of hyperthyroidism are present in patients with the 22q11.2 deletion. Overall, the associated predisposition to autoimmune disorders contributes to the wide phenotypic variability of the 22q11.2 deletion.

OTHER

In the series by McDonald-McGinn et al,[32] hematologic abnormalities included idiopathic thrombocytopenia and Bernard-Soulier syndrome, an autosomal recessive disorder of platelet function that maps to this chromosome region.[56] Further, in children with the 22q11.2 deletion, other findings included umbilical and inguinal hernia, accessory spleens, imperforate anus, cryptorchidism, hypospadias, significant constipation, bed-wetting, and leg pain.

NEUROPSYCHOLOGICAL

Developmental delays or learning disabilities have been reported in 90% to 100% of patients with the 22q11.2 deletion. Mental retardation was seen in 40% to 46% of the patients with 22q11.2 deletion described by Swillen et al[57] in the large Belgian series. In reports by Gerdes et al,[58,59] a wide range of expression of developmental and behavioral findings was observed in young children. In the preschool years, children with a 22q11.2 deletion were most commonly found to be hypotonic and developmentally delayed with language and speech difficulties. The more significantly delayed children are at high risk of subsequently receiving a diagnosis of mild or moderate mental retardation. Severe and profound retardation was not seen, and a few patients functioned within the average range. The studies by Gerdes et al[58,59] suggested that global delays and variations in intelligence were directly associated with the 22q11.2 deletion and were not explained by other physical anomalies or previous medical or surgical interventions.

In this same series, a history of mild to significant language delays was present in all the children. Solot et al[60] reported that two thirds of the study population with the 22q11.2 deletion were lacking in all verbal communication skills as late as 2 years of age. Furthermore, delays in expressive language were well beyond that expected for their developmental level. Voice quality disturbances, low facial tone, articulation errors, and dysarthria were present in many preschoolers. These findings highlight the need for early evaluation and intervention designed to develop alternative communication strategies best suited to the child's needs. In nonspeaking children, Solot et al[60,61] suggested that the use of alternative communication methods such as manual signs may reduce frustration, increase communicative competencies, and act as a bridge towards more conventional speech symbols.

Because all the preschool children studied by Gerdes et al[58,59] experienced some degree of delay, the use of early intervention strategies is suggested. The efficacy of early intervention in reducing the impact of a disability is well recognized. Because all children with the 22q11.2 deletion are at high risk for developmental disabilities, they would benefit from monitoring or special services. This would include occupational therapy, physical therapy, and speech therapy beginning at 1 year of age. Again, although this population demonstrates common findings of cognitive delays, language delays, and motor deficits, there is a wide range in the expression of the disabilities, from very mild to more significant disabilities. Early counseling for parents should emphasize this range and the individuality of their child. The intervention services should be directed at each child's areas of weakness and strengths beginning in infancy.

In terms of school-aged development, Moss et al[62,63] described 81 patients with the 22q11.2 deletion, older than 5 years, who underwent the age-appropriate Weschler IQ battery: 18% attained full-scale IQ scores in the average range, 20% in the low-average range; 32% in the borderline range; and 30% in the retarded range. However, detailed analysis of the battery became important. As an example, 1 patient had a verbal IQ of 111, which is above the average range, but a performance IQ of 65, which falls in the retarded range, bringing his full-scale IQ down to 87, in the low-average range. This split between verbal and performance IQ is consistent with a nonverbal learning disability. Rourke et al[64,65] described a pattern of behavioral, scholastic, and cognitive assets and deficits associated with nonverbal learning disabilities. Assets include innate rote verbal learning and phonemic awareness skills and higher verbal IQ scores. Deficits include fine motor delays, perceptual-motor integration difficulty, visual-spatial problems, and poor mathematics skills. Nonverbal learning disabilities have also been associated with a significantly increased risk for socialization deficits and internalizing psychiatric disorders such as depression or rage, and a slightly increased risk for suicide.[63] This nonverbal learning disability was present in 65% of these patients, with a mean split between verbal comprehension and perceptual organization of 12 points. Therefore, the full-scale IQ scores do not accurately represent many of these patients, and their verbal and performance IQ scores should be considered separately. These findings are of particular importance because there are direct ramifications for early intervention, including cognitive remediation, behavior management, and parental counseling, that are specific to this type of nonverbal learning disability. In addition, this is a rare type of learning disability as compared with that seen in the general population.[66]

PSYCHIATRIC

The 22q11.2 deletion is associated with a higher occurrence of psychiatric symptoms and disease, especially schizophrenia, than is found in the general population.[67,68] In a series by Jessani et al,[68] 24 children with the 22q11.2 deletion and their parents were evaluated by a child and adolescent psychiatrist and trained psychometricians. An increased frequency of psychiatric diagnoses, including attention-deficit/hyperactivity disorder, oppositional defiant disorder, separation anxiety disorder, specific phobias, generalized anxiety disorder, and depressive disorder, were found. Although in this young population, no increased frequency of bipolar affective disorder or schizophrenia was found, other studies have found an increased incidence of schizophrenia. Murphy and Owen[69] studied 50 adults with the deletion, of whom 24% fulfilled *Diagnostic and Statistical Manual of Mental Disorders, Fourth Edition (DSM-IV)* criteria for schizophrenia. Thus, a psychiatric component does seem to be associated with the 22q11.2 deletion in some patients. However, early childhood predictors and etiology remain to be defined.

DYSMORPHIA

Often the clinical suspicion of the 22q11.2 deletion in a patient with 1 or more of the above structural or functional findings is heightened, based on the presence of a characteristic facial appearance (Fig 1). Patients can present with only minimal findings of the 22q11.2 deletion but gain clinical attention when these findings are coupled with the characteristic craniofacial features. These typical facies include a prominent nasal root with a bulbous nasal tip and hypoplastic alae nasae, auricular abnormalities, and hooded eyelids (Fig 2). In the series by McDonald-McGinn et al,[46] a paucity of the latter findings in African American patients was recognized. For example, in the 370 patients with the 22q11.2 deletion, only 11% were African American, compared with the hospital-based population of 42%. The lack of characteristic facial features may lead to underrecognition in this population of patients, and therefore, the indcx of suspicion in patients who are not white may need to be changed to identify these individuals.

INHERITANCE PATTERN

Most patients identified with the 22q11.2 deletion do not have an affected parent. However, there are occasions where 1 parent has the deletion and has passed it on to his or her offspring at a rate of 50%. Twenty such nuclear families with the deletion were identified in a large cohort of 370 patients.[46] This suggests that the familial incidence of the 22q11.2 deletion is 6% when the number is adjusted to include only probands. However, there were adopted children within the cohort where the biological parent was suspect but not available for testing. There were also families in which both parents were not screened for the deletion. In a smaller subset of patients where both parents were screened (147 families), the familial incidence was 14%. However, this number may be inflated because parental testing was vigilantly pursued in those families where the parent was suspect, and was less aggressively sought in those situations where the parents had no medical

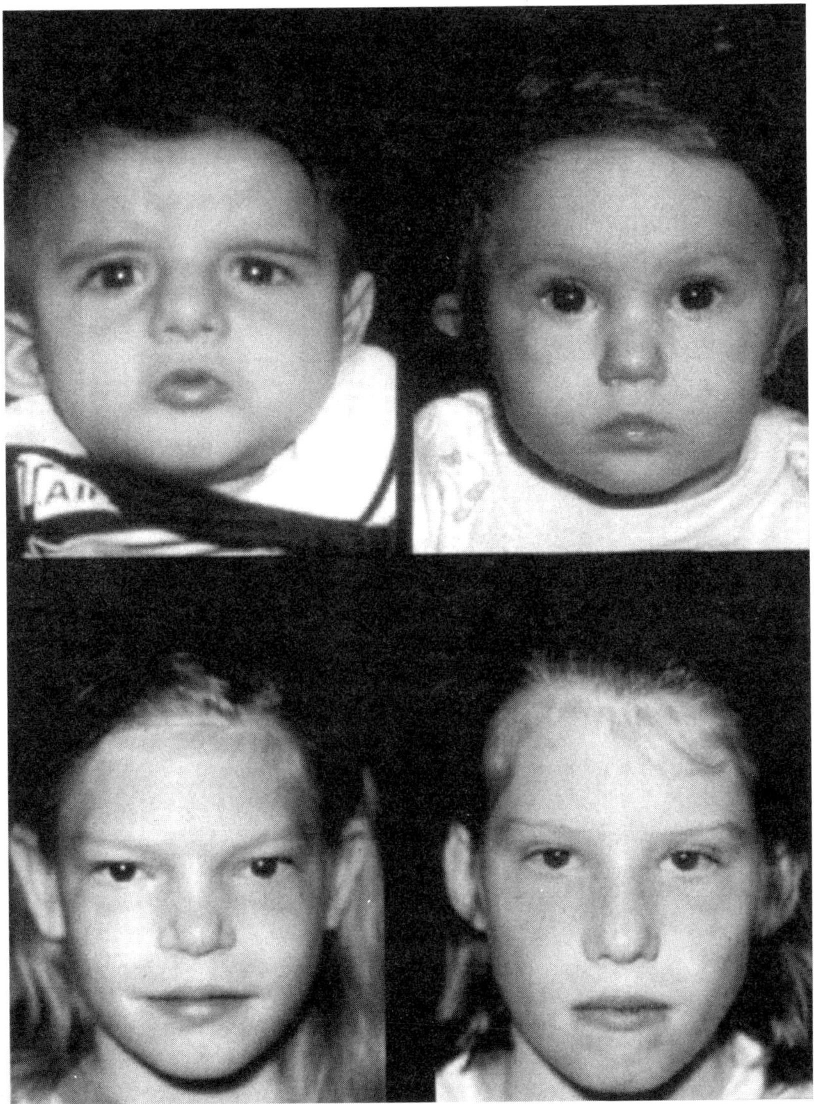

FIGURE 1.

Characteristic facies associated with chromosome 22q11.2 microdeletions. In the **upper row** are 2 young patients referred with features consistent with a diagnosis of DiGeorge syndrome. The 6-month old boy **(left)** and the 3-month-old girl **(right)** both have a bulbous nasal tip, small mouth, and protuberant ears. In the **lower row** are 2 preteens. The patient on the **right** demonstrates malar flatness, bulbous nasal tip, hypoplastic alae nasae; the patient on the **left** has typical "hooded eyelids" and protuberant ears.

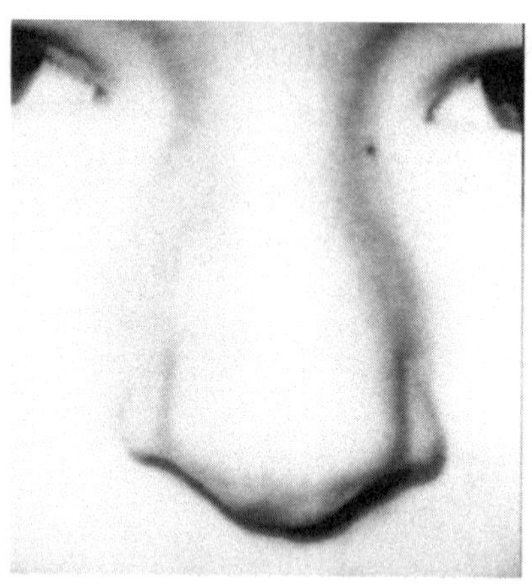

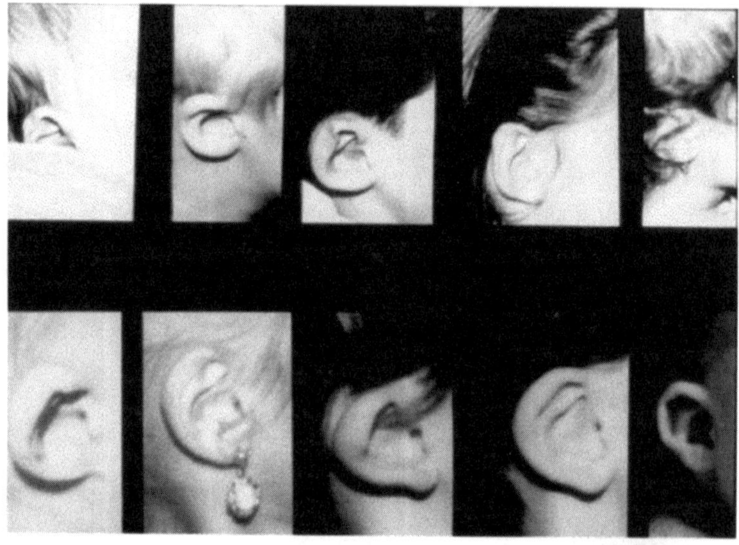

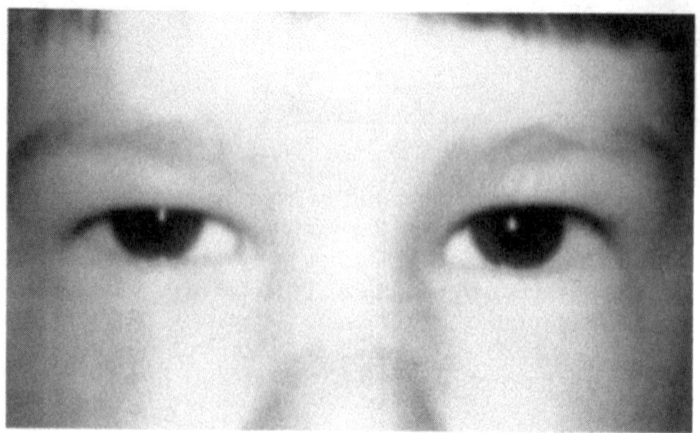

or learning issues and where third party reimbursement for the testing was uncertain. Thus, the true incidence of familial cases is more likely to be somewhere between these 2 numbers, approximately 10%.

INTERFAMILIAL AND INTRAFAMILIAL VARIABILITY

When McDonald-McGinn et al[46] examined the findings within the affected families, they noted wide intrafamilial variability. For example, one proband was ascertained because of his autism, short stature, and dysmorphic features. His family history was significant for a 12-year-old brother with a history of learning difficulty. Studies revealed that the brother, as well as the healthy father, carried the deletion. Similarly, another family came to attention after the identification of the 22q11.2 deletion in a neonate who died at 6 hours of age. At autopsy, heterotaxy, tracheal agenesis, an atrioventricular canal, and mild dysmorphic features were found, consistent with the deletion. The dysmorphia included a bulbous nasal tip and overfolded helices. During the postmortem parental conference, a paternal history of inguinal hernia, mild scoliosis, and the need for tutorial assistance in high school was obtained. Further studies revealed that the father also has the deletion.

To date, no explanation for this variability has been forthcoming. Most patients have the same large deletion; it remains unchanged with vertical transmission and is equally likely to occur on the chromosome derived from the mother or the father (see Molecular Studies; Parent of Origin). Still, great interfamilial and intrafamilial clinical variability occurs, making genotype-phenotype correlations difficult.[30,70,71]

Unselected Patients

In an effort to identify findings in an unselected and therefore unbiased population, McDonald-McGinn et al[44] described 31 patients with a 22q11.2 deletion who were identified only after the

---

FIGURE 2.

Characteristic facial features of the 22q11.2 deletion. **Top panel,** Hypoplastic alae nasae leading to the appearance of a bulbous nasal tip in a patient with a 22q11.2 deletion. **Middle panel,** Typical ear anomalies in patients with a 22q11.2 deletion including thick overfolded helices, "crumpled," protuberant, attached lobes, and microtia. In addition, preauricular tags have been seen. **Lower panel,** Typical "hooded eyelids" in a patient with a 22q11.2 deletion.

diagnosis in a relative. Nineteen were adults diagnosed after the diagnosis in their child, 8 were siblings of affected children, and 4 were affected co-twins. Only 5 of the 19 adult patients had come to medical attention before the diagnosis was established in their child. Two parents had overt cleft palate, one had hypocalcemic seizures, one had a laryngeal web, and one had received a diagnosis of schizophrenia. None had congenital cardiac anomalies. The "typical facial dysmorphia" associated with the 22q11.2 deletion only served to raise the index of suspicion in some adults with the deletion. When present, these findings most often included hooded eyelids, a prominent nasal root with a bulbous nasal tip, hypoplastic alae nasae, and auricular anomalies. In addition, the 12 previously undiagnosed children (8 males and 4 females) ranging in age from birth to 20 years often lacked phenotypic manifestations of the 22q11.2 deletion. Six were offspring of affected adults born before the identification of the deletion in their parent. One affected child was born subsequent to the identification of the 22q11.2 deletion in her father. One adult proband, who had come to attention as a teenager in the cleft clinic, had an affected child subsequent to her diagnosis. The latter 2 children were both identified prenatally via amniocentesis. Four other children received a diagnosis only after the identification of the deletion in their co-twins.

Many of the adults had completed high school, many with remedial assistance, and were functioning well in their jobs and relationships. Thus, analysis of this series of 31 patients, some with very mild manifestations of the deletion, allows examination of the outcome in individuals who had no specific remediations for this disorder. Further, it underscores the lack of familial concordance and the current lack of genotype-phenotype correlations in the disorder.

In conclusion, the phenotype of the 22q11.2 deletion syndromes is variable. Patients require significant medical surveillance and often specific interventions. An accurate diagnosis is essential to instituting an appropriate management plan. Thus, in Table 4, an approach to the clinical and laboratory studies relevant for evaluating patients for this disorder is presented.

MOLECULAR STUDIES

TYPES OF DELETIONS: STANDARD AND ATYPICALS

During the past few years, clinical and molecular studies have demonstrated that de novo deletions of chromosome 22 occur with a significant frequency, making the 22q11.2 deletion syndrome the

TABLE 4.
Suggested Evaluations for Patients With a 22q11.2 Deletion

Clinical Evaluations
- Standard:
  - Cardiology
  - Child psychology
  - ENT/audiology
  - Immunology
  - Plastic surgery/speech pathology
- Less Frequent:
  - Dental
  - Endocrine
  - Feeding team
  - Gastroenterology
  - Hematology
  - Neurology
  - Neurosurgery
  - Ophthalmology
  - Orthopedics
  - Psychiatry
  - Rheumatology
  - Urology

Laboratory/Diagnostic Studies
- Standard:
  - Renal ultrasound
- Standard depending on the age of the child:
  - Echocardiogram
  - Electrocardiogram
  - Immune profile
  - Ionized calcium
- Less Frequent:
  - Growth hormone studies
  - Hematologic profile
  - MRI (brain, spine)
  - Radiographs (chest, spine, limbs, etc)
  - VCUG

Abbreviations: ENT, Ear, nose, and throat; *MRI,* magnetic resonance imaging; *VCUG,* voiding cystourethrogram.

most common deletion in humans. In recent years, the development of sensitive fluorescence in situ hybridization (FISH) assays for diagnostic purposes has significantly improved detection of the deletion.[1-3] Analysis of a cohort of more than 200 deleted patients by FISH demonstrates a typically deleted region (TDR) of approximately 3 million base pairs or 3 megabases (Mb) in 80% to 90% of patients.[72-75] A minority of patients have variant deletion end points as depicted in Fig 3. These variant shorter deletions are nested within the large TDR.[76-80] The phenotypes of the patients with variant deletions appear to be similar to those with the approximately 3-Mb standard deletion.

In addition, several patients have been described with features of the 22q11.2 deletion syndrome and a microdeletion that falls outside the TDR and does not overlap with any of the known deletions. The first of these patients had craniofacial abnormalities and an interrupted aortic arch type B with truncus arteriosus, which emphasizes the likelihood that this 22q11.2-related phenotype probably does not result from defects involving a single gene within the TDR.[81] This finding has been further supported by the report of another patient with a novel deletion outside the TDR.[82] This second patient has a conotruncal defect (persistent truncus arteriosus), hypertelorism, micrognathia, bifid uvula, posteriorly rotated ears, hypospadias, and short stature. There was also evidence of hypocalcemia at birth and ongoing developmental delay. His deletion is also distal to the typical approximately 3-Mb deletion found in most patients with VCFS, and appears to overlap with the proximal portion of the deleted region (Fig 3) found in the patient described by Rauch et al.[81] Neither of these 2 variant deletions overlap with any of the previously described "minimal critical regions" for the 22q11.2 deletion. What is striking about these 2 patients is that they clearly demonstrate cardinal features of the 22q11.2 deletion, but appear to be deleted for a different set of genes than those thought to be responsible for the phenotypic features associated with the 22q11.2 deletion syndrome in the vast majority of patients.

DELETION MECHANISMS

The overwhelming majority of 22q11.2 deletions occur as de novo lesions, with less than 14% of deletions inherited from an affected parent. The prevalence of these de novo 22q11.2 deletions indicates an extremely high mutation or rearrangement rate within this genomic region (approximately 2.5×10^{-4}). Significant attention has recently been directed toward understanding

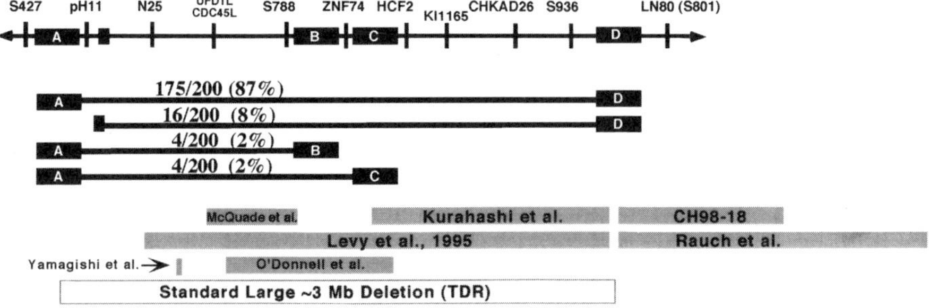

FIGURE 3.
Map of 22q11.2 illustrating the position of the standard deletion boundaries *(A-D)*. Individual duplicated sequence blocks are indicated as *A, B, C, D*. There are additional copies of the repeat blocks proximal and distal to the flanking markers (S427 and LN80 [S801]). Within the map, genes and markers used to identify cosmids used for fluorescence in situ hybridization (FISH) experiments to determine deletion size are indicated. The *lines immediately below the map* indicate the extent and frequency of recurrent deletions. The number of individual patients with particular deletion boundaries[74] are as indicated. The *bottom panel* shows the boundaries of variant deletions in several patients described in the text.

the molecular basis of such deletion or recombination "hot spots."[83,84] The high frequency of chromosome 22q11 meiotic abnormalities strongly suggests its genomic instability. In addition, the significant number of translocations and deletions associated with the 22q11.2 deletion syndrome phenotype[85] suggests that genomic instability may be related to the structure of this region.[72,74,75] Currently, little is known about the precise mechanisms involved in causing this instability. However, one important factor could be the presence of "recombination permissive" duplicated DNA sequences, low-copy chromosome 22–specific repeats or LCRs in 22q11.[72-75,86,87] Duplicated sequences allow for mispairing and unequal crossing over between homologues (interchromosomal) or allow intrachromosomal recombinations to take place within a single or between sister chromatids.[84]

CHROMOSOME 22–SPECIFIC LCRS

Through an extensive international collaboration, the complete sequence of 22q is now available.[87] As part of this effort, a contiguous set of cloned DNA segments, a contig, across the chromosomal region of the 22q11.2 deletion was completed.[74] These studies led to the description of complex modular blocks of duplicated DNA sequence, the 22-LCRs[74,75,87] within 22q11. These blocks are presumed to mediate the recombination events that lead to the rearrangements encountered in this region. The blocks of sequence are large and are composed of modular elements that have greater than 98% sequence identity with respect to one another. However, individual copies of these modular elements can be distinguished at the sequence level by single nucleotide polymorphisms.[74,75]

The typical 22q11.2 deletion interval (TDR) contains at least 4 of these large low-copy repeat blocks (22-LCRs) that coincide with the recurrent deletion end points and strongly implicate the 22-LCRs in the events leading to deletion. The 2 patients described above with deletions that do not overlap the TDR also appear to have deletion end points that coincide with additional distal copies of these repeat blocks. Thus, it appears that the structure of the genomic DNA in 22q11 predisposes it to a high rate of deletion and rearrangement, presumed to occur during meiotic recombination. Elucidating the mechanisms by which such chromosomal changes take place is currently an area of active investigation.

PARENT OF ORIGIN

Several other deletion-based genomic disorders show a specific bias with regard to the parent in whom the rearrangement takes place in meiosis. Parent-of-origin effects have been shown to be significant in the expression of the phenotype of the 15q11-q13 deletions of Prader-Willi and Angelman syndromes. This is primarily caused by the phenomenon of imprinting. For chromosome 22, data from several published studies differ with regard to the parent of origin of de novo 22q11.2 deletions, with 1 study[47] reporting that the majority are paternal in origin and 2 others[88,89] showing a maternal excess. When data for the patients from these 3 studies is combined, there are 33 maternal and 30 paternal deletions. Additional data derived from examination of 62 de novo standard deletion cases indicate 31 paternal and 31 maternal deletions.[90] Taken together, these data appear to provide limited evidence for major effects on the phenotype of the deleted individual as a result of imprinting in the 22q11.2 deletion. This is in agreement with the observation that both maternal and paternal uniparental disomy for chromosome 22 have been observed without obvious phenotypic effects.[91,92] Further, these findings underscore the instability of this chromosomal region in male as well as female meiosis.

MOUSE MODELS

In the past year, several exciting developments have occurred in studies of 22q11. One breakthrough was the release of the complete sequence of human chromosome 22q.[87] Through the efforts of a large international consortium, these data were accumulated, analyzed, and made available to all researchers. Although gaps still exist within the sequence, this massive effort has provided an unparalleled research tool for the study of the genomic structure and analysis of genes located within 22q11. Numerous groups have contributed to the characterization of the more than 30 genes encoded in the DNA sequence of the region. Of note is the observation that 1 of the sequence gaps falls within 1 of the low-copy repeats, LCR-B, lending further support to the concept of the genomic instability of the region.

A second major contribution to the research on the 22q11.2 deletion was the creation, in the mouse, of several genetically engineered deletions for a portion of the chromosomal region that is homologous to human 22q11.[93-95] There is extensive conservation of the genes from within the deleted region of human 22q11 in the mouse on the proximal portion of mouse chromosome 16.[93,96,97] Only a single gene found in humans, *CLTCL*, is not conserved in the mouse. However, the orientation of groups of genes on mouse chromosome 16 appears to be inverted when comparing the 2 species, and the organization between mouse and humans differs slightly (Fig 4). In the mouse models, a region of the TDR was targeted for deletion. By using *Cre-loxP*-based chromosome engineering,[98] several groups have generated heterozygously deleted mouse models of the 22q11.2 deletion. In each case, the amount of material deleted differs slightly from the others, allowing for comparisons among the mice.

The heterozygous mice produced by Lindsay et al[93] have a cardiovascular phenotype similar to humans. Lindsay et al further complemented their deletion with an engineered duplication of the region, and demonstrated that the phenotype could be "rescued." Thus, the phenotypic manifestations appear to be caused by haploinsufficiency of the genes deleted, rather than a "position effect" caused by creating the deletion itself. A homozygous deletion appears to confer embryonic lethality, implying the necessity of one or more of these genes in early embryonic development. The cardiovascular phenotypes observed in approximately 25% of the heterozygously deleted mice included interrupted aortic arch type B, VSDs, and most commonly an aberrant origin of the right subclavian artery. This particular type of interrupted aortic arch and anomalies of the subclavian artery are embryologically related through their origins from the fourth pharyngeal arch artery. Thus, the deletion demonstrated a profound, specific effect on the fourth

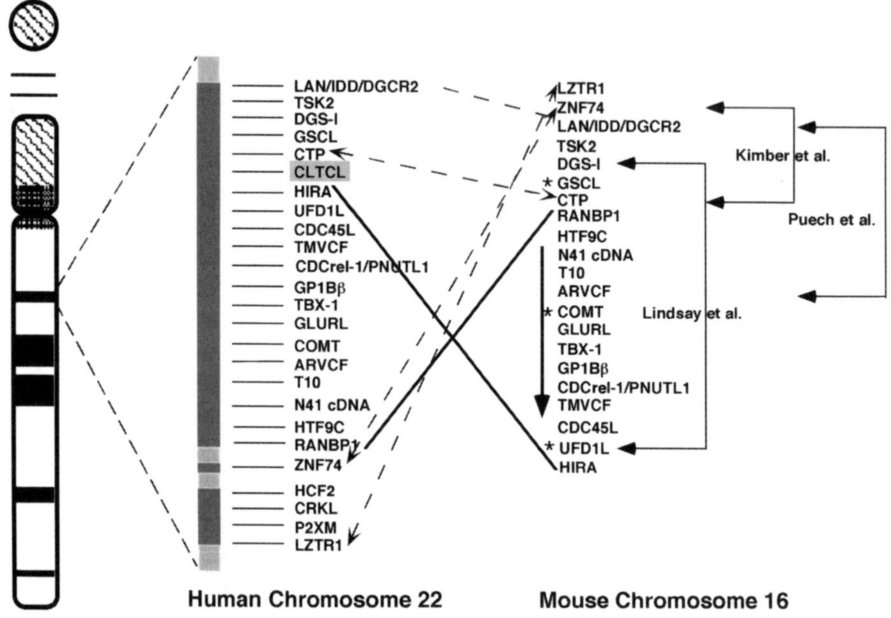

FIGURE 4.
Comparative human and mouse maps with deletion models. Human chromosome 22 is indicated to the **left** with the region of the deletion expanded alongside it as the *shaded box*. The blocks of duplicated sequence (LCRs) are shown as *lighter gray boxes*. The list of genes and their order in humans is shown to the **right**. **Further right** is the order of the genes on mouse chromosome 16. The *CLTCL* gene *(shaded box)* is not present in the mouse genome. The LCRs shown as *lighter shaded boxes* are not present in the mouse genome. *Broken lines with arrows* indicate the relative positions of individual genes in the mouse versus the human genome. The 3 deletions discussed in the text are indicated by the *brackets to the right*. Individual genes that have been "knocked out" in animal models are indicated by *asterisks*.

arch artery, which showed defective development ranging from mild hypoplasia to complete absence. Interestingly, the third and sixth arch arteries appeared normal, an especially striking finding in view of the role these arteries play in neural crest migration. These data provide evidence that the phenotype derived from deleting this group of genes in the TDR is not merely caused by a field defect of neural crest cells.

Although this particular mouse model has added important new insight into the 22q11.2 deletion, the answers it may provide are far from definitive. For example, the penetrance of the cardiovascular phenotype appears to be only 25%, whereas in humans it is closer to 85%. Certain conotruncal defects commonly seen in patients with the 22q11 deletion were not observed. These include persistent truncus arteriosus, which accounts for almost 20% of defects in humans with the deletion, and tetralogy of Fallot, which accounts for greater than 30% of defects. Further, in contrast to the findings in typical patients with the 22q11 deletion, no evidence of thymic dysplasia, T-cell immune dysfunction, craniofacial malformations, or calcium and parathyroid hormone dysregulation was observed. Whether this is a function of the differences in murine versus human development, or is related to the genes involved in the engineered deletion remains to be demonstrated. Further, mice heterozygous for a deletion that encompasses 16 of the genes deleted in the Lindsay mouse model are normal and do not have heart defects.[95] These findings led the authors to exclude these 16 genes as being completely or in combination responsible for the cardiac defects in the Lindsay model.

A third group of investigators[94] reported the creation of a mouse model with a smaller deletion than that of Lindsay.[93] This smaller deletion partially overlaps with that described by Lindsay,[93] but also includes several other genes (Fig 4) located both proximally and distally in the human TDR. This model does not demonstrate any of the phenotypic features described by Lindsay.[93] It does, however, display an abnormality of sensorimotor gating that is found in patients with schizophrenia. Although there is a significant prevalence of psychiatric disorders, including schizophrenia, among patients with the 22q11.2 deletion, the heterozygous deletion generated in this mouse model[94] did not appear to be sufficient to cause the developmental defects that are cardinal features of the 22q11.2 deletion.

There have been other attempts to elucidate the etiology of this disorder based on recent progress in outlining the basic molecular mechanisms that control cardiovascular development. Such studies have focused on targeted null mutations (knockouts) of single genes in murine models.[99,100] Several of these studies have included genes involved in neural crest migration based on their potential roles in production of conotruncal malformations. *HIRA* is a gene located within the TDR of 22q11 that encodes a protein which appears to interact with *PAX-3*.[101] *PAX-3* is a DNA- binding protein that maps to chromosome 2 and appears to be important for developmental patterning. Mice made homozygous null for *PAX-3* have a complete neural crest ablation phenotype and die in utero around embryonic day 14.[102] They often have persistent truncus arteriosus, aortic arch abnormalities, and thymic and parathyroid gland dysplasia.[103] Therefore, it is striking that *HIRA* antisense experiments using a chick model system demonstrated a prevalence of persistent truncus arteriosus.[104] Further, it is of interest to note that this gene was not deleted in the mouse models of Lindsay et al,[93] Kimber et al,[94] or Puech et al.[95] However, mutation analysis of *HIRA* in nondeleted patients with cardiac defects, including truncus arteriosus, has not revealed any mutations.[105] Thus, the role of *HIRA* in the 22q11 deletion phenotype remains unclear.

MUTATION ANALYSIS

Other efforts to identify a single gene as causative of the 22q11.2 deletion phenotype have been addressed by mutation analysis. These studies have, in part, been motivated by atypical deletions involving a limited number of genes that appear to represent "good candidates" for the disorder. A small 20-kb deletion within the TDR was reported in a patient with a classic *VCFS/DGS* phenotype.[80] This smaller deletion disrupts only the *UFD1L* and *CDC45L* genes, whose products have been suggested to play important roles in craniofacial and cardiac development resulting in the 22q11.2 deletion phenotype.[80,106] However, several of the aforementioned patients with variant deletions (some of whom have cardiac and craniofacial defects) have deletions that do not include the region containing *UFD1L* and *CDC45L*. Furthermore, a recent international collaborative study examined the *UFD1L* and *CDC45L* genes in patients with no deletion of chromosome 22q11.2 who have phenotypic features of the deletion, including conotruncal cardiac malformations. Mutation analysis in 57 patients was performed,[105] and no point mutations or microdeletions of these genes were found. Additionally, another 39 patients not deleted for 22q11 who had conotruncal defects were screened, and none were found to have mutations in *UFD1L* or *CDC45L* (M. Budarf, unpublished data). More significantly, in the studies described by Lindsay et al,[93] a mouse model with haploinsufficiency for *UFD1L* showed no evidence of a cardiac or any other phenotype. These observations suggest that genes other than *UFD1L* within the TDR may affect early craniofacial and cardiac morphogenesis.

Another attractive candidate gene is *TBX-1*, a member of the family of transcription factors that contain a "T-box" motif in its primary sequence.[107] This family of genes appears to play important roles in early pattern formation in the developing embryo, with mutations in *TBX-3* and *TBX-5* associated with the developmental defects found in ulnar-mammary syndrome and in Holt-

Oram syndrome. When a cohort of 16 patients with 2 or more of the major clinical features of VCFS/DGS and no demonstrable deletion of 22q11.2 were screened for mutations in the *TBX-1* coding sequence, none were found, although several polymorphisms or sequence variants were noted.[107] Studies to examine this gene in additional patients are ongoing. Therefore, at this time, no single gene has been implicated as causative of the 22q11.2 deletion phenotype.

Instead, the unique patients described by Rauch et al[81] and Saitta et al[82]—that is, patients with features of the deletion and microdeletions that fall outside the TDR—point to genes outside the TDR. The patient described by Rauch et al[81] had craniofacial abnormalities and an interrupted aortic arch type B with truncus arteriosus, the same defect seen in the patient described by Yamagishi et al.[80] That of Saitta et al[82] had persistent truncus arteriosus, VSD, hypertelorism, micrognathia, bifid uvula, posteriorly rotated ears, hypospadias, and short stature but was not deleted for *UFD1L, CDC45L, HIRA*, or any of the genes targeted in the mouse model of Lindsay et al.[93] It becomes apparent when studying such unique patients that delineating a minimal critical region as causal for the 22q11.2 deletion phenotype spectrum may be of limited applicability. These distal deletions, in fact, raise the possibility that 22q11.2-related defects could involve genes outside the TDR. For example, a developmental defect could arise as the result of haploinsufficiency of genes located in this distal deleted region, genes that might function with genes in the TDR in a common developmental pathway.

SUMMARY

Taken together, these data suggest that disruption of more than 1 gene most likely contributes to the 22q11.2 deletion phenotype. Definition of the mechanisms that lead to these deletions and the involvement of the duplicated sequence blocks found in the deleted region will enable a greater understanding of why these chromosomal deletions and their resulting phenotypes are so frequently encountered in this region.[72-75,86] They may also elucidate the role of specific DNA sequences on 22q11.2 in their etiology. Further, based on the many associated features listed here, it would seem likely that any or all systems could be affected by the 22q11.2 deletion. In light of the 50% recurrence risk, and the improved medical care of patients with congenital heart defects and other previously terminal conditions, an increased incidence of the deletion in the general population seems likely. With this in mind, pediatricians should consider broadening their index of suspicion for the 22q11.2 deletion in order to provide appropriate recurrence risk counseling, cognitive remediation, and medical management for these patients and their families.

REFERENCES

1. Driscoll DA, Budarf ML, Emanuel BS: A genetic etiology for DiGeorge syndrome: Consistent deletions and microdeletions of 22q11. *Am J Hum Genet* 50:924-933, 1992.
2. Driscoll DA, Spinner NB, Budarf ML, et al: Deletions and microdeletions of 22q11.2 in velo-cardio-facial syndrome. *Am J Med Genet* 44:261-268, 1992.
3. Driscoll DA, Salvin J, Sellinger B, et al: Prevalence of 22q11 microdeletions in DGS and VCFS: Implications for genetic counseling and prenatal diagnosis. *J Med Genet* 30:813-817, 1993.
4. Burn J, Takao A, Wilson D, et al: Conotruncal anomaly face syndrome is associated with a deletion within chromosome 22. *J Med Genet* 30:822-824, 1993.
5. Matsuoka R, Takao A, Kimura M, et al: Confirmation that the conotruncal anomaly face syndrome is associated with a deletion within 22q11.2. *Am J Med Genet* 53:285-289, 1994.
6. Goldmuntz E, Driscoll DA, Budarf ML, et al: Microdeletions of chromosomal region 22q11 in patients with conotruncal cardiac defects. *J Med Genet* 30:807-812, 1993.
7. McDonald-McGinn DM, Driscoll DA, Bason L, et al: Autosomal dominant "Opitz" GBBB syndrome due to a 22q11.2 deletion. *Am J Med Genet* 59:103-113, 1995.
8. Giannotti A, Diglio MC, Marino B, et al: Cayler cardiofacial syndrome and del 22q11: Part of the CATCH22 phenotype. *Am J Med Genet* 30:807-812, 1994.
9. Fryburg JS, Lin KY, Golden EF: Chromosome 22q11.2 deletion in a boy with Opitz oculo-genito-laryngeal syndrome. *Am J Med Genet* 62:274-275, 1996.
10. LaCassie Y, Arriaza MI: Opitz GBBB syndrome and the 22q11.2 deletion syndrome (letter). *Am J Med Genet* 62:318, 1996.
11. Burn J, Goodship J: Congenital heart disease, in Rimoin DL, Conner JM, Pyeritz RE, et al (eds): *Emery and Rimoin's Principles and Practice of Medical Genetics*, vol 1. London, Churchill Livingstone, 1996, pp 767-803.
12. DiGeorge AM: Discussion on a new concept of the cellular basis of immunology. *J Pediatr* 67:907, 1965.
13. Devriendt K, Swillen A, Fryns JP, et al: Renal and urological tract malformations caused by a 22q11 deletion. *J Med Genet* 33:349, 1996.
14. Nickel RE, Pillers D-AM, Merkens M, et al: Velo-cardio-facial and DiGeorge syndromes with meningomyelocele and deletions of the 22q11 region. *Eur J Pediatr Surg* 3:27-28, 1993.

15. Nickel RE, Pillers D-AM, Merkens M, et al: Velo-cardio-facial and DiGeorge syndromes with meningomyelocele and deletions of the 22q11 region. *Am J Med Genet* 52:445-449, 1994.
16. Nickel RE, Magenis RE: Neural tube defects and deletions of 22q11. *Am J Med Genet* 72:210-215, 1996.
17. Lammer EJ, Opitz JM: The DiGeorge anomaly as a developmental field defect. *Am J Med Genet* 29:113-127, 1986.
18. Scambler PJ, Carey AH, Wyse RK, et al: Microdeletions within 22q11 associated with sporadic and familial DiGeorge syndrome. *Genomics* 10:201-206, 1991.
19. Carey AH, Kelly D, Halford S, et al: Molecular genetic study of the frequency of monosomy 22q11 in DiGeorge syndrome. *Am J Hum Genet* 51:964-970, 1992.
20. Wilson DI, Cross IE, Goodship JA, et al: A prospective cytogenetic study of 36 cases of DiGeorge syndrome. *Am J Hum Genet* 51:957-963, 1992.
21. de la Chapelle A, Herva R, Koivisto M, et al: A deletion in chromosome 22 can cause DiGeorge syndrome. *Hum Genet* 57:253-256, 1981.
22. Kelley RI, Zackai EH, Emanuel BS, et al: The association of the DiGeorge anomalad with partial monosomy of chromosome 22. *J Pediatr* 101:197-200, 1982.
23. Greenberg F, Elder F, Haffner P, et al: Cytogenetic findings in a prospective series of patients with DiGeorge anomaly. *Am J Hum Genet* 43:605-611, 1988.
24. Mascarello JT, Bastian JF, Jones MC: Interstitial deletion of chromosome 22 in a patient with DiGeorge malformation sequence. *Am J Med Genet* 32:112-114, 1989.
25. Strong WB: Familial syndrome of right-sided aortic arch, mental deficiency and facial dysmorphism. *J Pediatr* 73:882-888, 1968.
26. Shprintzen RJ, Goldberg RB, Lewin ML, et al: A new syndrome involving cleft palate, cardiac anomalies, typical facies, and learning disabilities: Velo-cardio-facial syndrome. *Cleft Palate J* 15:56-62, 1978.
27. Goldberg R, Marion R, Borderon M: Phenotypic overlap between the velo-cardio-facial syndrome and DiGeorge syndrome. *Am J Med Genet* 37:54A, 1985.
28. Wilson TA, Blethen SL, Vallone A, et al: The DiGeorge anomaly with renal agenesis in infants of mothers with diabetes. *Am J Med Genet* 47:1076-1082, 1993.
29. Wulfsberg EA, Leana-Cox J, Neri G: What's in a name? Chromosome 22q abnormalities and the DiGeorge, velocardiofacial, and conotruncal anomaly face syndromes. *Am J Med Genet* 65:817-819, 1996.
30. McDonald-McGinn DM, LaRossa D, Goldmuntz E, et al: The 22q11.2 deletion: Screening, diagnostic workup, and outcome of results: Report on 181 patients. *Genet Testing* 1:99-108, 1997.
31. Thomas JA, Graham JM Jr: Chromosome 22q11 deletion syndrome: An update and review for the primary pediatrician. *Clin Pediatr (Phila)* 36:253-266, 1997.

32. McDonald-McGinn DM, Kirschner R, Goldmuntz E, et al: The Philadelphia story: The 22q11.2 deletion: Report on 250 patients. *Genet Couns* 10:11-24, 1999.
33. Takao A: Conotruncal anomaly face syndrome. Presented at Bringing the 22q11.2 Deletion into the 21st Century: Second International Conference for Families and Professionals, Philadelphia, June 22-25, 2000.
34. Goldmuntz E: Cardiac abnormalities in the 22q11 deletion syndrome. Presented at Bringing the 22q11.2 Deletion into the 21st Century: Second International Conference for Families and Professionals, Philadelphia, June 22-25, 2000.
35. Goldmuntz E, Clark BJ, Mitchell LE, et al: Frequency of 22q11 deletions in patients with conotruncal defects. *J Am Coll Cardiol* 32:492-498, 1998.
36. Kirschner RE: Palatal abnormalities associated with the 22q11.2 deletion. Presented at Bringing the 22q11.2 Deletion into the 21st Century: Second International Conference for Families and Professionals, Philadelphia, June 22-25, 2000.
37. Eicher PS, McDonald-McGinn DM, Fox CA, et al: Dysphagia in children with a 22q11.2 deletion: Unusual pattern found on modified barium swallow. *J Pediatr* 137:158-164, 2000.
38. Eicher PS: Feeding issues: Old challenges, new solutions. Presented at Bringing the 22q11.2 Deletion into the 21st Century: Second International Conference for Families and Professionals, Philadelphia, June 22-25, 2000.
39. Krantz ID, Piccoli DA, Spinner NB: Alagille syndrome. *J Med Genet* 34:152-157, 1997.
40. Lynch D: Neurological manifestations of patients with 22q11 deletions. Presented at Bringing the 22q11.2 Deletion into the 21st Century: Second International Conference for Families and Professionals, Philadelphia, June 22-25, 2000.
41. Lynch DR, McDonald-McGinn D, Zackai EH, et al: Cerebellar atrophy in a patient with velocardiofacial syndrome. *J Med Genet* 32:561-563, 1995.
42. Bingham P, Zimmerman RA, McDonald-McGinn DM, et al: Enlarged sylvian fissures in infants with interstitial deletion of chromosome 22q11. *Am J Med Genet* 74:538-543, 1997.
43. Ming JE, McDonald-McGinn DM, Megerian TE, et al: Skeletal anomalies in patients with deletions of 22q11. *Am J Med Genet* 72:210-215, 1997.
44. McDonald-McGinn DM, Laufer-Cahana A, Driscoll D, et al: The 22q11.2 deletion: Cast a wide fishing net! *Am J Hum Genet* 65:36A, 1999.
45. McDonald-McGinn DM, Kirschner R, Gripp K, et al: Craniosynostosis: Another feature of the 22q11.2 deletion syndrome. Presented at the 56th Annual Meeting of the American Cleft Palate-Craniofacial Association, Scottsdale, Arizona, April 13-18, 1999.

46. McDonald-McGinn DM: What Is the 22q11.2 deletion? Presented at Bringing the 22q11.2 Deletion into the 21st Century: Second International Conference for Families and Professionals, Philadelphia, June 22-25, 2000.
47. Ryan AK, Goodship JA, Wilson DI, et al: Spectrum of clinical features associated with interstitial chromosome 22q11 deletions: A European collaborative study. *J Med Genet* 34:798-804, 1997.
48. Canning DA: Urologic manifestations of 22q11.2 deletion. Presented at Bringing the 22q11.2 Deletion into the 21st Century: Second International Conference for Families and Professionals, Philadelphia, June 22-25, 2000.
49. Weinzimer SA: Endocrinology of the 22q11.2 deletion syndrome. Presented at Bringing the 22q11.2 Deletion into the 21st Century: Second International Conference for Families and Professionals, Philadelphia, June 22-25, 2000.
50. Weinzimer SA, McDonald-McGinn DM, Driscoll DA, et al: Growth hormone deficiency in patients with a 22q11.2 deletion: Expanding the phenotype. *Pediatrics* 101:929-932, 1998.
51. Kawame H, Adachi M, Tachibana K, et al: Graves disease in patients with a 22q11.2 deletion. Presented at Bringing the 22q11.2 Deletion into the 21st Century: Second International Conference for Families and Professionals, Philadelphia, June 22-25, 2000.
52. Sullivan KE, Jawad AF, Randall P, et al: The frequency and severity of immunodeficiency in chromosome 22q11.2 deletion syndromes (DiGeorge syndrome/velocardiofacial syndrome). *Clin Immunol Immunopathol* 86:141-146, 1998.
53. Smith CA, Driscoll DA, Emanuel BS, et al: Increased prevalence of immunoglobulin A deficiency in patients with the chromosome 22q11.2 deletion syndrome (DiGeorge syndrome/velocardiofacial syndrome). *Clin Diagn Lab Immunol* 5:415-417, 1998.
54. Sullivan KE, McDonald-McGinn D, Driscoll DA, et al: Longitudinal analysis of lymphocyte function and numbers in the first year of life in chromosome 22q11.2 deletion syndrome (DiGeorge/velocardiofacial syndrome). *Clin Diagn Lab Immunol* 6:906-911, 1999.
55. Sullivan KE, McDonald-McGinn DM, Driscoll DA, et al: JRA-like polyarthritis in chromosome 22q11.2 deletion syndrome (DiGeorge anomalad/velocardiofacial syndrome/conotruncal anomaly face syndrome). *Arthritis Rheum* 40:430-436, 1997.
56. Budarf ML, Konkle BA, Ludlow LB, et al: Identification of a patient with Bernard-Soulier syndrome and a deletion in the DiGeorge/velo-cardio-facial chromosomal region in 22q11.2. *Hum Mol Genet* 4:763-766, 1995.
57. Swillen A, Devriendt K, Vogels A, et al: Aspects of development: The cognitive-behavioural spectrum in 22q11 deletion: The "Leuven" experience. Presented at Bringing the 22q11.2 Deletion into the 21st Century: Second International Conference for Families and Professionals, Philadelphia, June 22-25, 2000.

58. Gerdes M, Solot C, Wang PP, et al: Cognitive and behavioral profile of preschool children with chromosome 22q11.2 Deletion. *Am J Med Genet* 85:127-133, 1999.
59. Gerdes M, Woodin M: Overview of developmental and educational needs. Presented at Bringing the 22q11.2 Deletion into the 21st Century: Second International Conference for Families and Professionals, Philadelphia, June 22-25, 2000.
60. Solot C, Knightly C, Handler S, et al: Communication disorders in the 22q11.2 microdeletion syndrome. *J Commun Disord* 33:87-204, 2000.
61. Solot CB: Communication issues. Presented at Bringing the 22q11.2 Deletion into the 21st Century: Second International Conference for Families and Professionals, Philadelphia, June 22-25, 2000.
62. Moss EM, Batshaw ML, Solot CB, et al: Psychoeducational profile of the 22q11.2 microdeletion: A complex pattern. *J Pediatr* 134:193-298, 1999.
63. Moss EM, Woodin MF, Wang PP, et al: Children and adolescents with chromosome 22q11.2 microdeletions: Aspects of development. Presented at Bringing the 22q11.2 Deletion into the 21st Century: Second International Conference for Families and Professionals, Philadelphia, June 22-25, 2000.
64. Rourke BP: *Nonverbal Learning Disabilities: The Syndrome and the Model.* New York, Guilford Press, 1979.
65. Rourke BP (ed): *Syndrome of nonverbal learning disabilities: Neurodevelopmental manifestations.* New York, Guilford Press, 1995.
66. Wang P, Solot C, Gerdes M, et al: Developmental presentation of 22q11.2 deletion. *Dev Behav Pediatr* 19:342-345, 1998.
67. Bassett AS, Chow EWC, Scutt L, et al: Psychiatric phenotype of 22q11 deletion syndrome in adults. Presented at Bringing the 22q11.2 Deletion into the 21st Century: Second International Conference for Families and Professionals, Philadelphia, June 22-25, 2000.
68. Jessani N, Weller E, Weller R: Psychiatric syndromes in children and adolescents with velo-cardio-facial syndrome. Presented at Bringing the 22q11.2 Deletion into the 21st Century: Second International Conference for Families and Professionals, Philadelphia, June 22-25, 2000.
69. Murphy KC, Owen MJ: Psychiatric issues: Evidence for association between polymorphisms of the catechol-o-methyltransferase (COMT) and monoamine oxidase (MAO) genes and schizophrenia in adults with velo-cardio-facial syndrome. Presented at Bringing the 22q11.2 Deletion into the 21st Century: Second International Conference for Families and Professionals, Philadelphia, June 22-25, 2000.
70. McLean SD, Saal HM, Spinner NB, et al: Velo-cardio-facial syndrome: Intrafamilial variability of the phenotype. *Am J Dis Child* 147:1212-1216, 1993.
71. Driscoll DA, Chen P, Li M, et al: Familial 22q11 deletions: Phenotypic variability and determination of deletion boundaries by FISH. *Am J Hum Genet* 57:92A, 1995.
72. Emanuel BS, Budard ML, Shaikh T, et al: Blocks of duplicated

sequence define the endpoints of DGS/VCFS 22q11.2 deletions. *Am J Hum Genet* 63:11A, 1998.

73. Emanuel BS, Goldmuntz E, Marcia L, et al: Blocks of duplicated sequence define the endpoints of DGS/VCFS 22q11.2 deletions, in Clark E, Nakazawa M, Takao A (eds): *Etiology and Morphogenesis of Congenital Heart Disease.* Armonk, NY, Futura, in press.
74. Shaikh TH, Kurahashi H, Saitta SC, et al: Duplicated sequence blocks and the 22q11.2 deletion syndrome: Genomic organization and deletion endpoint analysis. *Hum Mol Genet* 9:289-501, 2000.
75. Shaikh TH, Kurahashi H, Emanuel BS: Evolutionarily conserved low copy repeats (LCRs) in 22q11 mediate deletions, duplications, translocations and genomic instability: An update and literature review. *Genet Med* 3:6-13, 2001.
76. Levy A, Demczuk S, Aurias A, et al: Interstitial 22q11 deletions excluding the ADU breakpoint in a patient with DGS. *Hum Mol Genet* 4:2417-2418, 1995.
77. Kurahashi H, Nakayama T, Osugi Y, et al: Deletion mapping of 22q11 in CATCH22 syndrome: Identification of a second critical region. *Am J Hum Genet* 58:1377-1381, 1996.
78. O'Donnell H, McKeown C, Gould C, et al: Detection of an atypical 22q11 deletion that has no overlap with the DiGeorge syndrome critical region. *Am J Hum Genet* 60:1544-1548, 1997.
79. McQuade L, Christodoulou J, Budarf ML, et al: Patient with a 22q11.2 deletion with no overlap of the minimal DiGeorge syndrome critical region (MDGCR). *Am J Med Genet* 86:27-33, 1999.
80. Yamagishi H, Garg V, Matsuoka R, et al: A molecular pathway revealing a genetic basis for human cardiac and craniofacial defects. *Science* 283:1158-1161, 1999.
81. Rauch A, Pfeiffer RA, Leipold G, et al: A novel 22q11.2 microdeletion in DiGeorge Syndrome. *Am J Hum Genet* 64:659-667, 1999.
82. Saitta SC, McGrath JM, Mensch H, et al: A 22q11.2 deletion which excludes UFD1L and CDC45L in a patient with conotruncal and craniofacial defects. *Am J Hum Genet* 65:562-566, 1999.
83. Purandare SM, Patel PI: Recombination hot spots and human disease. *Genome Res* 7:773-786, 1997.
84. Lupski J: Genomic disorders: Structural features of the genome can lead to DNA rearrangements and human disease traits. *Trends Genet* 14:417-422, 1998.
85. Driscoll DA, Emanuel BS: DiGeorge and velocardiofacial syndromes: The 22q11 deletion syndrome. *Ment Retard Dev Disabil Res Rev* 2:130-138, 1996.
86. Edelmann L, Pandita RK, Morrow BE: Low-copy repeats mediate the common 3-Mb deletion in patients with velo-cardio-facial syndrome. *Am J Hum Genet* 64:1076-1086, 1999.
87. Dunham I, and the International Chromosome 22 Sequencing Consortium: The DNA sequence of human chromosome 22. *Nature* 402;489-495, 1999.

88. Demczuk S, Levy A, Aubry M, et al: Excess of deletions of maternal origin in the DiGeorge/velo-cardio-facial syndromes: A study of 22 new patients and review of the literature. *Hum Genet* 96:9-13, 1995.
89. Seaver LA, Pierpont JW, Erickson RP, et al: Pulmonary atresia associated with maternal 22q11.2 deletion: Possible parent of origin effect in the conotruncal anomaly face syndrome. *J Med Genet* 31:830-834, 1994.
90. Saitta SC, Driscoll DA, Rappaport EF, et al: The 22q11.2 deletion: Parental origin and meiotic mechanism. *Am J Hum Genet* 67:163S, 2000.
91. Schinzel AA, Basaran S, Bernasconi F, et al: Maternal uniparental disomy 22 has no impact on the phenotype. *Am J Hum Genet* 54:21-24, 1994.
92. Mimy P, Koppers B, Bogadanova N, et al: Paternal uniparental disomy 22. *Med Genetik* 2:216A, 1995.
93. Lindsay EA, Botta A, Jurecic V, et al: Congenital heart disease in mice deficient for the DiGeorge syndrome region. *Nature* 401:379-383, 1999.
94. Kimber WL, Hsieh P, Hirotsune S, et al: Deletion of 150 kb in the minimal DiGeorge/velocardiofacial syndrome critical region in mouse. *Hum Mol Genet* 8:2229-2237, 1999.
95. Puech A, Saint-Jore B, Merscher S, et al: Normal cardiovascular development in mice deficient for 16 genes in 550 kb of the velocardiofacial/DiGeorge syndrome region. *Proc Natl Acad Sci (U S A)* 97:10090-10095, 2000.
96. Lund J, Roe B, Chen F, et al: Sequence-ready physical map of the mouse chromosome 16 region with conserved synteny to the human velocardiofacial syndrome region on 22q11.2. *Mamm Genome* 10:438-443, 1999.
97. Lund J, Chen F, Hua A, et al: Comparative sequence analysis of 634 kb of the mouse chromosome 16 region of conserved synteny with the human velocardiofacial region on Chr 22q11.2. *Genomics* 63:374-383, 2000.
98. Ramirez-Solis R, Liu P, Bradley A: Chromosome engineering in mice. *Nature* 378:720-724, 1995.
99. Baldwin HS, Artman M: Recent advances in cardiovascular development: Promise for the future. *Cardiovasc Res* 40:456-468, 1998.
100. Baldwin HS: Advances in understanding the molecular regulation of cardiac development. *Curr Opin Pediatr* 11:413-418, 1999.
101. Magnaghi P, Roberts C, Lorain S, et al: *HIRA*, a mammalian homologue of *Saccharomyces cerevisiae* transcriptional co-repressors, interacts with *PAX-3*. *Nat Genet* 20:74-77, 1998.
102. Kirby ML: Contribution of neural crest to heart and vessel morphology, in Harvey R, Rosenthal N (eds): *Heart Development.* New York, Academic Press, 1999.
103. Conway SJ, Henderson DJ, Copp AJ: *PAX-3* is required for cardiac neural crest migration in the mouse: Evidence from the splotch mutant. *Development* 124:505-514, 1997.

104. Farrell MJ, Stadt H, Wallis KT, et al: *HIRA*, a DiGeorge syndrome candidate gene, is required for cardiac outflow tract septation. *Circ Res* 84:127-135, 1999.
105. Wadey R, McKie J, Papapetrou C, et al: Mutations of UFD1L are not responsible for the majority of cases of DiGeorge syndrome/velocardiofacial syndrome without deletions within chromosome 22q11. *Am J Hum Genet* 65:247-249, 1999.
106. Shaikh TH, Gottlieb S, Sellinger B, et al: Characterization of CDC45L: A gene in the 22q11.2 deletion region expressed during murine and human development. *Mamm Genome* 10:322-326, 1999.
107. Chieffo C, Garvey N, Roe B, et al: Isolation and characterization of a gene from the DiGeorge chromosomal region (DGCR) homologous to the mouse Tbx1 gene. *Genomics* 43:267-277, 1997.

CHAPTER 3

Wolf-Hirschhorn (4p-) Syndrome*

Agatino Battaglia, MD
Adjunct Professor of Child Neuropsychiatry, University of Pisa Medical School; Head, Center for the Study of Congenital Malformation Syndromes of Neuropsychiatric Interest, Stella Maris Clinical Research Institute, Pisa, Italy

John C. Carey, MD
Professor of Pediatrics, University of Utah; Attending Clinical Geneticist, Division of Medical Genetics, Department of Pediatrics, University of Utah Health Sciences Center, Salt Lake City

Tracy J. Wright, PhD
Postdoctoral Research Associate, Genomics Group, Life Sciences Division, Los Alamos National Laboratory, Los Alamos, NM, and Department of Human Genetics, University of Utah, Salt Lake City

ABSTRACT

Wolf-Hirschhorn syndrome (WHS) is a well-known congenital malformation syndrome caused by deletion of the short arm of chromosome 4 (4p-). In spite of more than 100 reported cases, information on its natural history remained very limited until recently. It was generally thought that these children had severe developmental disabilities and tended to be mere survivors devoid of personality. However, it is now evident that individuals with WHS are capable of more acquisition of developmental milestones than previously suggested. It is therefore very important to have guidelines for health supervision and anticipatory guidance of such patients. Although thought to affect 1 per 50,000 births, we believe that the syndrome is more common because of the many syndromes with which it is still misdiagnosed, and because only 58% of

*Supported in part by the International Program for Consultation and Research in Clinical Genetics of the University of Utah and Primary Children's Medical Center.

cases can be recognized on regular G-banding. The following discussion outlines the historical evolution of our recognition of the several complex aspects of this syndrome, from the very early description to the latest knowledge on clinical and cytogenetic/molecular genetic aspects. Its purpose is to draw the attention of professionals (particularly pediatricians and family practitioners) to a clinical disorder that probably affects many more individuals than previously thought. Accurate identification of such patients can lead to the organization of the most appropriate laboratory testing, to the prediction of the prognosis with relative certainty, to the development of the most appropriate health maintenance and educational plans, and to referral of the patient and the family to support groups.

In 1961, just 2 years after the chromosomal basis of Down syndrome was described, Herbert Cooper and Kurt Hirschhorn published a case report in the *Mammalian Chromosomal Newsletter* of a child with midline defects and an obvious deletion of the short arm of one of the B group chromosomes.[1] The partial monosomy in this patient represented the first example of such an observation in humans and consisted of a deletion of more than half of the p arm of the chromosome. In 1964, after the description of 3 patients with a deletion of a B group chromosome and a distinctive syndrome involving a characteristic cry (eventually known as the cri du chat syndrome), German et al[2] used autoradiography techniques to determine that these deletions were likely on 2 different B group chromosomes. Hence, the separation of chromosomes 4 and 5 in the B group. In 1965, Wolf and collaborators submitted a case report of a patient with 4p deletion to *Humangenetik* (now called *Human Genetics).* The editor, Dr Arno Motulsky, a pioneer in the field of medical genetics, recalled Cooper and Hirschhorn's report in the newsletter of 1961 and requested them to submit their case so that the reports could appear simultaneously in the journal. These 2 reports by Wolf et al[3] and Hirschhorn et al[4] brought Wolf-Hirschhorn syndrome (WHS) to the attention of the genetics community and confirmed the existence of human deletion (monosomy) syndromes. During the next 6 years, 18 additional patients were documented in the literature, mostly in the American pediatric literature, and the syndrome was introduced to the pediatric community.[5] By 1975, just over 40 cases of so-called 4p- had been described in the literature.[6] In the last 25 years, a number of notable series of patients with WHS have been published, and these have helped in the delineation and definition of this important condition.[7-10] Currently, more than 140 cases have been reported in varying degrees of detail. Through these reports, the phenotypic spectrum of WHS has been partly characterized, but only in recent years has a more complete continuum of the phenotype evolved.[9,10]

As indicated, the chromosomal basis of WHS consists of a deletion of the terminal portion of the short arm of chromosome 4. Early on in the history of the syndrome, the deleted segment of reported cases represented about one half of the short arm, occurring distal to the bands now called 4p15.1-15.2. With the development of banding techniques in the 1970s, smaller deletions could be detected, and it was determined that the phenotype of WHS was caused by monosomy of material within 4p16.[11] By 1981, the concept that the critical deletion of WHS was located within band 4p16 had become widely accepted. During the 1980s, patients with the WHS phenotype and apparently normal chromosomes were described.[12] By the end of that decade, advances in molecular techniques, including cytogenetic techniques, allowed for the ability to recognize that these cases had submicroscopic deletions. Then in the early 1990s, continued progression in the field led to the description of the smallest region of overlap of the microdeletions in these cases, and the boundaries of what is now known as the WHS critical region (WHSCR) began to be delimited.[13] The purpose of this chapter is to provide a current and comprehensive summary of the phenotypic and genotypic aspects of the WHS syndrome. The clinical features of WHS are reviewed, as well as the natural history of the disorder. The phenotypic part of the discussion will lay the foundation to propose health supervision guidelines for the care of the infant and child with the syndrome. The second half of the chapter summarizes the cytogenetic and molecular components of WHS and related disorders. An update on the state of knowledge surrounding the WHSCR and the phenotype/genotype correlations is presented.

PHENOTYPE

GENERAL CLINICAL DATA

The frequency of WHS is generally estimated to be about 1 per 50,000 births, with a female predilection of 2:1.[14] However, based on our experience and on literature reports,[9,10,15,16-18] we believe that this frequency rate is an underestimation because many patients are still misdiagnosed and unrecognized. Diagnoses that have been assigned incorrectly to patients with WHS include Seckel syndrome,[19] Pitt-Rogers-Danks syndrome,[12] CHARGE association,[20] partial trisomy 4p syndrome,[21] Smith-Lemli-Opitz syndrome,[22] Opitz-GBB syndrome,[23] Malpuech syndrome,[24] Lowry-MacLean syndrome,[25] Williams syndrome,[26] and Rett syndrome.[27] Misdiagnoses occur because of the difficulty of detecting very small deletions by standard cytogenetics, and the difficulty of recognizing the facial gestalt, particularly in older patients.

All individuals with WHS are born at term and are small for gestational age. In about one third, perinatal distress is observed. Decreased fetal movements are reported during pregnancy in almost all cases. The family history is generally noncontributory, and parental ages are similar to those found in the general population.

PHENOTYPIC FEATURES

From our experience,[15] standard cytogenetics (regular G-banding) can detect only 58% of WHS cases, and clinical diagnosis can sometimes be difficult. Therefore, it is extremely important that clinicians become familiar with the WHS clinical phenotype, so to pursue high-resolution banding and fluorescence in situ hybridization (FISH) studies that can confirm the provisional clinical diagnosis. In a recent photo essay,[28] we showed how individuals with WHS have a characteristic facial appearance in infancy and early childhood that changes with age but shows a typical pattern at each period.

Craniofacial Features

The most striking feature is represented by the "Greek warrior helmet appearance" of the nose—that is, the broad bridge of the nose continuing to the forehead. This is easily recognizable in all WHS individuals from birth to childhood, becoming much less evident at puberty.[28] In addition, microcephaly, high forehead, prominent glabella, hypertelorism, epicanthal folds, high-arched eyebrows, short philtrum, distinct mouth, and micrognathia are present in all patients (Figs 1-4).[7,9-11,15] The nose has a flattened, sometimes beaked tip, with occasional triangular or asymmetric nares. The eyebrows give the appearance of beginning over the center of the eye, because the medial hairs slant upward and are sparse. In some patients, the upper lip is full and appears to be pulled up in the middle and curled downward at the corners in a way that gives the mouth a distinctive appearance, similar to that seen after cleft lip repair. The facial features of WHS are currently proposed as the minimum criteria for its clinical diagnosis.[11] Some degree of craniofacial asymmetry is seen in almost 60% of cases. The ears are

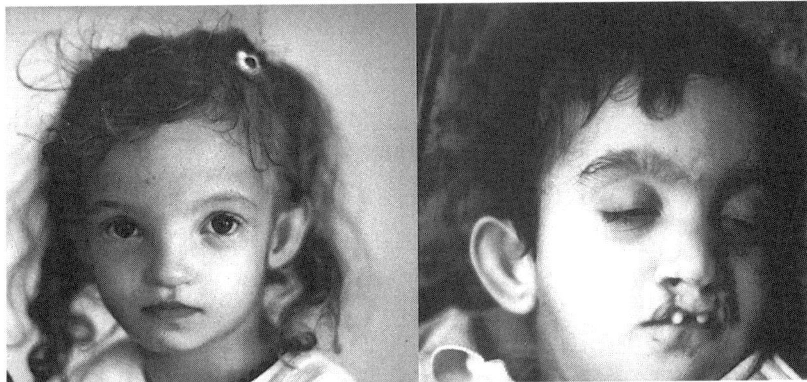

FIGURE 1.
A $3^{3}/_{12}$-year-old girl (left) and a $4^{9}/_{12}$-year-old boy (right) with classic picture of Wolf-Hirschhorn syndrome. Note the "Greek warrior helmet" appearance of the nose, hypertelorism, short philtrum, and, on the right, repaired bilateral cleft lip and distinctive ears with no cartilage.

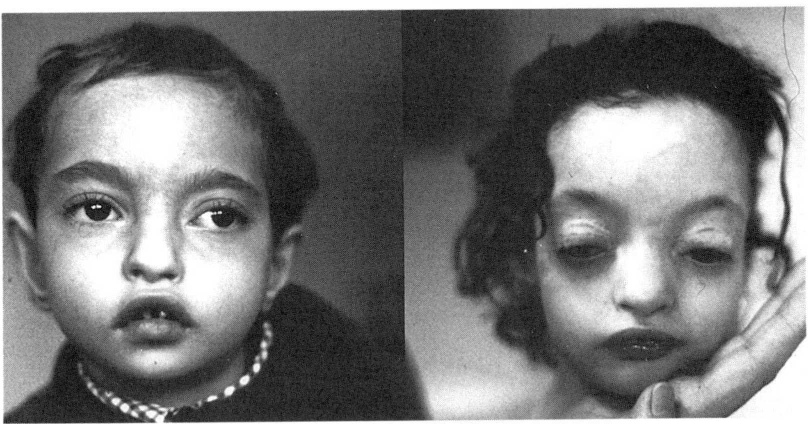

FIGURE 2.
A 5-year-old boy (left) and a $7^{1}/_{2}$-year-old girl (right) with classic picture of Wolf-Hirschhorn syndrome. Note the "Greek warrior helmet" appearance of the nose, hypertelorism, short philtrum, distinct mouth with downturned corners (left), highly arched eyebrows, and skin graft for eyelid hypoplasia (right).

poorly differentiated, posteriorly angulated, or low set, and may have lobeless pinnae. In many cases, the cartilage of the outer ear is extremely underdeveloped and may even be absent. Pits and tags are frequently present. These ear anomalies have been observed in more than 80% of patients with WHS. Cleft lip (unilateral or bilateral) and palate are reported in slightly more than one third of patients. Forty percent have eye/optic nerve defects, mainly coloboma. Glaucoma, at times severe, can be a serious clinical challenge, although it is infrequent in such patients. Ptosis of the eyelid, usually bilateral, can be present in as many as 50% of cases, and eyelid hypolasia, requiring a skin graft, has been observed occasionally.[15] Facial angiomas are recognized in almost 50% of patients. Midline scalp defects seem to be an occasional finding in WHS; their frequency varies considerably in different samples, from 0% to 50%.[7,9,10,29,30]

Growth

Marked growth deficiency of prenatal onset is seen in all WHS individuals, who continue to show short stature and slow weight

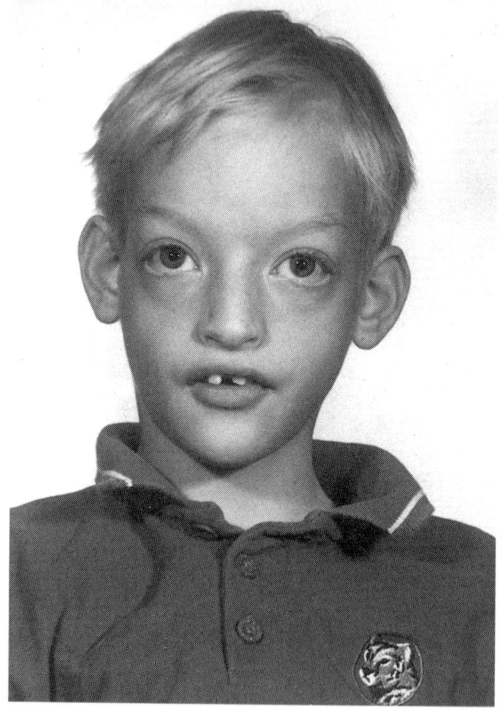

FIGURE 3.
Eight-year-old boy with Wolf-Hirschhorn syndrome showing highly arched eyebrows, somewhat prominent eyes, short philtral length, anteverted ears, and distinct mouth. Note how the "Greek warrior helmet" appearance of the nose is still quite a hallmark.

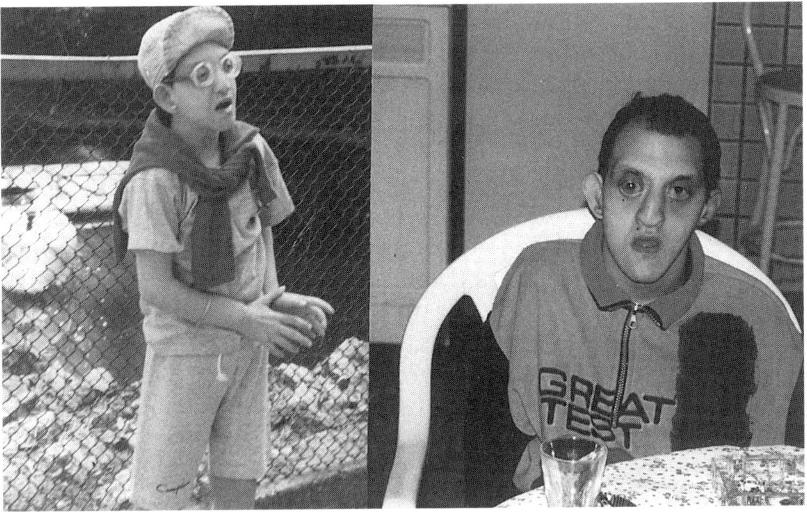

FIGURE 4.
Male patient with Wolf-Hirschhorn syndrome at ages 10 years (left) and 15 years (right). Note how the "Greek warrior helmet" appearance of the nose becomes less evident over the years, and how the facial features tend to coarsen over time.

gain (less than third percentile) later in life, despite adequate caloric and protein intake.[9-11,15,31] This may result from a number of factors such as oral facial clefts with related difficulty in sucking (almost 50%); poorly coordinated swallow with consequent aspirations; and gastroesophageal reflux. Although gastroesophageal reflux seems common (1/300 to 1/1000) and is usually transitory in infancy, it may persist and result in failure to thrive and respiratory diseases in infants with WHS.

Skeletal Anomalies

A large variety of skeletal anomalies are found in 60% to 70% of individuals with WHS.[9,10,15,32] These consist of craniostenosis with brachycephalic skull, underdevelopment of ossification centers in the cervical spine, anomalies of sternal ossification, split hand, clinodactyly, fingerlike appearance of the thumb, thin fingers with bilateral overriding of the second finger onto the third, absence of the ossification nucleus for the ulnar styloid apophysis, proximal radioulnar synostosis, severely delayed bone age, club feet, malformed toes (double first phalanx of the first ray), scoliosis and kyphosis, small iliac alae with coxa valga subluxans, hip dislocation, and lack of pubic bone ossification. Malformed vertebral bodies and accessory or fused ribs have also been reported.[33,34] When counting the infants who die during the perinatal period and are not seen by clinical geneticists, it seems that orthopedic deformities can be noted in 82% of patients with WHS.[35]

Abnormal Tooth Development

Altered tooth development seems to be present in more than 50% of the patients.[15] This usually consists of agenesis of lower lateral incisors or upper canines, peg-shaped teeth, delayed teeth eruption with persistence of deciduous teeth, and taurodontism in the primary dentition.[15,36] However, it is possible that the number of WHS patients with abnormal teething is higher, since only a minority of children are being checked for dental changes.

Skin Changes

Skin changes can be observed in approximately 70% of patients with WHS.[15] They are characterized by cutis marmorata, dry skin, and hemangiomas mainly of the forehead. Sacral dimples seem to be an almost constant feature,[7] whereas tufts of hair on the back are much rarer. Midline scalp defects, described in the original patient,[1] seem to be a rare finding.

Heart Defects

The most frequent congenital heart malformation in individuals with WHS is atrial septal defect, followed by pulmonary stenosis, ventricular septal defect, patent ductus arteriosus, and aortic insufficiency.[15] Tetralogy of Fallot has also been reported.[7] Congenital heart lesions are noted in about 30% to 50% of the children[7,9,10,15,31] but are usually not complex and can be easily surgically repaired, if needed.

Genitourinary Tract Defects

Genitourinary tract malformations are observed in almost one quarter of individuals with WHS.[15] The renal abnormalities are heterogeneous, including renal agenesis, either unilateral or bilateral, cystic dysplasia/hypoplasia, and oligomeganephroma.[11,35,37,38] An apparently high incidence of vescicoureteric reflux has been found by Grisaru et al,[39] associated with unilateral renal agenesis, renal malrotation, horseshoe kidney, small rudimentary kidney, cystic kidney, and hyperechocity with loss of corticomedullary differentiation on ultrasonography. In addition, bladder extrophy and obstructive uropathy were reported in 2 of 48 patients.[15] Renal tubular acidosis can occasionally also be seen in these children.[40]

Abnormalities of the genitalia include hypospadias and cryptorchidism in almost 50% of boys,[15] and absent uterus and streak gonads in a number of females.[35,41,42]

Hearing Defects

Hearing loss can be detected in more than 40% of patients with WHS.[15] This is most often of the conductive type, it is caused by chronic serous otitis media, and it is of a degree that can potentially affect language acquisition and educational achievement. In a series of 48 patients,[15] 5 showed sensorineural hearing loss, a finding previously described in only 2 other patients with WHS.[43,44] These data are not surprising, because one (DFNA6) of the more than 25 genes responsible for nonsyndromic hearing impairment has been mapped to chromosome 4p16.3.[45]

Antibody Deficiency

Antibody deficiencies have been reported in 9 (69%) of 13 children with WHS.[46] These consist of common variable immunodeficiency, IgA and IgG2 subclass deficiency, isolated IgA deficiency, and impaired polysaccharide responsiveness. T-cell immunity appears to be normal. These findings would suggest the presence of a regulatory gene within the deleted chromosome region, affecting the B-cell system.

Occasional Abnormalities

Different types of congenital defects have been reported in a minority of WHS cases. These include partial or complete malrotation of the gut; abnormal liver lobulation and absent gallbladder; diaphragmatic herniation with upward displacement of viscera; esophageal atresia; severe diaphragmatic defect with displacement of the abdominal viscera into the chest; bilateral lung hypoplasia; bilateral bilobed or trilobed lungs, and aneurysmal dilatation of the ascending aorta.[11,34,38,47,48]

NEUROLOGIC FINDINGS

One of the major concerns for parents and professionals caring for children with WHS is seizures/epilepsy. A rather characteristic finding is represented by distinctive electroencephalographic (EEG) abnormalities. Generalized hypotonia is present in all patients with WHS, accompanied, in most of them, by muscle hypotrophy, mainly involving the lower legs. The latter may presumably be caused by the reduced movements in utero; results of electromyography, nerve conduction velocities, and muscle biopsy are normal.

Seizures/Epilepsy

According to different reports, seizures occur in 50% to 100% of children with WHS.[5,9,10,29,30,33] On the basis of our experience with 48 patients with WHS, we estimate that seizures occur in 95.8% (46/48) of these children.[15] The seizures start between 3 and 23 months of age, with a peak incidence at 9 to 10 months. They are either unilateral clonic or tonic, with or without secondary generalization, or generalized tonic-clonic from the onset. Varying degrees of fever (most often around 37.5°C) frequently trigger such seizures, which, at times, last longer than 15 minutes and often occur in clusters. On several occasions, unilateral or generalized clonic or tonic-clonic status epilepticus occurs in 58% of patients, during the early years, in spite of adequate antiepileptic treatment.[15] In addition, more than 60% of patients have atypical absences, with onset between 1 and 5 years of age. These fits are accompanied often by a myoclonic component, mainly involving the eyelids and, less frequently, the eyeballs and the upper limbs. In 33% of cases, seizures stop by 2 to 13 years of age, and 16.6% of patients studied[15] are currently off medication.

Electroencephalography

Distinctive EEG abnormalities were found in 70% of patients studied by Battaglia et al.[15] These children had received serial EEG studies over time (up to 18 years follow-up), most often during wakefulness and sleep. The abnormal EEG findings included frequent, ill-defined, usually diffuse or generalized, high-amplitude, sharp element spike/wave complexes at 2 to 3.5 Hz, occurring in long bursts (lasting up to 25 seconds), activated by slow-wave sleep; and frequent high-amplitude spikes, polyspikes/wave complexes at 4 to 6 Hz, over the posterior regions of the brain, often triggered by eye closure.[49] The diffuse/generalized abnormalities were most often associated with atypical absences, whereas the ones localized posteriorly could still be seen for many years after seizures had stopped.

Neuroimaging/Neuropathology

Neuroimaging studies of the brain (magnetic resonance imaging [MRI], computed tomography [CT]), carried out in more than 60% of patients studied by Battaglia et al,[15] show thinning of the corpus callosum as the most frequent abnormality. In a few cases, this is associated with other abnormal findings, such as diffusely decreased volume of the white matter, or marked hypoplasia or agenesis of the posterior lobes of both cerebellar hemispheres.

Neuropathologic findings have only been reported in a minority of cases, and include hypoplasia of the brain with narrow gyri, shortening of the H2 area of Ammon's horn, arhinencephaly, and dystopic dysplastic gyri in the cerebellum.[35]

Stereotypies

Different kinds of stereotypies can be observed in as many as 40% of the children with WHS.[15] These consist of holding both hands in front of the face, hand washing or flapping, patting self on chest, rocking, head shaking, and stretching of legs.

Sleeping Problems

During the early years, sleeping problems are rather common in children with WHS but seldom constitute a real concern.[15] The children usually wake up between midnight and 4 AM, start crying, and then generally stop when mother arrives in their bedroom. Then they are usually allowed to lay in front of the television, or watch a videotape of favorite cartoons, or play with their favorite toys. On occasion, cuddling is sufficient for them to settle down. When subsequently put back to bed, they either cry again or go quietly to sleep. Such behavior tends to modify spontaneously, and most children are able to achieve a satisfactory overnight sleep. However, on occasion, there may be need for the so-called extinction procedure.[50]

DEVELOPMENTAL FINDINGS

In the literature, it is commonly stated that individuals with WHS are severely to profoundly mentally retarded and that typically they do not develop speech and have minimal communication skills.[7,11,29,33,51,52] These patients have even been defined by some professionals as "mere survivors devoid of any personality."[40] In a survey we have just completed on 48 children and adolescents with WHS,[15] we found mental retardation to be severe in only 66.6% of them, whereas it was moderate in 25% and mild in 8.3%. In most patients, expressive language was limited to guttural or disyllabic sounds that were occasionally modulated in a communicative way. In 3 patients, language was at the level of simple sentences. Comprehension was limited to simple orders or to a specific context. In 6 (12.5%) of 48 patients, intention to communicate appeared to be poor or absent in the early years. For example, these patients did not smile in response to seeing their mother, did not look at her while being breast-fed, did not follow with their eyes, and often reacted to both the human face and voice by crying. However, it is now clear that communication skills improve over time in all cases, with extension of the gesture repertoire and reduction of isolation and anxiety. Most individuals with WHS interact and relate to their families and, generally, to the people they meet or know (such as the professionals taking care of them, and their peers and teachers). Sphincter control, by day, is achieved in 10% of the patients, at 8 to 14 years of age.[15] Although generally stated by many professionals that children with WHS would never learn to walk, 45.8% of our sample were able to walk; 13 (27.1%) of 48 were able to walk independently by 2 to 7 years of age, and 9 (18.7%) of 48 were able to walk with support by 2 to 12 years of age. They usually walk with a broad-based gait, which tends to improve over time, and with poor swinging movements of the upper limbs. By 4 to 12 years of age, 10.4% of the children become self-feeders, and by 8 to 14 years, 18.7% help with food. Some individuals with WHS (18.7%) help in dressing and undressing themselves. Others (18.7%) do simple household tasks, such as setting and clearing the dinner table, putting dirty clothes in hampers, cleaning rooms, and cleaning up dust. Their graphic abilities overall are limited to scribbling. All patients show slow but constant improvement over time, with an initial differentiation of the "I" processes, and improved adaptation to new situations. These children usually show a rather distinctive adhesive approach toward adults in an attempt to draw their attention.

MEDICAL MANAGEMENT, HEALTH SUPERVISION, AND ANTICIPATORY GUIDANCE

Recent studies of the natural history of WHS allow for the development of guidelines for medical management and health supervision.[9,10,15] In our experience, the 2 most consistent medical problems occurring in children with WHS are major feeding difficulties and seizures.

Gastrostomy, occasionally associated with gastroesophageal fundoplication, seems to be the best way of dealing with feeding difficulties. In our study,[15] 21 (43.7%) of 48 patients underwent this surgical procedure, which was followed by a satisfactory weight gain and improvement in the general health status. As a consequence, the children became more responsive to stimuli and more alert and interested in their surroundings, with an improvement in motor abilities. This procedure is also helpful in protecting the airway and in coping with gastroesophageal reflux. On the basis of our experience, gained from interviewing the families and through filled-out questionnaires sent to families of WHS children nationwide in the United States and Italy, we would encourage decision making about this therapeutic procedure. On many occasions, the decision appears to be very difficult, both for parents and professionals, because of the critical clinical status of the child.

Seizures, although difficult to control in some patients during the early years, eventually tend to disappear with age, provided they are treated with the most appropriate antiepileptic drugs.[9,10,31] Because of the subtleness of many episodes of atypical absences, it is extremely important that waking/sleeping video-EEG-polygraphic studies be carrried out in such patients, both in infancy and childhood, for the best characterization of seizures. Furthermore, because almost 95% of children with WHS have multiple seizures, most often triggered by fever accompanying frequent infections, and because almost 60% later show atypical absences (responsive to valproic acid), it seems appropriate to suggest the administration of valproic acid soon after the first seizure.

Atypical absences, difficult to detect in many of these children because of their clinical subtleness, are well controlled by the combination of valproic acid and ethosuximide. Because we have found that patients with WHS show distinctive EEG abnormalities not necessarily associated with seizures, and still present for many years after seizures have stopped, it seems appropriate to withdraw antiepileptic medications gradually in all those who have not had seizures for 5 years.[53]

Even today some parents are asked by professionals why surgery should be performed to correct the clubfeet of a child who will never learn to walk. We now are aware that almost 46% of children with WHS will learn to walk either unassisted or with support.[15]

Again, some parents are still asked why surgery should be performed to correct the scoliosis/kyphosis of a child who has severe mental retardation. We now are aware that more than 30% of children with WHS have only a moderate-to-mild cognitive deficit.[15] Skeletal anomalies in WHS are highly variable and need to be addressed on an individual basis. We would therefore suggest offering early referral for adequate evaluation, along with early intensive physical therapy and full biomechanical assessment, and surgery when appropriate. This approach would maximize the children's chances of realizing their full potential.

Congenital heart defects are usually not complex in WHS, and can be easily repaired, if appropriate. In some instances, the septal defects will close. A focused examination of the heart, including auscultation, electrocardiography, and echocardiography, is indicated in infancy.

Hearing loss seems to be a frequent finding in children with WHS. Although most frequently of the conductive type, it may also be sensorineural or mixed. Comprehensive audiologic and otologic evaluation should be carried out as early as possible, particularly when bearing in mind that all children with WHS have communication skills, and a few are also able to communicate through simple sentences. Even difficult-to-test children with WHS can be studied with brainstem auditory-evoked responses (BAER), otoacoustic emissions, or both. The advantage of BAER testing over auditory field examination is the ability to rule out frequency-specific or unilateral sensorineural hearing loss. It is well known that early diagnosis of hearing impairment is of the utmost importance to allow the most appropriate interventions that facilitate the development of communication skills and of speech and language.

Children with WHS can have kidney disorders, but these do not seem to be a major concern. However, because silent kidney disease is possible in an apparently healthy child, and because some authors[39] have reported a high incidence of vescicoureteric reflux (4/6 patients) in WHS, it is worth carrying out renal function testing and renal ultrasonography in infancy, because antibiotic prophylaxis for urinary tract infections may be indicated. If the bladder extrophy observed in 2 of our patients[15] is related to a particular gene defect within the WHSCR, it still remains to be clarified. Ocular abnormalities are present in almost 50% of children with WHS; thus, ophthalmology consultation is suggested in infancy, even if the child has no iris coloboma or obvious abnormality.

The occurrence of antibody deficiency in WHS[46] explains why many of these children have recurrent respiratory tract infections and otitis media. Because these children may benefit from intravenous immunoglobulin infusions or continuous antibiotics, it seems appropriate to test all patients with WHS for immunodeficiency. Sleeping problems in WHS are usually mild and can be easily overcome with the "extinction procedure."[50] Most children, however, outgrow them.

The most relevant data of our experience[15] are that individuals with WHS do not invariably have severe to profound mental retardation, contrary to the information found in the medical literature. Indeed, 33.3% of individuals with WHS studied by us[15] show a cognitive deficit of mild to moderate degree; 6.4% are able to pronounce simple sentences; and communication skills are satisfactory in all. This latter finding is extremely important with regard to the possibility of teaching these children international sign language, which does not inhibit the appearance of speech. In all cases, a slow but constant improvement in psychomotor development occurs, which in most patients, proceeds farther than ever reported. The belief that individuals with this condition show no progression or development must be dropped. Each child with WHS should receive appropriate psychometric, speech, and motor evaluation. We would stress the need to enroll these patients in a personalized rehabilitation program, which should cover motor aspects (oral motor and feeding therapy included), cognition, communication, and social skills. Early intervention and, later, appropriate school placement are mandatory.

Referring the patient and the family to support groups is an important strategy for helping parents to cope with a child with disabilities. There are 2 support organizations in North America for families of children with WHS: The Wolf-Hirschhorn Syndrome Network and The Support Organization for Trisomy 18, 13, and Related Disorders (SOFT). Also, several national support groups are located in many countries in Europe (Italy, United Kingdom, France, Holland, Germany/Austria). All of these groups can be contacted through the Internet.

WHS is said to have a high postnatal mortality rate; apparently, one third of patients die during infancy.[54] However, based on our experience, we believe that this figure is overestimated, perhaps because of selection bias. The lifespan of individuals with WHS seems to be similar to that of the general population. We are aware of at least 12 adults, aged 24 to 50 years, who have WHS.[55-59] Besides endocarditis and Raynaud phenomenon plus liver hemangioma, reported in 2 of them, no other particular clinical concerns seem to arise in adulthood. More systematic follow-up of adults with WHS is needed to understand more thoroughly the natural history of the syndrome.

GENOTYPE

CYTOGENETICS

4p Deletion

As mentioned above, WHS is caused by a deletion located in the distal portion of the short arm of chromosome 4. In the original cases and in the patients described in the prebanding era before 1970, the monosomy comprised about one half of the 4p. By 1980, with knowledge of about 100 cases, Lurie et al[14] indicated that the full phenotype was present even if only the distal G negative band, 4p16, is deleted. Soon after, the notion of a critical region contain-

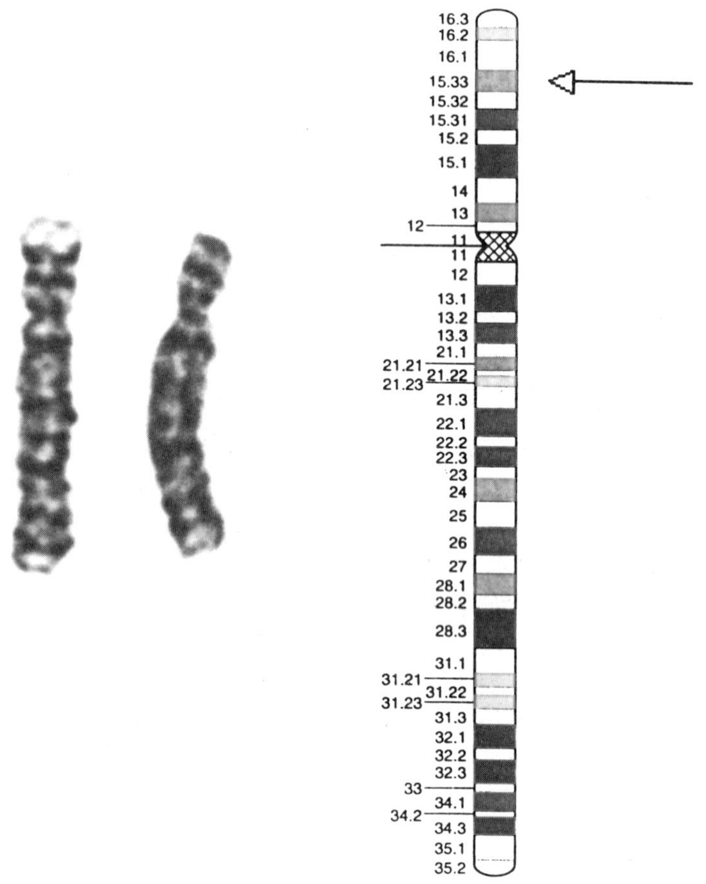

FIGURE 5.
4p deletion. This abbreviated karyotype shows the two 4 chromosomes in a patient with Wolf-Hirschhorn syndrome. The normal 4 is on the left whereas the right is deleted at band 4pt5.3 (band level 550). The *arrow* designates the breakpoint of the deletion. The standard bands of chromosome 4 are shown next to the ideogram (band level 850). (Courtesy of Monica Hale and Aurelia Meloni.)

ing genes important in the production of the WHS phenotype became established and accepted.[60,61]

Figure 5 depicts an abbreviated karyotype showing a typical visible deletion of 4p15.3 at the 550 band level in a patient with typical WHS. As discussed above, in our recent series of patients ascertained from cases in Italy and the United States,[15] only 58% of cases are detected by standard cytogenetic techniques (ie, G-banding at the 400-500 band level). Thus, at this time in the history of the definition of WHS, about 40% of patients would require high-resolution banding (>550 bands) or FISH with cosmid probes from the region to confirm the diagnosis of the syndrome. This observation accounts for some of the delay in making the diagnosis described above; unless a cytogenetics laboratory is capable of performing state-of-the-art testing with the appropriate FISH probes, the diagnosis will be missed or not confirmed. In fact, the FISH probe used commercially in the mid-1990s is now known to be telomeric to the WHS critical region and thus will not detect all cases.[62]

Translocations

In a review of cytogenetically confirmed cases as of 1980, Lurie et al[14] reported that about 75% of patients with WHS will have a de novo uncomplicated deletion of 4p; about 12% will have an unusual cytogenetic situation, such as a ring 4 chromosome, mosaicism of the 4p-, or a sporadic unbalanced translocation. The remaining 13% of cases will have the 4p deletion as a derivative chromosome 4 in an unbalanced parental translocation. This article still remains the most comprehensive review of this issue. At present, there are at least 20 reports of inherited aberrations in patients with 4p-.[63,64]

In almost two thirds of the translocation cases, the mother carries the rearrangement.[65] The unbalanced translocation cases are of great importance because in those situations, the parents are at increased risk to have another child with an aneuploidy syndrome, either WHS or 4p trisomy (with monosomy of the other involved chromosome) depending on the malsegregation of derivative chromosomes. It is always recommended to perform karyotypes on the parents of a child with 4p-, looking for the possibilty of a translocation (or other less common rearrangment such as an inversion) in a parent. In fact, in an apparently de novo deletion (where parental chromosomes are normal), whole chromosome painting of chromosome 4 is suggested to exclude a cryptic unbalanced translocation. In recent years with the refinement of techniques, cryptic translocations have been increasingly described in cases of WHS,[64,66] most interestingly in familial cases. Of note, the addition of material from another chromosome in an unbalanced translocation does not usually modify the WHS phenotype.[63-65] Theoretically, this partial trisomy of chromosomal material from the other chromosome could produce additional features; this possibility should be considered in all patients with WHS who have atypical manifestations.

Parent of Origin of the De Novo Deletion

From studies that use DNA probes in the deleted region to determine the parent of origin of the deletion in de novo cases, 17 of 19 patients documented in the literature had paternal origin of the deletion.[67,68] Adding this figure to other DNA techniques to discern the parent of origin in sporadic 4p-, Dallapiccola[68] showed that the origin was paternal in 24 and maternal in 5. This figure of about 85% paternal origin is similar to the paternal origin of the deletion in 5p-/cri du chat syndrome.[68] The fact that the unbalanced translocations are more often maternally inherited and that the de novo cases are paternal in origin speaks against the notion that imprinted genes play a role in phenotypic expression in WHS.[68]

Whether size of the deletion is a factor in determining the phenotype in WHS is a point of much discussion. Most reports suggest that the size is not correlated with severity of manifestations.[9-11,13,15] This is based primarily on the observation that patients with the classic syndrome can exhibit an easily visible deletion by standard techniques or can have a microdeletion detectable only by FISH. This has been our experience with the series of patients from the United States and Italy.[69] However, a recent report by Zollino et al[70] suggests that deletion size predicts clinical outcome. These investigators scored the severity of the condition and suggested that patients who had visible deletions by usual cytogenetics showed a more serious picture than those detected only by FISH. Further work will be required on more cases before this issue can be resolved. It will be important to score cases in detail with objective techniques in any correlation of genotype and phenotype.

Related Disorders

Two related syndromes are important to discuss in the context of a review of the genotype and phenotype of WHS: the syndrome of proximal 4p deletion and the Pitt-Rogers-Danks syndrome (PRDS). Deletions of 4p in WHS are generally terminal but also include interstitial deletions, and invariably involve the 4p16 region, often just the 4p16.3 distal sub-band. Since the report by Francke et al[71] in 1977, there have been several patients documented with an interstitial deletion of 4p, usually involving bands 4p12-15 and proximal to the critical region for WHS described below. The pattern seen in these patients with this more proximal deletion is distinct from WHS; they usually have normal stature and a facial appearance very different from the craniofacial manifestations of WHS. The face is long with upslanted palpebral fissures and a normal head circumference. Major congenital malformations are uncommon in the proximal interstitial deletion syndrome. The degree of developmental disability is clearly milder than that present in the typical patient with WHS. This disorder is a discrete syndromic condition[72,73] separate from WHS. Of note, the deletion in these cases is variable in location and in size and ranges from bands 4p12 to 4p16. Some patients have interstitial deletions that border on the 4p16.3 band, and the cases that have this more distal involvement (but do not have the WHS phenotype) have been crucial in defining the centromeric boundary of the WHS critical region (see below). In clinical practice, if a patient is said to have a 4p- but does not have the WHS phenotype, this condition needs to be considered. Monosomy in this region (ie, 4p14-16), rather than in the near-terminal portion of 4p16.3 of WHS, is 1 potential explanation for an apparent difference in phenotype in a patient labeled as having a 4p deletion. Other mechanisms (ie, unbalanced translocation and size of the WHS deletion) are discussed elsewhere in this chapter

The other related condition is the so-called PRDS. This syndrome was described in 4 patients, including 2 sisters, in 1984.[12] By 1996, 4 additional patients had been described in the literature.[74] The syndrome consists of intrauterine growth retardation, short stature, a characteristic face, microcephaly, seizures, and mental retardation. In 1996, Clemens et al[74] described a distal 4p microdeletion identical to that seen in WHS in 2 new cases, as well as in the siblings in the original report. The siblings from the original report were found to have a paternally inherited 4;8 translocation. Lindeman-Kusse et al[75] detected this same microdeletion in 2 other previously unreported cases. Both groups used FISH probes isolated from the 4p16.3 region to diagnose the microdeletion of WHS. The clinical similarities of PRDS and WHS are striking, and in retrospect, it appears that patients with WHS evolve into the PRDS phenotype; there were so few cases of older persons with WHS that the clinical picture was not recognized, making it understandable that PRDS was felt to be its own discreet syndrome. More detailed molecular techniques with multiple probes have shown that the microdeletion in patients with WHS and PRDS are highly similar (see below).

The narrowing of the critical region of WHS during the last decade raises the hypothesis that most of the WHS phenotype results from a single gene or from only a few contiguous genes.

MOLECULAR BASIS OF WHS

Defining the Critical Region for WHS

Because of the complex and variable expression of WHS, it is thought that this disorder is a contiguous gene syndrome with an undefined number of genes contributing to the phenotype. The critical region for a segmental aneusomy is defined as the minimum region that is deleted in all patients. In 1994, the minimal molecular deletion resulting in WHS was defined as 2.2 Mb between D4F26 and D4S43.[60-62] The abundant cloned resources from this region led to the identification of a large number of potential coding sequences.[76-79] Overall, this region is gene dense and, in addition to the potential coding sequences, includes sequences encoding *FGFR3*,[80] *PDEß*,[81] *MYL5*,[82] *ZNF141*,[83] *LETM1*,[84] and *IDUA*.[85] In an attempt to reduce the size of the WHSCR, and therefore the number of known genes and coding sequences to be analyzed, a series of "landmark" cosmids were used. These clones were chosen from an extensive 4p16 physical map, and they spanned a 4.5-Mb region of chromosome 4p16.3, extending from *MSX1* to the 4p telomere (Fig 6).[86,87] The use of landmark cosmids for FISH in patient cell lines expedites the localization of deletion breakpoints. In cell lines that are not deleted for a specific cosmid, signal can be detected on both chromosome 4s (Fig 7, A), and in cell lines that are deleted for a cosmid, signal can be detected on only 1 chromosome 4 (Fig 7, B). A second round of FISH can be carried out by using a series of overlapping cosmids that map between the landmarks. This allows fine mapping of the breakpoints to a specific cosmid within the region. These cosmids were used to analyse several patient cell lines.[21,86,88-90] To define the critical region, cell lines from 2 patients were used. The first patient, CM, was described initally in 1992.[61] She was born after a full-term uncomplicated pregnancy. She weighed 1.96 kg with Apgar scores of 9 at both 1 and 5 minutes. When born, she was small and microcephaly was noted; during the neonatal period, she had a poor suck and feeding difficulties. Developmental delay was documented, and she developed a seizure disorder at 1 year. At 15 months, she had a broad forehead with a prominent glabella and mild facial asymmetry. She had relative hypertelorism, arched eyebrows, and upslanting fissures. The nose was broad with a wide prominent nasal bridge, and there was a short philtrum with thin lips and a downslanting carplike mouth. Her ears were mildly posteriorly angulated with minimal lobes. In addition, she had hypoplastic nipples, clinodactyly, and small, slender, tapered fingers. Initial high-resolution chromosome analysis and FISH analysis detected a

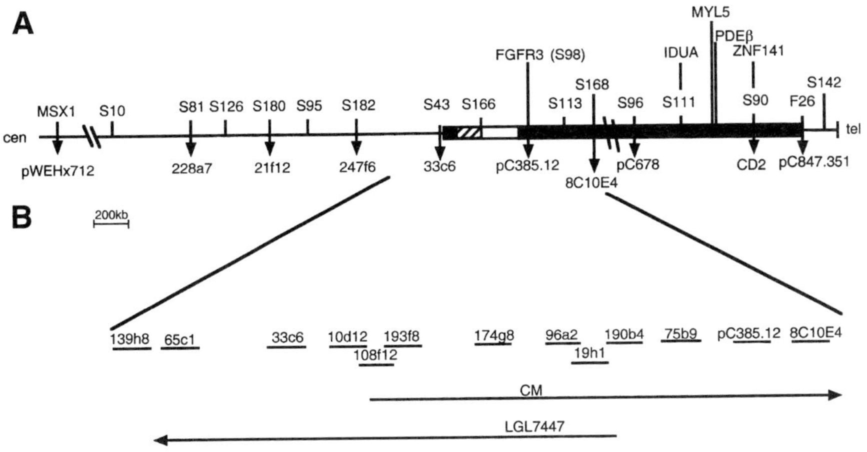

FIGURE 6.

A, Physical map of 4p16. The loci utilized in this and previous studies are shown *above the line,* and the probes used in this study are shown *below the line.* The distance from D4S81 to the telomere is approximately 4.5 Mb. The genetic distance between *MSX1* and D4S10 is 3 cM.[108] The previously published critical region is depicted by *solid boxes* flanking the critical region defined by the patients with Wolf-Hirschhorn syndrome described in this study and depicted by an *open box.* The *crosshatched portion of the open bcx* is the area that can be excluded when considering the 4p- syndrome patient.[93] **B**, Second tier cosmids used in fluorescence in situ hybridization (FISH) analysis determine the breakpoints in the patients defining the critical region. Cosmids are denoted by plate and row by column coordinates in the Los Alamos chromosome 4 library array. The *continuous horizontal lines* indicate the extent of the deletion in the designated patient, *arrowheads* indicate that the deletion continues either telomeric *(CM)* or centromeric *(LGL7447).* (Modified from Altherr MR, Wright TJ, Denison K, et al: Delimiting the Wolf-Hirschhorn syndrome critical region to 750 kilobase pairs. *Am J Med Genet* 71:47-53. Copyright 1997, Wiley-Liss, Inc, a subsidiary of John Wiley & Sons, Inc. Courtesy of Wright TJ, Ricke DO, Denison K, et al: A transcript map of the newly defined 165kb Wolf-Hirschhorn syndrome critical region. *Hum Mol Genet* 6:317-324, 1997. Published by permission of Oxford University Press.)

subtle deletion in 4p16.[61] The cell line from the second patient, LGL7447, was derived from a previously described WHS patient.[91] She was described as having triangular facies, broad and prominent forehead, hypertelorism, antimongoloid slanting of the eyes, high nasal bridge with a broad nose, and short philtrum. She had growth retardation and moderate developmental delay. Prometaphase studies showed a deletion between 4p15.32 and 4p16.3. FISH analysis showed that the loci D4F26 and D4S96 were intact in this patient. The analysis of cell lines from these patients, CM

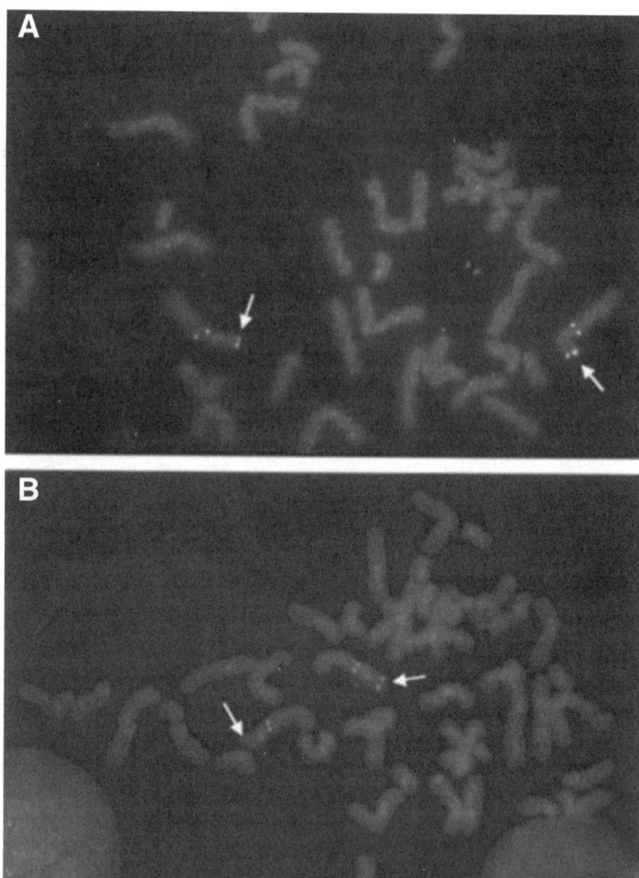

FIGURE 7.
Metaphase spreads from the patient cell line were cohybridized with a 4q specific cosmid 135E11(D4S762) and the 4p test cosmids pC385.12 and pC678. **A**, Partial metaphase spread showing hybridization of 135E11 and pC678 (D4S96) on both chromosome 4 homologues. **B**, Partial metaphase spread showing hybridization of 135E11 to both homologues and pC385.12 *(FGFR3)* hybridization to only 1 homologue.

and LGL7447, using the landmark and second tier cosmids, defined the WHSCR to 260 kb flanked by the markers D4S132 (defined by the cosmid 108f12) and D4S3327 (defined by the cosmid 190b4)[86] (Fig 6). The reduction of the WHSCR to 260 kb excluded all the characterized genes from the region. The 260-kb region maps entirely within a 2-Mb cosmid contig whose sequence was generated by the Sanger Centre, United Kingdom. This sequence was used to identify potential coding sequences that, when deleted, may be involved in this syndrome. Sequences from the cosmids within the WHSCR and flanking region were aligned to form a contiguous sequence of the region. The genomic sequence of the WHSCR was analysed through BLAST, Fasta, and GRAIL by using the program Sequence Comparison ANalysis (SCAN).[92] These programs identify any significant similarities between the WHSCR sequence and known genes or proteins in the databases, as well as predicting possible exons and exon clusters. A total of 42 cDNA clones were identified in dbEST (expressed sequence tag). Alignment of both the 5' and 3' sequences in combination with the analysis of the position of the 3' sequence and the direction of transcription identified a total of 9 distinct sequences (Fig 8). Localization of the cDNA clones back to the cosmids provides a transcript map for the WHSCR. Analysis of the sequences, and putative translation products, of the 9 cDNA clones showed no significant similarity to any members of DNA or protein databases (with the exception of dbEST).

Of the 9 cDNA clones, transcriptional orientation could not be determined for 2 of them, HFBEP10 and HHCJ43, because the sequences were cloned in nondirectional vectors. Of the remaining

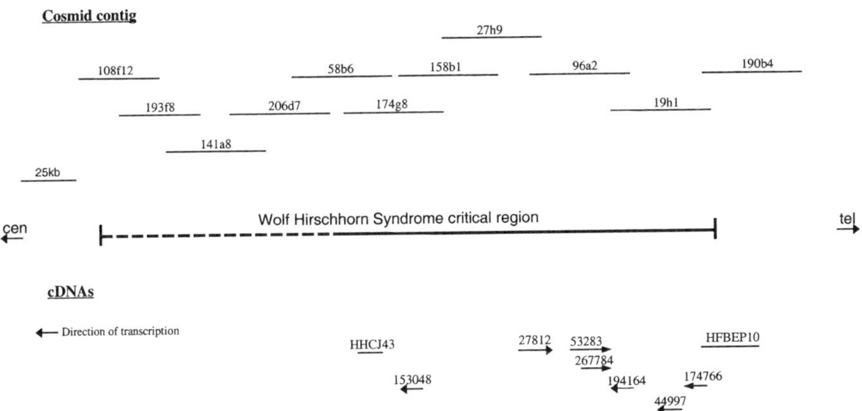

FIGURE 8.
Transcription map of the Wolf-Hirschhorn syndrome critical region (WHSCR). A cosmid contig of the WHSCR and region immediately flanking is shown. The *horizontal line* indicates the position of the WHSCR. The position and direction of transcription, where known, of cDNAs is shown below the WHSCR. The *broken line* represents the region that can be excluded when considering the 4p- syndrome patient.[93] (Courtesy of Wright TJ, Ricke DO, Denison K, et al: A transcript map of the newly defined 165kb Wolf-Hirschhorn syndrome critical region. *Hum Mol Genet* 6:317-324, 1997. Published by permission of Oxford University Press.)

7 cDNA clones, 3 are transcribed centromere to telomere, and 4 are transcribed towards the centromere (Fig 8). GRAIL analysis of this region predicted a total of 109 exons. As eukaryotic gene organization typically includes multiple exons, GRAIL gene predictions are most reliable when clusters of exons are observed along a segment of genomic DNA sequence. Seven clusters of GRAIL-predicted exons were identified in the WHSCR. Three of the 7 clusters of GRAIL-predicted exons were identified on the centromere-to-telomere strand, whereas 4 of the 7 clusters of GRAIL-predicted exons were identified on the telomere-to-centromere strand. Only in 1 case did the exon cluster overlap with regions of EST homologies (cDNA clones 53283 and 267784).[86]

The WHSCR was further reduced by considering the analysis of a patient with diagnosed proximal 4p- syndrome.[93] This clinically distinct abnormality is caused by an interstitial deletion of the proximal short arm of chromosome 4.[71] Cytogenetic analysis of this patient revealed an interstitial deletion involving band 4p14-4p16.1.[93] Molecular characterization of a cell line derived from this patient determined the distal breakpoint to lie within D4S166.[94] Because this patient does not have the "typical" anomalies associated with WHS,[93] it is possible to exclude the region of overlap between this patient and the WHSCR. This region is from D4S132 to D4S166, and therefore it is excluded from the WHSCR (Fig 6). Therefore, the critical region based on patients with WHS alone is 260 kb, but including this 4p- patient reduces the WHSCR to 165 kb. Interestingly, this reduction excluded only 1 of the 7 clusters of GRAIL-predicted exon, and it did not exclude any of the 9 cDNA clones.

Characterization of Two Candidate Genes Mapping Into the WHSCR

The transcript map shown in Fig 8 provides the starting point for further characterization of the role of these clones in both WHS and normal human development. It is important to determine whether the 9 cDNA clones identified in the WHSCR by silica cloning encode for genes. Secondly, it is important to characterize any genes identified in the WHSCR to determine their role in both normal human development and in WHS.

To date, 2 genes have been characterized that fall totally or partially into the WHSCR.[95,96] *WHSC1* (Wolf-Hirschhorn syndrome candidate 1) is a novel gene that spans a 90-kb genomic region, two thirds of which maps in the telomeric end of the WHSCR.[95] Analysis of cDNA and EST clones, as well as products amplified by using RACE (rapid amplification of cDNA ends), shows that *WHSC1* is a 25-exon gene that encompasses the cDNAs HFBEP10 (exons 7-11b) and 194164 (exon 25a) from the transcript map (Fig 8). This 25-exon gene encodes an 8-kb cDNA that is transcribed from telomere to centromere. Therefore, in the patient LGL7447, who defines the telomeric breakpoint of the WHSCR, the gene is either truncated or forms a fusion transcript. *WHSC1* is a complex gene with multiple splice variants involving exons located in the 5' untranslated region (exons 2 and 3), the coding region (exons 11, 11a, 11b, 12a, 12b) and the 3' untranslated region (exons 25 and 25a). Between exons 4 and 25, *WHSC1* contains a 4095-bp open reading frame encoding a putative protein of 136 KDa. Alternative splicing in exons 11a and 11b would yield a 62-KDa protein, and alternative splicing in exon 12 would yield a 64-KDa protein. Both of the proteins generated by alternative splicing would contain novel amino acids when compared with the full length *WHSC1* protein.

To determine the expression profile for *WHSC1,* Northern blot analysis was carried out by using probes across the gene on RNA derived from different adult and fetal tissues. A complex pattern emerged with at least 5 different transcripts detected in fetal tissues and 3 transcripts detected in adult tissues. Because of the complex nature of this gene, it will be important to generate antibodies to different parts of *WHSC1* to examine the protein expression with Western blots.

In an attempt to determine the function of the *WHSC1* protein, the putative amino acid sequence was used to search available databases. Identity to 4 different protein families was found. A PWWP (proline-tryptophan-tryptophan-proline) domain was located in exons 5 and 6, an HMG box in exons 7 and 8, a PHD-type zinc finger domain in exons 16 and 17, and a SET domain in exons 21 to 24.[95,97] HMG boxes are classified into 3 families (HMG-1/-2, HMG-14/-17, and HMG-I[Y]) and found in many proteins including the mammalian testis-binding factor SRY.[98] These proteins facilitate DNA binding. The SET domain genes are a highly conserved family including the human proteins ALL1 (acute lymphocytic leukemia) and HRX (human homolgue of Trithorax).[99,100] The SET domain-containing proteins influence transcription by changing chromatin-mediated regulating mechanisms, leading to secondary effects on developmental programs. These data suggest that the *WHSC1* protein may play a role in transcription regulation of genes involved in embryonic development.

It is important to determine whether *WHSC1* is expressed early in development in the tissues that are affected in WHS. Because this cannot be easily carried out in human embryos, it is necessary to move to a model organism. Therefore, to study the developmental expression pattern of *WHSC1*, mouse cDNA clones corresponding to exons 9 to 12a and 20 to 25a of *WHSC1* were used to perform in situ hybridization on mouse embryo sections.[95] The expression pattern was analyzed at 13.5 dpc (days postcoitum), which is equivalent to approximately 49 to 53 days (Carnegie stage 20-21) of human development.[101] Expression was detected in the telencephalon and rhombencephalon, spinal and trigeminal ganglia, the anlage region of the jaw, the frontal face region including the developing upper and lower lips, to intestinal and lung epithelium, the liver, the adrenals, and the urogenital region. The temporal and spatial expression of *WHSC1* in early development and the protein domain identities, including the SET domain, suggest that *WHSC1* may play a significant role in normal development. In addition, the deletion of *WHSC1* is likely to be involved in WHS. This role may include the transcriptional regulation of genes involved in early embryonic development.

The second gene from the WHSCR that has been characterized was named *WHSC2* (Wolf-Hirschhorn syndrome candidate 2).[96] This gene was identified after the analysis of cDNA clone 53283 (Fig 8). *WHSC2* spans a 26.2-kb genomic region which is all contained within cosmid 96a2 (Fig 8). Sequence from cDNA clone 53283, in combination with 5' RACE, detected an 11-exon gene containing a 1584-bp open reading frame. The gene is transcribed from centromere to telomere and, interestingly, the 3' end of *WHSC2* lies just 523 bp from the 3' end of *WHSC1*. However, *WHSC2* differs from *WHSC1* in several ways. It is a simple gene that contains no splice variants and no similarity to known proteins, and analysis of Northern blots showed that *WHSC2* is expressed in all human fetal and adult tissues examined. To determine the role of this gene in early embryonic development, the mouse homologue was identified. *WHSC2h* has a 93% identity to *WHSC2* across the open reading flame, suggesting that it is the mouse homologue of *WHSC2*. To analyse the expression of this gene, Northern blot and in situ hybridizations were carried out. Northern blot hybridization showed that *WHSC2h* was expressed at all embryonic developmental stages examined and in all adult tissues studied.

It is possible that expression of this gene was spatially, not temporally, restricted during embryonic development, and this was analyzed by using whole-mount in situ hybridization to mouse embryos between 10.5 and 13.5 dpc.[102] At 10.5 dpc, most of the organs have formed in the developing embryo, and by 13.5 dpc, patterning of the embryo is almost complete. This is equivalent to

Carnegie stages 14 to 21 of human embryonic development.[101] These experiments confirmed that the gene was ubiquitously expressed. It is difficult to associate function with a gene when no obvious indications are provided by database similarities or expression patterns. However, the location of this gene in the WHSCR and the identification of a mouse homologue, *WHSC2h,* suggests that *WHSC2* encodes a protein that may play a role in WHS. To date, 2 genes have been characterized in the 165-kb WHSCR. It is important to characterize any remaining genes in this region and to identify the function of *WHSC1* and *WHSC2* in both normal development and in WHS.

WHS and PRDS Represent the Clinical Spectrum Associated With a Single Syndrome

A second segmental aneusomy is located on chromosome 4p16. PRDS is a multiple congenital abnormality syndrome.[12] A t(4;8) was detected in the father of the sisters originally described by Pitt et al,[12] and the derivative chromosome 4 was identified in the sisters by using a probe to locus D4S96.[103] A study of 7 patients with PRDS, including the original sibling pair, has shown that all are deleted for D4S96.[74,75,104] Clinically, PRDS has been described as consisting of prenatal and postnatal growth retardation, mental retardation, characteristic facial appearance, microcephaly, and seizures.[12] WHS and PRDS were thought to be similar, yet clinically distinct, conditions. It has been suggested that PRDS generally tends to be clinically less severe than WHS.[75] To determine whether PRDS and WHS were caused by similar deletions of 4p16, Kant et al[105] studied 4 patients with diagnosed PRDS by using a series of probes extending from D4F26 to D4S1582. All 4 patients were deleted for the WHSCR, but in all cases, the deletion was terminal and was larger than the smallest deletion seen in WHS.[105] The smallest deletion detected in these patients extended from telomeric to D4F26 to centromeric to D4S126 (see Fig 6 for locus locations).

To further study the molecular similarities between PRDS and WHS, 3 patients, 1 with WHS and 2 with PRDS, were analyzed by using the series of landmark cosmids.[89] The patient with diagnosed WHS (cell line MA110 was derived from this patient) was delivered by an elective cesarean section at 36 weeks, and the birth weight was 1.56 kg. The infant spent 6 weeks in the intensive care unit, and the principal problem on discharge was difficulty feeding and poor weight gain.

Significant developmental delay was present; at 12 months, she was able to sit against a cushion, and she sat unaided at 20 months.

By 3 years and 3 months, she could walk independently. However, she was unable to get up once she had fallen until approximately 5 years of age. Between 2 and 3 years she was able to use single words. As a child, she had febrile convulsions and received sodium valproate (Epilim) from 3 to 10 years of age. On clinical examination at 14 years, her height was 133.3 cm and her head circumference was 49 cm (both measurements well below the 3rd percentile). She had 2 hair whorls. No evidence of cutis aplasia was present. Her palpebral fissures were level with an inner canthal distance of 2.75 cm; these measurements confirmed a clinical impression of hypertelorism. She had mild myopia. Her ears were low set with attached lobes; no ear pits were present. She had a short philtrum that measured 1 cm and a small chin. Her fingers appeared slender and tended to deviate to the right. She had a mild scoliosis concave to the left. Her heart sounds were normal. She was able to hold a simple conversation, and she could copy printed sentences.

The first patient with diagnosed PRDS (cell line MA115 was derived from this patient) was born at 40 weeks' gestation, but she was small at birth with a weight of 2.1 kg (<10th percentile).[74] She could sit at 9 months but was unable to attain a sitting position by herself. She walked at 3 years 1 month and began using single words at 2 years. She began to use full sentences at 5 years of age. At 11 years, her weight, height, and head circumference were well below the 5th percentile. She has febrile seizures and has been tried on 2 medications but is allergic to both of these. The shape of her skull is normal, but she has a prominent forehead and proptotic eyes resulting from hypoplastic orbits. She has micrognathia, a hypoplastic maxilla, and a narrow arched palate. Her ears are large with hypoplastic lobes and open helices. She has a short philtrum. She has long, lean limbs with hyperextensible joints. However, her fingers are unremarkable. The palmar and digital flexion creases are normal with an extra flexion crease on the thumb.

To identify and characterize the molecular defect in these patients, the series of "landmark" cosmids were used (Fig 9). Hybridization to chromosome spreads derived from cell lines MA110 and MA115 with cosmids including, and centromeric to, 112a12 detected fluorescence on both chromosome 4 homologues (Fig 9).

All cosmids including, and telomeric to, 70d1 exhibited a hemizygous pattern of inheritance (Fig 9). Therefore, both patients have an approximately 4-Mb terminal deletion that differs by a maximum of 70 kb (the distance between the ends of 112a12 and 70d1; Fig 9).

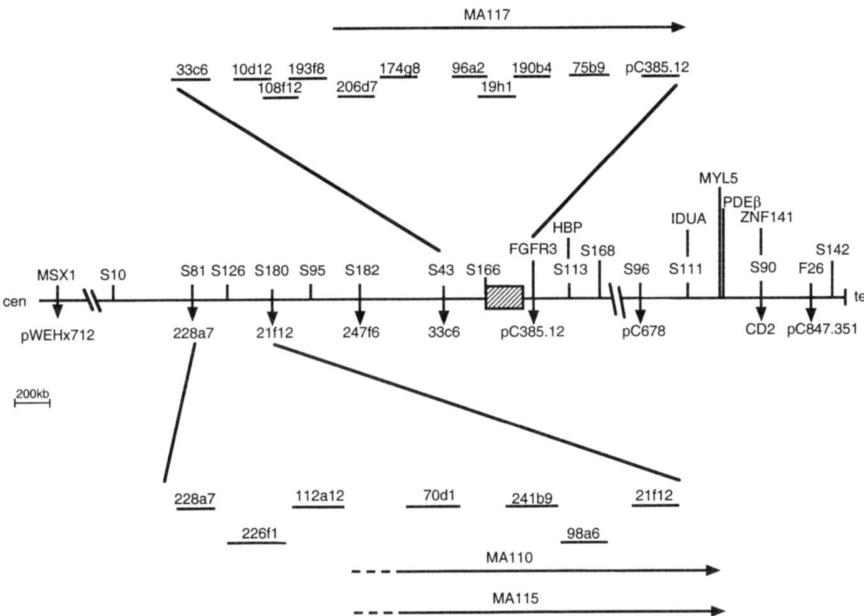

FIGURE 9.
Deletion in Wolf-Hirschhorn patient MA110 and Pitt-Rogers-Danks patients MA115 and MA117. The loci used in this and previous studies are shown *above the line,* and the probes used in this study are shown *below the line.* The *hatched box* indicates the location of the Wolf-Hirschhorn syndrome critical region. The expanded region above the loci designations shows the names and relative locations of the second tier cosmids used for fluorescence in situ hybridization (FISH) in cell line MA117. The *solid line* shows the breakpoint position and cosmids deleted in this patient. The expanded region below the probe names shows the names and relative locations of the second tier cosmids used for FISH in cell lines MA110 and MA115. The *solid line* shows cosmids deleted in the patients MA110 and MA115; the *dashed line* indicates the position of the breakpoint region. (Courtesy of Wright TJ, Clemens M, Quarrell O, et al: Wolf-Hirschhorn and Pitt-Rogers-Danks syndromes caused by overlapping 4p deletions. *Am J Med Genet* 75:345-350. Copyright 1998, Wiley-Liss, Inc, a subsidiary of John Wiley & Sons, Inc.)

The second patient with diagnosed PRDS (cell line MA117 was derived from this patient)[74,89] was born at 41 weeks' gestation, but she was small at birth with a weight of 2.3 kg (<10th percentile) and a length of 48 cm (<10th percentile). She had a grand mal seizure at 6 months of age and has since had a seizure disorder. Developmental delay was noted, and at 6 years of age she was well below the 5th percentile for weight (13.1 kg), length (100 cm), and occipitofrontal circumference (42 cm). She walked at 28 months and began to "babble" at 4 to 5 years of age. Facially, she has a short lower facial height, wide mouth, short philtrum, maxillary hypoplasia, and slightly beaked nose. Her ears are slightly low set and simple. Her eyes are prominent but lacking true hypertelorism. Her limbs are normally proportioned with mildly hyperextensible joints. Her palmar flexion creases are bridged with extra palmar creases bilaterally.

To determine the size and location of the deletion in this patient, FISH was carried out by using the "landmark" cosmids (Fig 9). Hybridization to chromosome spreads derived from cell line MA117 with cosmids including, and centromeric to, 193f8 detected fluorescence on both chromosome 4 homologues. All cosmids including, and telomeric to, 206d7 exhibited a hemizygous pattern of inheritance. These results show that this patient has a terminal deletion that is approximately 2.8 Mb (Fig 9). This localizes the centromeric boundary for the PRDS critical region just 40 kb from the centromeric boundary for the WHSCR. In addition, the telomeric boundary of the PRDS critical region has been placed at D4S96 after the identification of 2 patients who are not deleted for this locus.[104,106] The striking phenotypic similarities between PRDS and WHS in combination with the similarities in the sizes of the critical region for the 2 syndromes suggest that WHS and PRDS represent the clinical similarity associated with a single syndrome.

CORRELATION OF PHENOTYPE WITH GENOTYPE

As discussed in the phenotype section of this chapter, a wide range of findings and manifestations occur in WHS (Box 1). Major congenital malformations such as cleft lip/palate, hypospadias, or heart defects are each seen in 50% of patients or less, whereas the nonspecific findings of developmental disability and growth delay are consistent features, occurring in all patients. As we have addressed, some patients with WHS show a milder degree of mental retardation than previously reported. How then do we explain the variability of phenotype within the syndrome? One obvious explanation has been discussed above: could a smaller size of the deletion account for a milder case presentation? Battaglia et al[9] reviewed the literature and discussed this point in a recent report. Most investigators in the field have concluded that the size of the deletion and the severity of developmental disability are not correlated. However, as mentioned, Zollino et al[70] suggested that a correlation exists based on a clinical scoring system of severity of manifestations. Wieczorek et al[107] also proposed that the question of deletion size influencing phenotype is still open. These investi-

BOX 1.
Frequency of Main Characteristics of Wolf-Hirschhorn Syndrome

Exceeding 75%
- Greek warrior helmet appearance of the nose
- Microcephaly
- Hypertelorism
- High-arched eyebrows
- Distinct mouth
- Short philtrum
- Micrognathia
- Mental retardation
- IUGR/postnatal growth retardation
- Hypotonia
- Muscle hypotrophy
- Seizures
- Feeding difficulties
- Simple/angulated ears/pits/tags

50% to 75%
- Distinctive EEG abnormalities
- Skin changes
- Skeletal anomalies
- Craniofacial asymmetry
- Abnormal teething
- Ptosis
- Antibody deficiency

25% to 50%
- Heart defects
- Hearing defects
- Eye/optic nerve defect
- Stereotypies
- Cleft lip/palate
- Structural brain anomalies
- Genitourinary tract defects

Below 25%
- Liver/gallbladder/gut/diaphragm/esophagus/lung/aorta anomalies

Abbreviations: IUGR, Intrauterine growth retardation; *EEG,* electroencephalogram.

gators studied 13 cases, 4 of which had submicroscopic deletions. Major malformations, oral-facial clefts, and heart defects were only present in patients with larger deletions (>10 Mb), suggesting the presence of some correlation of phenotype and deletion size. Although the number of patients with smaller deletions is too small for statistical comparison, they felt that patients with small deletions had better development. In our experience, we have evaluated patients with the classic syndrome, including profound mental retardation, who are detected only by FISH, indicating that a submicroscopic deletion accounts for their severe WHS phenotype. In contrast, we have also examined patients with a relatively large deletion detected by standard techniques who have moderate to mild mental retardation.[69] Future studies with larger samples of patients that use objective techniques for categorizing the degree of severity of developmental disability will be necessary to sort this out. The essential criterion to diagnose the WHS phenotype is the craniofacial appearance.[11] However, this assessment is fraught with subjectivity as well. Application of standardized anthropometric techniques to the study of the facial phenotype could bring some objectivity to the question. In the future, cases that are detected with the WHS phenotype who have no detectable deletion become very important in the study of candidate genes. Objective determination of phenotype will be vital in deciding whether such patients actually have WHS.

In regards to the notion that WHS is or can be a contiguous gene syndrome, Estabrooks et al[13] performed a study to determine a preliminary phenotypic map. In this investigation, the finding of hypospadias only occurred with the larger deletions, suggesting that the presence of that feature may require deletion of material centromeric to the WHSCR. The same idea may apply to scalp defects: although observed in early cases with presumed large deletions, detected in the prebanding era, scalp defects are uncommon in recent series.[9,15]

Other genetic factors that can potentially affect the phenotype are imprinting and the presence of additional material in an unbalanced translocation, causing a partial trisomy. Dallapiccola et al[68] suggested that the parent of origin does not play a role in WHS. However, evaluation of phenotypic variability where maternally derived cases are compared with paternally derived cases has not been accomplished. Again, objective methods of defining phenotype need to be applied. Regarding the other issue—that is, the presence of an accompanying partial trisomy—the idea that the other chromosome piece does not contribute to phenotype is simply a matter of ascertainment. If a patient were to have an unbalanced translocation with a rather large piece of additional material, there could be additional features in the patient caused by the trisomy.

SUMMARY AND CONCLUSIONS

In the 4 decades since the original description, knowledge of the clinical phenotype, natural history, and cytogenetics of WHS has increased, especially in the last 10 years. Recent work has led to the documentation of a wider range of developmental skills and abilities in children with the syndrome than was previously thought. A rational plan for routine health supervision and anticipatory guidance has emerged to assist the primary care practitioner in the care of individuals at all ages with WHS. Advances in molecular cytogenetics allow for diagnosis of patients with submicroscopic deletions. Current efforts are focused in clarifying the critical region within 4p16.3 that contains the gene (or genes) important in causing the WHS phenotype. These genes may provide insight into the developmental pathogenesis of numerous congenital malformations.

ACKNOWLEDGMENT

We thank the families of the children with WHS who kindly participated in our project, and who have taught us so much.

REFERENCES

1. Cooper H, Hirschhorn K: Apparent deletion of short arms of one chromosome (4 or 5) in a child with defects of midline fusion. *Mamm Chrom Nwsl* 4:14, 1961.
2. German J, Lejeune J, Macintire MN, et al: Chromosomal autoradiography in the cri du chat syndrome. *Cytogenetics* 3:347, 1964.
3. Wolf U, Reinwein H, Porsch R, et al: Defizienz am den kurzen Armen eines chromosoms nr. 4. *Humangenetik* 1:397, 1965.
4. Hirschhorn K, Cooper H, Firschein IL: Deletion of short arms of chromosome 4-5 in a child with defects of midline fusion. *Humangenetik* 1:479-482, 1965.
5. Guthrie RD, Aase JM, Asper AC, et al: The 4p- syndrome. *Am J Dis Child* 122:421-425, 1971.
6. Johnson VP, Mulder RD, Hosen R: The Wolf-Hirschhorn (4p-) syndrome. *Clin Genet* 10:104-112, 1976.
7. Wilson MG, Towner JW, Coffin GS, et al: Genetic and clinical studies in 13 patients with the Wolf-Hirschorn syndrome [del(4p)]. *Hum Genet* 59:297-307, 1981.
8. Preus M, Ayme S, Kaplan P, et al: A taxonomic approach to the del (4p) phenotype. *Am J Med Genet* 21:337-345, 1985.

9. Battaglia A, Carey JC, Cederholm P, et al: Natural history of Wolf-Hirschhorn syndrome: Experience with 15 cases. *Pediatrics* 103:830-836, 1999.
10. Battaglia A, Carey JC, Cederholm P, et al: Storia naturale della sindrome di Wolf-Hirschhorn: Esperienza con 15 casi. *Pediatrics* (ed italiana) 11:236-242, 1999.
11. Estabrooks LL, Roy Breg W, Hayden MR, et al: Summary of the 1993 ASHG ancillary meeting "Recent research on chromosome 4p syndromes and genes." *Am J Med Genet* 55:453-458, 1995.
12. Pitt DB, Rogers JG, Danks DM: Mental retardation, unusual facies and intrauterine growth retardation: A new recessive syndrome? *Am J Med* Genet 19:307-313; 1984.
13. Estabrooks LL, Rao KW, Driscoll DA, et al: Preliminary phenotypic map of chromosome 4p16 based on 4p deletions. *Am J Med Genet* 57:581-586, 1995.
14. Lurie IW, Lazjuk CL, Ussova YL, et al: The Wolf-Hirschhorn syndrome: I. Genetics. *Clin Genet* 17:375-384, 1980.
15. Battaglia A, Carey JC: Update on the clinical features and natural history of Wolf-Hirschhorn syndrome (WHS): Experience with 48 cases. *Am J Hum Genet* 6:127, 2000.
16. Battaglia A: Sindrome di Wolf-Hirschhorn (4p-): Una causa di ritardo mentale grave di difficile diagnosi. *Riv Ital Pediatr (IJP)* 23:254-259, 1997.
17. Battaglia A, Carey JC: Wolf-Hirschhorn syndrome and Pitt-Rogers-Danks syndrome. *Am J Med Genet* 75:541, 1998.
18. Wright TJ, Altherr MR, Callen D, et al: Reply to the letter to the editor by Partington and Turner, Wolf-Hirschhorn and Pitt-Rogers-Danks syndromes. *Am J Med Genet* 82:89-90, 1999.
19. Seckel HPG: *Bird Headed Dwarfs.* Springfield, Ill, CC Thomas, 1960.
20. Pagon RA: Coloboma, congenital heart disease and choanal atresia with multiple anomalies. CHARGE association. J *Pediatr* 99:223-227, 1981.
21. Zollino M, Wright TJ, Di Stefano C, et al: "Tandem" duplication of 4p16.1p16.3 chromosome region associated with 4pl6.3pter molecular deletion resulting in Wolf-Hirschhorn syndrome phenotype. *Am J Med Genet* 82:371-375, 1999.
22. Smith DW, Lemli L, Opitz JM: A newly recognized syndrome of multiple congenital anomalies. *J Pediatr* 64:210-217, 1964.
23. Opitz JM, Summit RL, Smith DW: The G syndrome of multiple congenital anomalies. *Birth Defects* 5:161-166, 1969.
24. Malpuech G, Demecocq F, Palcoux JB, et al: A previously undescribed autosomal recessive multiple congenital anomalies/mental retardation (MCA/MR) syndrome with growth failure, lip/palate cleft(s), and urogenital anomalies. *Am J Med Genet* 16:475-480, 1983.
25. Lowry RB, MacLean JR: Syndrome of mental retardation, cleft palate, eventration of diaphragm, congenital heart defect, glaucoma, growth failure and craniosynostosis. *Birth Defects* 13:203-228, 1977.

26. Williams JCP, Barrat-Boyes BG, Lowe JG: Supravalvular aortic stenosis. *Circulation* 24:1311-1318, 1961.
27. Rett A: Uber ein eigenartiges hirmarrophes syndrom bei hyperammoneumie im kindesalter. *Wien Med Wischr* 110:723, 1966.
28. Battaglia A, Carey JC, Viskochil DH, et al: Wolf-Hirschhorn syndrome (WHS): A history in pictures. *Clin Dysmorphol* 9:25-30, 2000.
29. Centerwall WR, Thompson WP, Allen IE, et al: Translocation 4p- syndrome. *Am J Dis Child* 129:366-370, 1975.
30. De Grouchy J, Tufieau C: *Clinical Atlas of Human Chromosomes,* ed 2. New York, John Wiley, 1984.
31. Battaglia A, Carey JC: Health supervision and anticipatory guidance of individuals with Wolf-Hirschhorn syndrome. *Am J Med Genet (Semin Med Genet)* 89:111-115, 1999.
32. Magill HL, Shackelford GD, McAlister WH, et al: 4p-(Wolf-Hirschhorn) syndrome. *Am J Roentgenol* 135:283-288, 1980.
33. Stengel-Rutkowski S, Warkotsch A, Schimanek P, et al: Familial Wolf's syndrome with a hidden 4p deletion by translocation of an 8p segment. Unbalanced inheritance from a maternal translocation (4;8) (p15.3;p22.). Case report, review and risk estimates. *Clin Genet* 25:500-521, 1984.
34. Sergi C, Schulze BRB, Hager HD, et al: Wolf-Hirschhorn syndrome: Case report and review of the chromosomal aberrations associated with diaphragmatic defects. *Pathologica* 90:285-293, 1998.
35. Lazjuk GI, Lurie IW, Ostrowskaja TI, et al: The Wolf-Hirschhorn syndrome: II. Pathologic anatomy. *Clin* Genet 18:6-12, 1980.
36. Breen GH: Taurodontism, an unreported dental finding in Wolf-Hirschhorn (4p-) syndrome. J *Dent Child* 65:344-345, 1998.
37. Park SH, Chi JB: Oligomeganephroma associated with 4p deletion type chromosomal anomaly. Pediatr *Pathol* 13:731-740, 1993.
38. Tachdijan G, Fondacci C, Tapia S, et al: The Wolf-Hirschhorn syndrome in fetuses. *Clin Genet* 42:281-287, 1992.
39. Grisam S, Ramage IJ, Rosenblum ND: Vesicoureteric reflux associated with renal dysplasia in the Wolf-Hirschhorn syndrome. *Pediatr Nephrol* 14:146-148, 2000.
40. Schaefer BG, Kleimola CN, Stenson C, et al:. *Wolf-Hirschhorn Syndrome (Deletion 4p): A Guidebook for Families.* Omaha, Neb, SOFT 18,13, and RD and Meyer Rehabilitation Institute, University of Nebraska Medical Center, 1996.
41. Fryns JP: The 4p- syndrome, with a report of two new cases. *Humangenetik* 19:99-109, 1973.
42. Gonzales CH, Capelozzi VL, Vajntal A: Brief clinical report: Pathologic findings in the Wolf-Hirschhorn (4p-) syndrome. *Am J Med Genet* 9:183-187, 1981.
43. Lesperance MM, Grundfast KM, Rosenbaum KN: Otologic manifestations of Wolf-Hirschhorn syndrome. *Arch Otol Head Neck Surg* 124:193-196, 1998.
44. Estabrooks LL, Lamb AN, Ayslworth AS, et al: Molecular characteri-

zation of chromosome 4p deletions resulting in Wolf-Hirschhorn syndrome. J Med Genet 31:103-107, 1994.
45. Petit C: Genes responsible for human hereditary deafness. *Nat Genet* 14:385-391, 1996.
46. Hanley-Lopez J, Estabrooks LL, Steihm ER: Antibody deficiency in Wolf-Hirschhorn syndrome. *J Pediatr* 133:141-143, 1998.
47. Eiben B, Leipoldt M, Schubbe I, et al: Partial deletion of 4p in fetal cells not present in chorionic villi. *Clin Genet* 33:49-52, 1988.
48. Verloes A, Schaaps JP, Herens C, et al: Prenatal diagnosis of cystic hygroma and chorioangioma in the Wolf-Hirschhorn syndrome. *Prenat Diagn* 11:129-132, 1991.
49. Battaglia A, Carey JC, Tliompson JA, et al: EEG studies in the Wolf-Hirschhorn (4p-) syndrome. *Electroencephalogr Clin Neurophysiol* 99:324, 1996.
50. Curfs LMG, Didden R, Sikkema SPE, et al: Management of sleeping problems in Wolf-Hirschhorn syndrome: A case study. *Genet Couns* 10:345-350, 1999.
51. Jones KL: *Smith's Recognizable Patterns of Human Malformation.* Philadelphia, WB Saunders, 1997, pp 38-39.
52. O'Brien G, Yule W: *Behavioural Phenotypes.* London, Cambridge University Press, 1995.
53. Dean JC, Penry JK: Discontinuation of antiepileptic drugs, in Levy RH, Mattson RH, Meldrum BS (eds): *Antiepileptic Drugs.* New York, Raven Press, 1995, pp 201-208.
54. Schinzel A: *Catalogue of Unbalanced Chromosome Aberrations in Man.* New York, de Gruyter, 1984, p 163.
55. Opitz JM: Twenty-seven-year follow-up in the Wolf-Hirschhorn syndrome. *Am J Med* Genet 55:459-461, 1995.
56. Wheeler PG, Weaver DD, Palmer CG: Familial translocation resulting in Wolf-Hirschhorn syndrome in two related unbalanced individuals: Clinical evaluation of a 39-year-old man with Wolf-Hirschhorn syndrome. *Am J Med Genet* 55:462-465, 1995.
57. Ogle R, Sillence DO, Merrick A, et al: The Wolf-Hirschhorn syndrome in adulthood: Evaluation of a 24-year-old man with a rec (4) chromosome. *Am J Med Genet* 65:124-127, 1996.
58. Lanters LT: *Nieuwsbrief Wolf-Hirschhorn.* 6:1-2, 2000.
59. Battaglia A, unpublished observations.
60. Estabrooks LL, Lamb AN, Kirkman HN, et al: A molecular deletion of distal chromosome 4p in two families with a satellited chromosome 4 lacking the Wolf-Hirschhorn syndrome phenotype. *Am J Hum Genet* 51:971-978, 1992.
61. Gandelman K-Y, Gibson L, Meyn MS, et al: Molecular definition of the smallest region of deletion overlap in the Wolf-Hirschhorn syndrome. *Am J Hum Genet* 51:571-578, 1992.
62. Johnson VP, Altherr MR, Blake JM, et al: FISH detection of Wolf-Hirschhorn syndrome: Exclusion of D4F26 as critical site. *Am J Med Genet* 52:70-74, 1994.

63. El-Rifai W, Leisti J, Kahkonen M, et al: A patient with Wolf-Hirschhorn syndrome originating from translocation t(4;8) (p16.3;q24.3)pat. *J Med Genet* 32:65-67, 1995.
64. Reid E, Morrison N, Barton L, et al: Familial Wolf-Hirschhorn syndrome resulting from a cryptic translocation: A clinical and molecular study. *J Med Genet* 33:197-202, 1996.
65. Bauer K, Howard-Peebles PN, Keele D, et al: Wolf-Hirschhorn syndrome owing to 1:3 segregation of a maternal 4;21 translocation. *Am J Med Genet* 21:351-356, 1985.
66. Altherr MR, Bengtsson U, Elder FFB, et al: Molecular confirmation of Wolf-Hirschhorn syndrome with a subtle translocation of chromosome *4. Am J Hum Genet* 49:1235-1242, 1991.
67. Tupler R, Bortotto L, Buhler E, et al: Paternal origin of denovo deleted chromosome 4 in Wolf-Hirschhorn syndrome. *J Med Genet* 29:53-55, 1992.
68. Dallapiccola B, Mandich P, Bellone E, et al: Parental origin of chromosome 4p deletion in Wolf-Hirschhorn syndrome. Am *J Med Genet* 47:921-924,1993.
69. Meloni A, Shepard RR, Battaglia A, et al: Wolf-Hirschhorn syndrome: Correlation between cytogenetics, FISH, and severity of disease. *Am J Hum Genet* 67:149, 2000.
70. Zollino M, Di Stefano C, Zampino G, et al: Genotype-phenotype correlations and clinical diagnostic criteria in Wolf-Hirschhorn syndrome. *Am J Med Genet* 94:254-261, 2000.
71. Francke U, Arias DE, Nyhan WL: Proximal 4p- deletion: Phenotype differs from classical 4p- syndrome. *J Pediatr* 90:250-252, 1977.
72. Chitayat D, Ruvalcaba RHA, Babul R, et al: Syndrome of proximal interstitial deletion 4p15: Report of three cases and review of the literature. *Am J Med Genet* 55:147-154, 1995.
73. White DM, Pillers DM, Reiss JA, et al: Interstitial deletions of the short arm of chromosome 4 in patients with a similar combination of multiple minor anomalies and mental retardation. *Am J Med Genet* 57:588-597, 1995.
74. Clemens M, Martsolf JT, Rogers JG, et al: Pitt-Rogers-Danks syndrome: The result of a 4p microdeletion. *Am J Med Genet* 66:95-100, 1996.
75. Lindeman-Kusse MC, Haeringen AV, Hoorweg-Nijman JJG, et al: Cytogenetic abnormalities in two new patients with Pitt-Rogers-Danks phenotype. *Am J Med Genet* 66:104-112, 1996.
76. Gilliam TC, Bucan M, MacDonald ME, et al: A DNA segment encoding two genes very tightly linked to Huntington's disease. *Science* 238:950-952, 1987.
77. John RM, Robbins CA, Myers RM: Identification of genes within CpG-enriched DNA from human chromosome 4p16.3. *Hum Mol Genet* 3:1611-1616, 1994.
78. Rommens JM, Lin B, Hutchinson GB, et al: A transcription map of the region containing the Huntington disease gene. *Hum Mol Genet* 2:901-907, 1993.

79. Snell RG, Doucette-Stamm KA, Gillespie KM, et al: The isolation of cDNAs within the Huntington disease region by hybridisation of yeast artificial chromosomes to a cDNA library. *Hum Mol Genet* 2:305-309, 1993.
80. Thompson LM, Plummer S, Schalling M, et al: A gene encoding a fibroblast growth factor receptor isolated from the Huntington disease gene region of human chromosome 4. *Genomics* 11:1133-1142, 1991.
81. Collins C, Hutchinson G, Kowbel D, et al: The human [3-subunit of rod photoreceptor cGMP phosphodiesterase: Complete retinal cDNA sequence and evidence for expression in brain. *Genomics* 13:698-704, 1992.
82. Andrew S, Theilmann J, Hedrick A, et al Nonrandom association between Huntington disease and two loci separated by about 3Mb on 4p16.3. *Genomics* 13:310-311, 1992.
83. Tommerup N, Aagaard L, Lund CL, et al: A zinc-finger gene ZNF141 mapping at 4p16.3/D4S90 is a candidate gene for the Wolf-Hirschhorn (4p-) syndrome. *Hum Mol Genet* 2:1571-1575, 1993.
84. Endele S, Fuhry M, Pak SJ, et al: LETM1, a novel gene encoding a putative EF-hand Ca(2+)-binding protein, flanks the Wolf-Hirschhorn syndrome (WHS) critical region and is deleted in most WHS patients. *Genomics* 60:218-225, 1999.
85. Scott HS, Ashton LJ, Eyre HJ, et al: Chromosomal localization of the human α-L-iduronidase gene *(IDUA)* to 4p16.3. *Am J Hum Genet* 47:802-807, 1990.
86. Wright TJ, Ricke DO, Denison K, et al: A transcript map of the newly defined 165kb Wolf-Hirschhorn syndrome critical region. *Hum Mol Genet* 6:317-324, 1997.
87. Baxendale S, MacDonald ME, Mott R, et al: A cosmid contig and high resolution restriction map of the 2 megabase region containing the Huntington's disease gene. *Nat Genet* 4:181-186, 1993.
88. Altherr MR, Wright TJ, Denison K, et al: Delimiting the Wolf-Hirschhorn syndrome critical region to 750 kilobase pairs. *Am J Med Genet* 71:47-53, 1997.
89. Wright TJ, Clemens M, Quarrell O, et al: Wolf-Hirschhorn and Pitt-Rogers-Danks syndromes caused by overlapping 4p deletions. *Am J Med Genet* 75:345-350, 1998.
90. Fang YY, Bain S, Haan EA, et al: High resolution characterization of an interstitial deletion of less than 1.9Mb at k4p16.3 associated with Wolf-Hirschhorn syndrome. *Am J Med Genet* 71:452-457, 1997.
91. Somer M, Peippo M, Keinanen M: Controversial findings in two patients with commercially available probe D4S96 for the Wolf-Hirschhorn syndrome. *Am J Hum Genet* 57:A127, 1995.
92. Ricke DO, Mundt MO, Buckingham JM, et al: Whole genome sequence sampling and gene analysis and annotation of megabases of low redundancy human chromosome 16p13 sample sequencing comparison analysis (SCAN). *Microb Comp Genomics* 1:264, 1996.
93. White DM, Pillers D-AM, Reiss JA, et al: Interstitial deletions of the

short arm of chromosome 4 in patients with a similar combination of multiple minor anomalies and mental retardation. *Am J Med Genet* 57:588-597, 1995.

94. Whaley WL, Bates GP, Novelletto A, et al: Mapping of cosmid clones in Huntington's disease region of chromosome 4. *Somat Cell Mol Genet* 17:83-91, 1991.
95. Stec I, Wright TJ, van Ommen G-JB, et al: WHSC1, a 90kb SET domain-containing gene, expessed in early development and homologous to a *Drosophila* dysmorphy gene maps in the Wolf-Hirschhorn syndrome critical region and is fused to *IgH* in t(4;14) multiple myeloma. *Hum Mol Genet* 7:1071-1082, 1998.
96. Wright TJ, Costa JL, Naranjo C, et al: Comparative analysis of a novel gene from the Wolf-Hirschhorn/Pitt-Rogers-Danks syndrome critical region. *Genomics* 59:203-212, 1999.
97. Stec I, Nagl SB, van Ommen GJ, et al: The PWWP domain: A potential protein-protein interaction domain in nuclear proteins influencing differentiation? FEBS Lett 473:1-5, 2000.
98. Baxevanis AD, Landsman D: The HMG-1 box protein family: Classification and functional relationships. *Nucleic Acids Res* 23:1604-1613, 1995.
99. Tkachuk DC, Kohler S, Cleary ML: Involvement of a homolog of *Drosophila trithorax* by 11q23 chromosomal translocations in acute leukemias. *Cell* 71:691-700, 1992.
100. Gu Y, Nakamura T, Alder H, et al: The t(4;11) chromosome translocation of human acute leukemias fuses the ALL-1 gene, related to *Drosophila trithorax,* to the AF-4 gene. *Cell* 71:701-708, 1992.
101. Moore KL, Persaud TVN: *The Developing Human: Clinically Oriented Embyrology.* Philadelphia, WB Saunders, 1998.
102. Wilkinson DG: Whole mount *in situ* hybridization of vertebrate embryos, in Wilkinson DG (ed): *In Situ Hybridization: A Practical Approach.* New York, Oxford University Press, 1993.
103. Clemens M, McPherson EW, Surt U: 4p microdeletion in a child with Pitt-Rogers-Danks syndrome. *Am J Hum Genet* 57:A85, 1995.
104. Donnai D: Pitt-Rogers-Danks syndrome and Wolf-Hirschhorn syndrome (editorial). *Am J Med Genet* 66:101-103, 1996.
105. Kant SG, van Haeringen A, Bakker E, et al: Pitt-Rogers-Danks syndrome and Wolf-Hirschhorn syndrome are caused by a deletion in the same region on chromosome 4p16.3. *J Med Genet* 34:569-572, 1997.
106. Zollino M, Bova R, Neri G: From Pitt-Rogers-Danks syndrome to Wolf-Hirschhorn syndrome and back? *Am J Med Genet* 66:113-115, 1996.
107. Wieczorek D, Krause M, Majewski F, et al: Effect of the size of the deletion and clinical manifestation in Wolf-Hirschhorn syndrome: Analysis of 13 patients with a de novo deletion. *Eur J Hum* Genet 8:519-526, 2000.

CHAPTER 4

The Prolonged QT Syndrome

Julien I. E. Hoffman, MD, FRCP
Professor of Pediatrics (Emeritus), Attending Pediatric Cardiologist, University of California, San Francisco

The QT interval of the electrocardiogram is the duration from the onset of the Q wave to the end of the T wave. The interval may be abnormally prolonged in some families,[1-4] by myocardial disease or by certain drugs.[5-11] Patients with prolonged QT intervals may have a distinctive form of ventricular tachycardia termed *torsades de pointes* that may develop into ventricular fibrillation and cause sudden death. Because autopsy examination in these patients shows no gross pathologic changes, some investigators have postulated that the sudden infant death syndrome (SIDS) might be secondary to a long QT interval.[5-8]

This review describes the basic electrophysiology that determines the QT, followed by a listing of the factors that prolong the QT interval. Then the clinical features, diagnosis, and treatment of the heritable long QT syndrome are presented. Finally, the relationship of the long QT interval to SIDS and the issues about screening for the long QT interval are discussed.

BASIC ELECTROPHYSIOLOGY

The QT interval encompasses the duration of electrical activity from the onset of depolarization (the beginning of the septal Q wave) to the end of repolarization marked by the end of the T wave. Because at normal heart rates depolarization occupies only a small part of this interval, changes in repolarization are the main determinants of the QT interval.

The ventricular transmembrane potential has 5 phases (Fig 1). The resting transmembrane potential (phase 4) is –80 to –90 mV. With activation, the transmembrane potential rapidly becomes positive (phase 0) because of a sudden increase in sodium con-

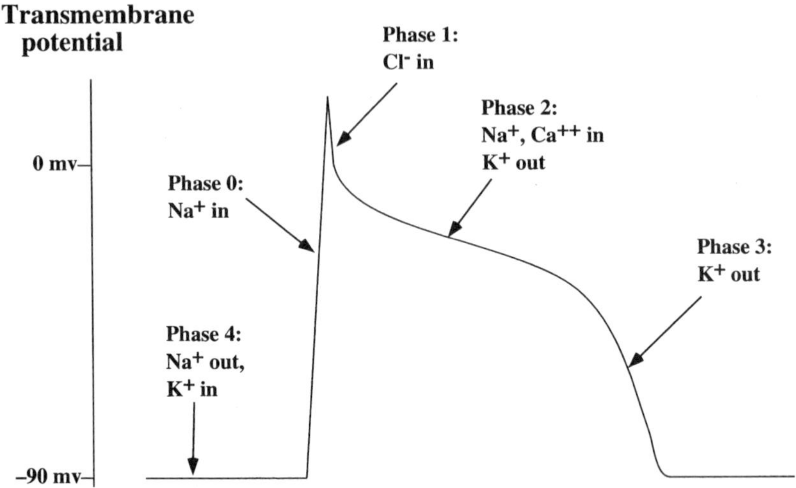

FIGURE 1.
Diagram of main ion movements during a typical ventricular muscle action potential. The potassium movements are given in more detail in Figures 2 and 3.

ductance and influx of positively charged sodium ions into the cell. In phase 1, the potential returns rapidly to near zero as sodium conductance suddenly decreases and there is an influx of negatively charged chloride ions. Then a plateau (phase 2) occurs in which the potential gradually becomes more negative, resulting from a slow inward movement of sodium and calcium almost balanced by a slow outward movement of potassium. Finally, there is a rapid decrease in potential to its resting level (phase 3) because of an increased potassium conductance. In phase 4, the negative potential is stable as sodium is pumped out of the cell in exchange for potassium.

The major ion channels responsible for depolarization and repolarization are associated with potassium, sodium, and calcium; several channels exist for each ion (Fig 2).

POTASSIUM CHANNELS

There are 3 main types of potassium channels that carry potassium-induced currents[9] (Fig 3): the inward rectifier current (I_{K1}), the transient outward current (I_{to}), and the delayed rectifier current (I_K). The inward rectifier K^+ channels allow inward potassium current at positive potentials, but after repolarization has brought membrane potential below about –20 mV, they permit outward

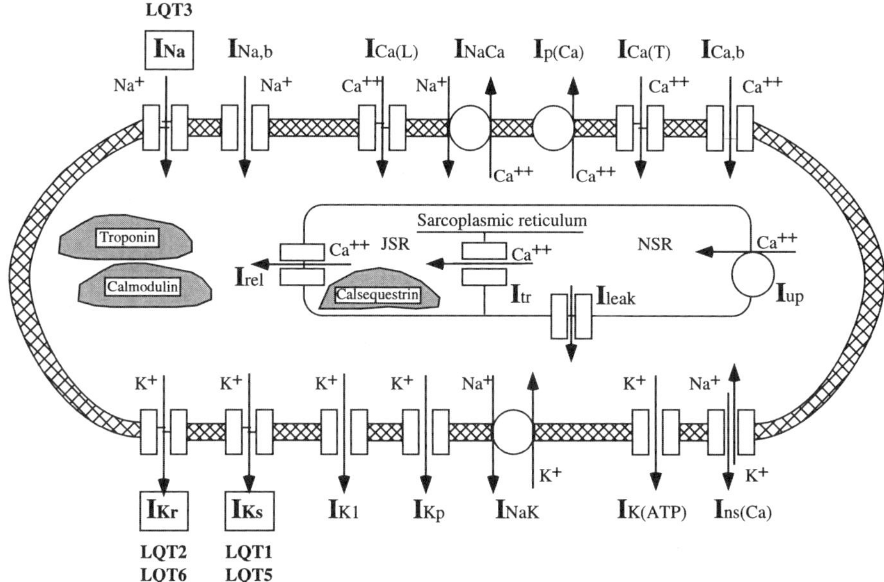

FIGURE 2.
Diagram of mammalian ventricular cell to show ion channels. *Abbreviations:* $I_{Ca(L)}$, Calcium current through L-type calcium channel; $I_{Ca(T)}$, calcium current through T-type calcium channel; $I_{Ca,b}$, calcium background current; $I_{K(ATP)}$, ATP-sensitive potassium current; I_{Kp}, plateau potassium current; I_{K1}, inward rectifier potassium current; I_{Kr}, fast component of delayed rectifier current; I_{Ks}, slow component of the delayed rectifier current; I_{leak}, calcium leakage from NSR to myoplasm; I_{Na}, fast sodium current; $I_{Na,b}$, sodium background current; I_{NaCa}, sodium-calcium exchange current; I_{NaK}, sodium-potassium pump; $I_{ns(Ca)}$, non-specific calcium-activated current; $I_{p(Ca)}$, calcium pump in the sarcolemma; I_{rel}, calcium release from junctional sarcoplasmic reticulum; I_{tr}, calcium translocation from NSR to JSR; I_{up}, calcium uptake from the myoplasm to network sarcoplasmic reticulum (NSR); *JSR,* junctional sarcoplasmic reticulum; *NSR,* network sarcoplasmic reticulum. *LQT1, LQT2, LQT3* are the three main forms of the long QT syndrome, and they and *LQT5* and *LQT6* are positioned opposite the channels that are involved in them. LQT5 and LQT6 are added to the published figure. (Courtesy of Viswanathan PC, Rudy Y: Pause induced early afterdepolarizations in the long QT syndrome: A simulation study. *Cardiovasc Res* 42:530-542. Copyright 1999, with permission from Elsevier Science.)

potassium efflux that peaks towards the end of phase 2. The transient outward K^+ channels open a few milliseconds after membrane depolarization but close very rapidly, and so do not contribute to phase 2. Finally, the delayed rectifier current K^+ channels produce an outward current that develops slowly during phase 2 and opposes the inward calcium and sodium/calcium exchange currents. These channels are responsible for the slow depolarization in phase 2 until the membrane potential reaches about –20 mV, after which the inward rectifier current (above) rapidly increases and returns the membrane potential to its resting level of about –80 mV.

The delayed rectifier is composed of 2 different channels that are responsible for the I_{Kr} (rapid) and I_{Ks} (slow) potassium currents, with the major potassium currents responsible for the duration of the action potential. The I_{Ks} channel is formed from an α subunit encoded by a gene termed KvLQT1 on chromosome 11, and a β subunit formed by the smallest potassium channel protein known (hence the name minK), the gene for which has been cloned and is found on chromosome 21. The I_{Kr} channel is encoded by a gene

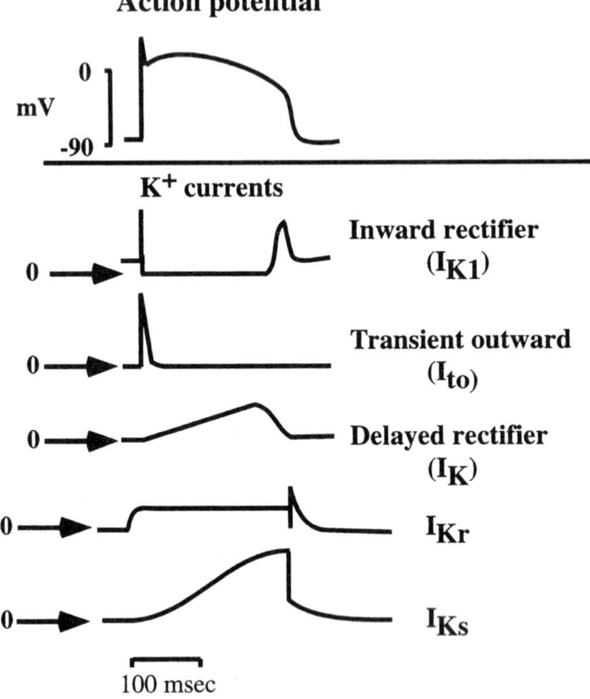

FIGURE 3.
Diagram of the action potential **(above the line)** and the main potassium currents **(below the line)**. The delayed rectifier current I_K has two components: I_{Kr} and I_{Ks}. (Adapted from Sanguinetti MC, Keating MT: Role of delayed rectifier potassium channel in cardiac repolarization and arrhythmias. *News in Physiological Sciences* 12:152-157, 1997, with permission.)

termed HERG, named after its similarity to the *ether-a-go-go* gene first cloned from *Drosophila*; this gene is on chromosome 7. The channel is a tetramer formed from 4 HERG α subunits. Recently, minK-related peptide 1 (MiRP1) has been identified as a protein partner for HERG.[10,11] Blockade of the I_{Kr} channel by drugs like sotalol reduces potassium efflux and prolongs the action potential and thus the QT interval. Conversely, stimulation of this channel by isoproterenol increases potassium efflux and shortens the action potential.

The distribution of these various potassium channels is not constant throughout the heart. In particular, cells in the midmyocardium of the left ventricle, the M cells, have a much lower density of I_{Ks} channels than in the subepicardium or subendocardium. As a result, as compared with these other layers, M cells have a prolonged action potential duration, a greater dependence of the action potential on heart rate, and a greater sensitivity to interventions that decrease repolarizing currents or enhance depolarizing currents.[12] In addition, there are also adenosine triphosphate (ATP)-dependent and plateau potassium channels that produce $I_{K(ATP)}$ and I_{Kp} currents, respectively.

SODIUM CHANNELS

There are 4 sodium channels. Two exchange sodium for calcium or potassium, producing the I_{NaCa} and I_{NaK} currents, respectively. One is responsible for the background sodium current, $I_{Na,b}$. The most important, from our point of view, is the channel for the fast sodium current, I_{na}, its protein encoded by a gene termed SCN5A on chromosome 3.

CALCIUM CHANNELS

Calcium enters the myocardial cell through 3 channels that produce the $I_{Ca(T)}$ (transient), $I_{Ca(L)}$ (long lasting), and background ($I_{Ca,b}$) currents, and is pumped out of the cell by the sarcolemmal pump and the sodium-calcium exchanger, giving the $I_{p(Ca)}$ and I_{NaCa} currents, respectively.

Because of the importance of these ion channels, changes in serum electrolyte concentrations have large effects on the QT interval.[13] An increase in serum potassium shortens the QT interval by increasing the efflux of potassium by the I_{Kr} channel. By contrast, hypokalemia lengthens the QT interval. A long QT interval with a prolonged isoelectric ST segment is characteristic of hypocalcemia, and hypercalcemia tends to shorten the QT interval. Hypomagnesemia also lengthens the QT interval.[14]

MODULATION OF QT INTERVAL

During phase 2 of the action potential, the myocyte is completely refractory to stimulation; it is partially refractory in phase 3, and regains full responsiveness only in phase 4. Refractoriness prevents ventricular contraction from interrupting the filling of the ventricle. Such a mechanism must adapt to changes in heart rate: the action potential must shorten to allow more beats when tachycardia is needed, and must lengthen to allow more ventricular filling during bradycardia.

Although measurement of the QT interval is of obvious importance because of the relationship between long QT interval and sudden death, measurement of the QT interval to determine disease risk is not straightforward. The simplest way of deciding if the QT interval is normal for a given heart rate is to examine a table of the range of normal QT intervals at specified heart rates[15] or a graph of that relationship.[16-18] If the data are obtained from a large enough study, then percentiles of the QT interval at each heart rate can be shown (Fig 4).[19] Because evaluating the QT interval involves having the appropriate tables or figures at hand, many investigators have developed empirical formulas for relating the QT interval to the heart rate. This was done first in 1920 when Bazett[20] found the QT interval to be proportional to the square root of the preceding RR interval; that is, the ratio $QT/\sqrt{RR}$ was con-

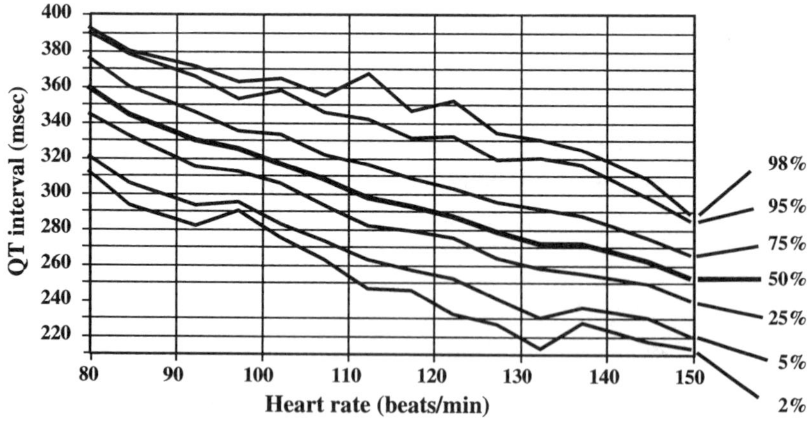

FIGURE 4.
Percentile chart for QT intervals at different heart rates. (Adapted from Davignon A, Rautaharju P, Boiselle E, et al: Normal ECG standards for infants and children. *Pediatr Cardiol* 1:121-152, 1980, with permission.)

stant. This ratio, originally called K, is now called QTc (corrected QT interval). The ratio has an average value of 0.40 and a narrow normal range of 0.36 to 0.44. Bazett's study has many limitations. He studied only 15 men aged 14 to 36 years, 19 women aged 21 to 30 years, and 5 infants over a range of heart rates from 40 to 200 beats per minute, of which only two had less than 70 beats per minute. Over the years, additional studies have shown that Bazett's formula overadjusts the QT interval at high heart rates (ie, the QTc is too high) and underadjusts the QT interval at low heart rates (ie, the QTc is too low).

In the same year, Fridericia[21] introduced a slightly more complicated formula used extensively in Europe. He found that the QT interval was related to the cube root of the RR interval if both were measured in hundredths of a second:

$$QT = k\sqrt[3]{RR}$$

where k = 8.45 in young men and 8.51 in middle-aged men according to some investigators,[22] although Fridericia used 8.22 as the constant. His sample size was also low: 9 children older than 2 years, 19 men and 15 women aged 28 to 40 years, and 3 men and 3 women older than 40 years, for a total of 50 patients and at heart rates from 51 to 135 beats per minute. His formula gives a QTc interval that is too low at high heart rates.

Since those 2 formulas were introduced, there have been many attempts to provide and compare better formulas.[15,16,23-29] Investigators have explored linear, logarithmic, and power functions, with 1, 2, or 3 parameters in each. A recent linear formula for corrected QT interval (QTlc) based on 5018 healthy persons comes from Framingham[15]:

$$QTlc = QT + 0.154(1 - RR)$$

Sarma et al[29] used an exponential formula:

$$QTc = a - be^{-cRR}$$

Unfortunately, the constants a, b, and c differ in different studies. Rautaharju et al[28] in a study of 17,139 patients ranging in age from birth to 75 years provided a relationship of predicted QT (QTp) to heart rate (HR):

$$QTp = 656/(1 + 0.01HR)$$

All of these formulas and the observed data agree closely between heart rates of 60 and 120 beats per minute, but less well at faster and slower rates.

EFFECT OF AGE AND GENDER

In 1919, Lombard and Cope[30] observed that mechanical systole was longer in women than in men. Bazett[20] confirmed that the difference applied also to the QT interval; in fact, his constant K was 0.37 for men and 0.40 for women. Gender differences in QT interval were well recognized by others[17,31] and have recently been examined in detail.[32-34] In young children, the QT interval does not differ in boys and girls, but after puberty there is a 20-millisecond shortening of the corrected QT interval in males relative to females. The QT interval in males gradually increases in length to equal that in women by about 60 years of age. Rautaharju et al[32] modified their predictive formula to take account of gender and age. For males 15 to 50 years of age, their formula was:

$$QTp = [656/(1 + 0.01HR)] + 0.4age - 23$$

In addition, they corrected for QRS duration by the formula:

$$QTp = [600/(1 + 0.01HR)] + 0.4QRS$$

where QRS is the QRS duration in milliseconds. For males between 15 and 50 years of age, the formula is:

$$QTp = [600/(1 + 0.01HR)] + 0.4QRS + 0.4age - 25$$

MECHANISMS OF HEART RATE CHANGES

Heart rate depends on the balance of vagal and sympathetic nerve effects on the sinuatrial node. The increased rate with exercise is caused mainly by increased sympathetic nerve stimulation, and the heart rate slowing with sleep is caused mainly by sympathetic withdrawal.

Vagal Influence on the QT Interval

In human volunteers, blocking the vagi with atropine (with or without concomitant propranolol administration) shortened the QT (and QTc) interval while the heart rate was fixed by atrial pacing.[35,36] An increase in heart rate after parasympathetic blockade with atropine changed the QT interval according to a cube root formula,[37] whereas after exercise a square root relationship was noted; the difference was possibly caused by changes in sympathetic tone with exercise. Stimulating vagal reflexes by immersing the face in water (diving reflex) decreased heart rate by 40 beats per minute, barely changed the QT interval, and consequently decreased the QTc interval by about 85 milliseconds.[38]

Sympathetic Influence on the QT Interval

The history of sympathetic cardiac nerves and their imbalance has been discussed by Schwartz,[39] who has contributed much of our understanding to this field. The basic features are summarized in Fig 5.[39] The right and left stellate ganglia inhibit each other directly and also communicate with the central nervous system. Each ganglion innervates its appropriate ventricle, with the left-sided effects larger than those from the right side. The nerves from the right stellate ganglion increase heart rate and right ventricular contractility, whereas the nerves from the left stellate ganglion increase left ventricular contractility. Yanowitz et al[40] showed in cats that right stellate ganglionectomy or left stellate ganglion stimulation prolonged the QT interval and accentuated the positive T waves, whereas right stellate ganglion stimulation or left stellate ganglionectomy did not change the QT interval but made the T waves negative. In anesthetized cats paced at a fixed heart rate, Abildskov[41] found that left stellate ganglion stimulation gave a longer QT interval but shorter refractory periods, and concluded that the stimulation had caused greater dispersion of recovery times. He also observed that a long QT interval could be produced by brief left stellate ganglion stimulation or a rapid catecholamine infusion, whereas prolonged stimulation or infusion either did not change the QT interval or even shortened it slightly. He concluded that the effect of rapid stimulation caused a localized effect, but that prolonged stimulation caused a more widespread effect on recovery times.

Schwartz et al[42-44] found that in dogs, left stellectomy decreased excitability, whereas right stellectomy shortened the refractory period and increased excitability. These sympathetic effects were antagonized by tonic vagal stimulation.[43] Stramba-Badiale et al,[45] and others have also shown that vagal or right stellate ganglion removal or left stellate ganglion stimulation increases the likelihood of ventricular fibrillation.

These findings have been confirmed in humans. When there is myocardial ischemia, left stellate ganglion stimulation produces ventricular arrhythmias[46] in humans as it does in animals. In controls and patients treated with stellectomy for Raynaud syndrome,[47] a submaximal exercise test produced ventricular arrhythmias in 1 (3%) of 32 controls, 6 (18%) of 34 patients with a right stellectomy, 1 (5%) of 19 patients with a left stellectomy, and 0 of 18 patients with bilateral stellectomy.

With exercise, the QTc interval remains almost unchanged.[48] The effects of heart rate and autonomic tone have been studied by comparing the effects on the QT interval of exercise, atrial pacing,

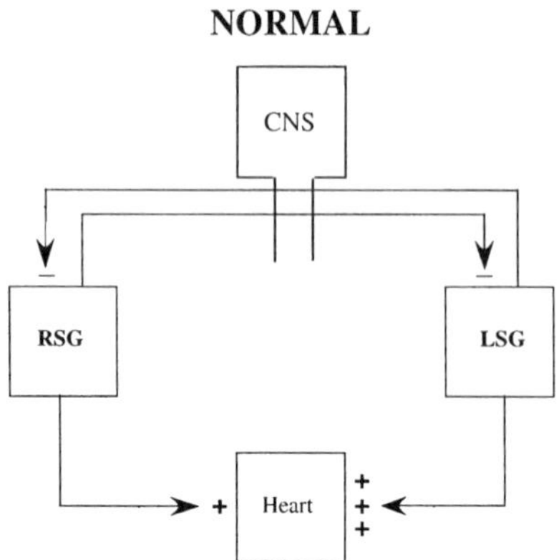

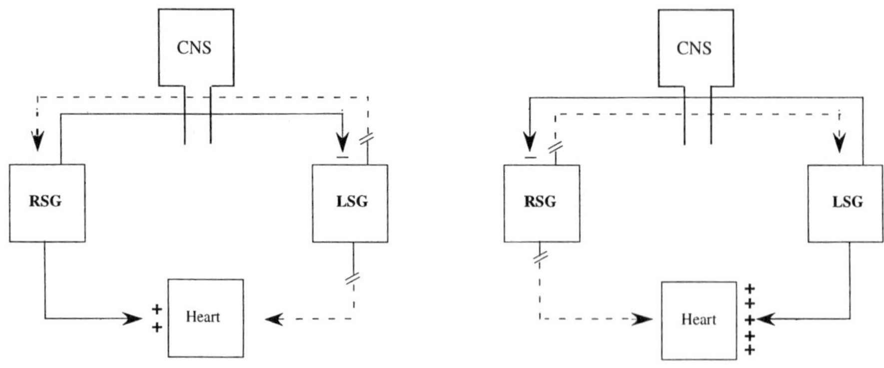

FIGURE 5.

Left and right sympathetic interaction. **Upper panel,** In the normal state, the left stellate ganglion *(LSG)* and the right stellate ganglion *(RSG)* inhibit each other directly. There are also interactions with the central nervous system *(CNS)*. Inhibition is indicated by *minus signs*. Stimulation is indicated by *plus signs*. Left cardiac sympathetic innervation has more effect on the left ventricle than right cardiac sympathetic innervation has on the right ventricle, either because of the greater muscle mass or an increased receptor density. **Left lower panel,** Left stellectomy removes the inhibition of the right stellate ganglion, so that right-sided sympathetic stimulation increases, and also removes direct effects on the heart from the left stellate ganglion *(dashed lines)*. This is beneficial in preventing arrhythmias. **Right lower panel,** Right stellectomy removes inhibition of the left stellate ganglion, increases left-sided sympathetic stimulation, decreases the effect of the right stellate ganglion on the heart *(dashed lines)*, and increases the tendency to ventricular arrhythmias. (From *Nervous Control of Cardiovascular Function,* in Randall WC (ed). New York, Oxford University Press, 1984. Copyright 1984 by Oxford University Press, Inc. Used by permission of Oxford University Press, Inc.)

and exercise during fixed rate ventricular pacing[49-52]; with fixed rate ventricular pacing, the QT interval is related to the atrial rate, an indicator of autonomic nerve activity. During atrial pacing at rest, the QT interval shortened as heart rate increased, although the QTc interval became longer at the higher rates.[50] With exercise and normal atrioventricular conduction, the QT interval shortened much more for a given increase in heart rate. With exercise at a fixed ventricular paced rate of 70 beats per minute, the QT interval still shortened as atrial rate increased, but did so much less than when ventricular rate also increased. Therefore, shortening of the QT interval is partly caused by the change in heart rate and partly independent of rate and presumably caused by autonomic nerve influences. Clearly a change in heart rate is only one of the factors responsible for a change in the QT interval with exercise.[53]

The sympathetic nerve component should be tested easily by examining the effects of β-adrenergic blockade, but studies of this subject are not in agreement. Fananapazir et al[49] found that intravenous atenolol almost completely abolished the shortening of the QT interval as heart rate increased with exercise. Rickards and Norman[51] found the relationship of QT interval to heart rate unchanged by intravenous propranolol, whereas Milne et al[50] found that intravenous propranolol lengthened the QT interval at a fixed heart rate. When heart rate was allowed to vary, propranolol lengthened the QT interval but shortened the QTc interval. Basic studies on cat papillary muscles[54] have also demonstrated both rate-dependent and rate-independent shortening of the action potential, and this fits with the observation by Bazett[20] that the change in QT lagged considerably behind the change in heart rate when exercise started.

Measurement of the QT interval is not always accurate. The onset of the Q wave can be determined precisely, but the T wave often ends with a gentle curve that reaches the baseline asymptotically. Some investigators measure to the junction of the T wave and the baseline, whereas others measure to the initial change in slope at the end of the rapid downstroke of the T wave. These 2 measurements can differ by as much as 0.04 seconds.[55] Other investigators believe it better to avoid any influence of QRS duration on the QT interval by measuring the JT interval instead of the QT interval.[56-59] This could be particularly important at high heart rates or with bundle branch block, in both of which the QRS duration becomes a significant part of the QT interval.[56,60]

There is a diurnal variation to the QTc interval. Morganroth et al[61] noted that in healthy men, the QTc interval varied by 35 to 108 (average, 76) milliseconds over 24 hours. The QTc interval is about 19 to

23 milliseconds longer during deep sleep than when awake,[62-64] and Bexton et al[64] observed a sudden shortening of the QTc interval on waking. They also noted that the QTc interval was only about 9 milliseconds longer during sleep in patients with heart transplants, and found no diurnal change in a group of diabetic patients. These diurnal changes are therefore associated with variations in autonomic tone and the activity of the receptors.

Some investigators have recommended that the QT interval be measured in lead II, others in leads V_2 or V_5, and some choose the lead with the longest QT interval. In fact, QT intervals vary from lead to lead, a phenomenon known as QT dispersion. Some of the differences in QT duration result from the fact that in a given lead, the onset or offset of the action potential might be isoelectric,[65] but in the main the differences reflect dispersion of recovery times throughout the ventricles.[66,67] The difference between the longest and the shortest QT intervals in any electrocardiogram averages about 43 ± 12 milliseconds in healthy people, and the QTc interval varies about 0.05 ± 0.02 milliseconds.[68] Some of the differences are transmural. The subepicardial muscle is the first to repolarize, and the peak of the T wave marks the completion of subepicardial repolarization. Then the subendocardial muscle begins to depolarize, giving rise to the descending limb of the T wave. Finally, the M cells in the midmyocardium depolarize, giving rise to the last segment of the T wave.[69] In addition, there are anteroposterior and apico-basal differences in action potential duration, and corresponding differences in recovery times of monophasic action potentials in different parts of the right ventricle[70] and the left ventricle[71] have been shown.

CONSEQUENCES OF A LONG QT INTERVAL

A long QT interval does not affect cardiac function other than by the propensity to cause cardiac arrhythmias. (However, about half of the patients with the long QT syndrome by echocardiography reach half-maximal systolic contraction more rapidly than controls, and spend more time at a very low thickening rate.[72]) The pathognomonic arrhythmia is the torsades de pointes, a form of ventricular tachycardia in which the pointed ends of the QRS complexes cycle from pointing upwards to pointing downwards, and then upwards again (Fig 6). Not only does this rapid arrhythmia decrease cardiac output, but it also often progresses to ventricular fibrillation. As a consequence, people with long QT intervals may have dizziness, syncope, or sudden death. These complications do not depend on the cause of the long QT interval.

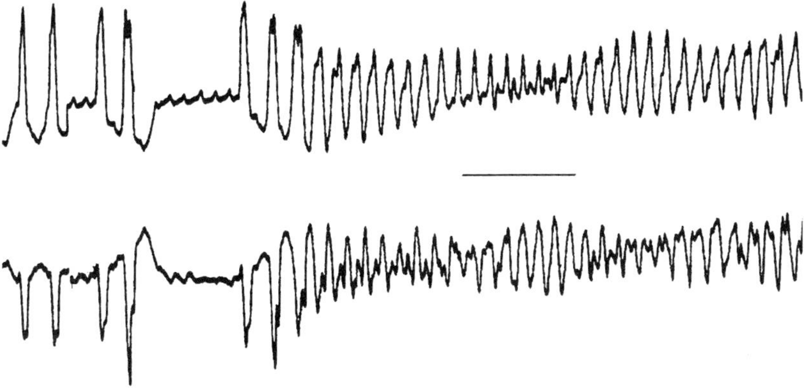

FIGURE 6.
Torsades de pointes. Two simultaneously recorded strips of an electrocardiogram show a premature beat followed by a long pause (there is atrial fibrillation, but this is irrelevant) that initiates a long run of polymorphous ventricular tachycardia—that is, a ventricular tachycardia in which successive complexes have different shapes. Characteristic of torsades de pointes is that the sharp ends of some complexes point upward, and others point downward. In addition, the sinusoidal-like increasing and decreasing size of the complexes is typical of torsades. *Horizontal line* shows that recording is at 25 mm/s. (Electrocardiogram provided courtesy of Dr Melvin Scheinman.)

Two main mechanisms have been proposed for initiation of the arrhythmias. One is increased QT temporal dispersion. Normally when a premature impulse occurs, all the ventricular muscle depolarizes, and the recovery period is relatively homogeneous. If there is considerable dispersion of the action potential, then an early premature beat depolarizes those muscle cells with a short action potential but does not affect those muscle cells with a long action potential (and long refractory period). The latter cells, when they become responsive again, may be stimulated by cells that have just been activated, and microcircuits may be set up that result in a ventricular tachycardia.[73]

The second mechanism involves early afterdepolarizations that have been recorded in patients with the long QT syndrome.[70,74,75] Decreases in outward potassium currents or increases in inward sodium currents lead to increased entry of calcium into the cell, perhaps involving the Na/Ca and the Ca/K exchangers. As a result of the increased intracellular calcium, early after depolarizations develop,[73,76] some of which may reach the threshold for depolarizing other muscle cells and setting up a malignant arrhythmia.

Interestingly, catecholamines and left stellate ganglion stimulation enhance the development of afterdepolarizations.[74,77-80]

Torsade de pointes characteristically occurs when a long RR interval is followed by a short RR interval, the "long-short" sequence.[14,81,82] The long RR interval may result from a transient bradycardia or in the pause after an ectopic beat. This prolongs the action potential. (In other patients, the QT interval is prolonged without a preceding pause or change in heart rate.[81]) As model studies have shown,[76] after a pause, the M cells develop afterdepolarizations, probably caused by increased calcium entry into the cell. These depolarizations in the setting of increased temporal QR dispersion cause torsades de pointes. It is noteworthy that patients with the long QT syndrome tend to have lower-than-normal basic heart rates[83] as well as increased QT interval dispersion.[57,68,84,85]

CAUSES OF A LONG QT INTERVAL

The causes of a long QT interval are listed in Box 1. The most common causes of a long QT interval are drugs, with agents from many different classes being possible causes. The drugs mentioned below have been associated with a long QT interval and torsades de pointes.

1. Antiarrhythmic agents.
   - *Class I drugs* such as quinidine, procainamide (Pronestyl), disopyramide (Norpace), moricizine (Ethmozine), and flecainide (Tambocor) are sodium channel blockers used to treat

BOX 1.

Causes of a Prolonged QT Interval

Drugs
Genetic long QT syndrome
Sympathetic nervous system imbalance
Severe myocardial disease
  Myocarditis
  Cardiomyopathy
Electrolyte abnormalities
  Low calcium, potassium, or magnesium
Neurologic and endocrine abnormalities
  Brain trauma, subarachnoid hemorrhage, hypothyroidism, pheochromocytoma

various arrhythmias. Unfortunately, they may also affect potassium channels and thereby prolong the QT interval.

- *Class III drugs* such as sotalol (Betapace), ibutilide (Corvert), dofetilide (Tikosyn), and amiodarone (Cordarone) act by blocking potassium channels and deliberately prolonging the action potential. This decreases automaticity and slows atrioventricular (AV) nodal conduction, but decreasing heart rate and prolonging the QT interval may lead to early afterdepolarizations.
- *Class IV drugs* act by blocking calcium channels. One of them, bepridil (Vascor), can prolong the QT interval.

2. Gastrointestinal agents. Cisapride (Propulsid) was used extensively to stimulate gastrointestinal motility in children with gastroesophageal reflux. The risk of torsades de pointes caused this drug to be withdrawn in the United States, although it can still be obtained for compassionate use. This agent may be no more dangerous than many other agents that lengthen the QT interval; in most of the reports of fatalities, cisapride was combined with another drug or risk factor known to prolong the QT interval.
3. Antihistamines. Terfenedine (Seldane) and astemizole (Hismanal) can prolong the QT interval, probably by blocking potassium channels. Diphenhydramine, fexofenadine, and clemastine also prolong the QT interval.
4. Antifungal drugs. Ketoconazole (Nizoral), fluconazole (Diflucan), and itraconazole (Sporanox).
5. Psychotropic drugs.
   - *Tricyclic antidepressants:* Amitriptyline (Elavil), imipramine (Tofranil), desimipramine (Norpramin), doxepin (Sinequan), etc.
   - *Phenothiazines:* Prochlorperazine (Compazine), trifluoperazine (Stelazin), chlorpromazine (Thorazine), thioridizine (Mellaril), etc.
   - *Miscellaneous:* Haloperidol (Haldol), risperidone (Risperdal), and carbamazine (Tegretol).
6. Antibiotics. Macrolides such as erythromycin, azithromycin, and clarithromycin occasionally prolong the QT interval; so may pentamidine, trimethoprim/sulfamethoxazole, amantadine, chloroquine, and clindamycin.
7. Diuretics. Indapamide; any that produce severe hypokalemia.
8. Miscellaneous. Epinephrine, probucol (Lorelco), fludrocortisone, and tamoxifen.

Many of these drugs have been shown to block the I_{Kr} channel in the M cells,[69,86-91] although blockade of other potassium channels is also possible. Because it is difficult to tell whether a new drug affects potassium channels, it is prudent to check existing recommendations, and to use any drugs that block potassium channels cautiously, if at all, whenever a patient already has a long QT interval.

THE LONG QT SYNDROME

INCIDENCE

In 1957, Jervell and Lange-Nielsen[1] reported the familial (autosomal recessive) association of congenital deafness, prolonged QT interval on the electrocardiogram, and sudden death, and a similar patient was described soon afterwards by Levine and Woodworth.[2] An association between sudden death and a prolonged QT interval in the absence of deafness (with autosomal dominant inheritance) was reported independently by Romano et al[3] and by Ward.[4] These 2 syndromes are often referred to as the Jervell and Lange-Nielsen and the Romano-Ward syndromes, respectively. Initial theories about mechanisms concentrated on sympathetic nerve imbalance,[92-95] and were supported by the apparent effectiveness of therapy with propranolol[92,96] and left stellectomy.[97,98] Nevertheless, Schwartz[83,99] and Moss[100] recognized early that there could be an additional intracardiac abnormality, even going so far as to postulate abnormal regulation of the outward potassium current during phase 3 of the action potential. In the last decade, emphasis has indeed been placed on genetic defects of myocardial cell ion channels.[101-110] These heritable long QT syndromes have a population incidence of 1 case per 10,000 to 15,000 people.[111,112] This makes them much rarer than sickle cell disease (1 per 600 African Americans), or cystic fibrosis (1 per 2550 white Americans), and of the same order of magnitude as hemophilia (1 per 10,000 white males). The disorder may be more frequent than cited because many people with it have no symptoms and may even have normal QT intervals.[11] Schwartz has concluded that the incidence may be between 1 per 3000 and 1 per 5000 births (personal communication).

CLINICAL FEATURES

The cardinal clinical features of the disorder are syncope, seizures, and sudden cardiac arrest and death. In a multinational registry, Moss et al[113] followed up 328 probands and 3015 family members for many years. The presenting features were mainly syncope associated with fright or anger (47%), vigorous exercise (excluding swimming) (41%), on awakening (19%), while swimming (15%), and with auditory stimulation (8%). The incidence of symptoms is increased during menstruation[114] and in the postpartum period.[115]

About 85% of the probands had an affected family member, suggesting that the disorder arises spontaneously in not more than 15%. Other studies suggest that in about 30% of long QT patients the disease is sporadic.[116] Convulsions are relatively frequent in this syndrome, and lead to the most common misdiagnosis, that of epilepsy. In a similar study confined to 287 patients younger than 21 years, Garson et al[117] found that 45% presented with severe symptoms: 9% with cardiac arrest, 26% with syncope, and 10% with seizures. Another 6% presented with palpitations. Of those with symptoms, 67% had symptoms associated with exercise, 18% with exercise and emotion, 7% with emotion alone, 3% with a loud noise and emotion, and 2% with anesthesia. There are some differences between studies depending on how the patients come to medical attention. In general, about 60% of these patients are diagnosed because of symptoms, 30% because of a suggestive family history, and 10% are detected after an electrocardiogram is done for some other purpose.

NATURAL HISTORY

In the multinational study, 147 (45%) of 328 probands died, all under 50 years of age, with the mean age at death being 21 years. Some of these were receiving some type of treatment. Ackerman[111] cites a mortality rate in probands of 50% within 10 years of presentation in the absence of treatment, and Viskin et al[81] observed in untreated patients a mortality rate of 53% within 15 years of the first syncopal episode.

ETIOLOGY

Specific mutations have been found in many patients with heritable forms of the long QT syndrome.[10,102-106,110,111,118-130] Those identified so far are shown in Table 1. The potassium channel mutations are loss-of-function mutations; haploinsufficiency leads to reduction in the amount of protein made or an interfering protein, so that there are fewer potassium channels and therefore decreased potassium efflux from the cell, thereby keeping it positive for a longer time. The sodium channel mutation is a gain-of-function mutation; a mutant protein is made that is incorporated into the sodium channels, makes them leaky, and allows too much sodium to enter the cell, again keeping it positive for too long.

The Jervell and Lange-Nielsen syndrome is rare (affecting 1-6 patients per million population and only about 1% of patients with congenital deafness) and is caused by defects in KvLQT1 or minK.[107,108,131] The I_{Ks} potassium channel encoded by these genes

TABLE 1.
Genetic Defects in Long QT Syndrome

Syndrome Name	Chromosome	Gene	Affected Function
LQT1	11p15.5	KVLQT1*	I_{Ks} potassium channel
LQT2	7q35-36	HERG	I_{Kr} potassium channel
LQT3	3p21-24	SCN5A	I_{Na} sodium channel
LQT4	4q25-27	?	?
LQT5	21q22.122.2	minK	KCNE1-β-subunit of I_{Ks} potassium channel
LQT6	21q22.122.2	MiRP1	KCNE2 associated with HERG and the I_{Kr} potassium channel

*Most common cause of the syndrome.[154]

is also found in the inner ear. In heterozygotes, with 1 normal gene, the dominant effect expresses itself as the Romano-Ward syndrome: a long QT interval without deafness. In homozygotes with both genes defective there is deafness as well, so that the deafness is inherited as a recessive trait. Because of this, both parents are obligate carriers of the mutant genes. However, not all homozygous mutations in KvLQT1 cause deafness, and the Romano-Ward syndrome can occasionally be recessive.[132]

The described gene defects identify only about 50% to 60% of those with the syndrome. In some with apparently normal genes, examination of portions of the gene not previously explored (the C-terminal end) may reveal an abnormality.[133] Other patients could have defects in other ion channels, or even in cyclic nucleotides or other messengers.

Each chromosomal abnormality includes a wide range of variations, some of which may predispose to less severe phenotypic expression.[133-135] Zareba et al[136] found that the incidence of a cardiac event was highest for patients with LQT1 (63%) than for LQT2 (46%) or LQT3 (18%). On the other hand, those with LQT3 were more likely to have a lethal cardiac event (20%) as compared with 4% for the other 2 channel defects. Consequently, the cumulative probability of death was similar (5% to 6%) in all groups by 40 years of age. These figures are below the 50% mortality cited above because the patients included those receiving treatment or those who had not yet had any symptoms.

DIAGNOSIS

The hallmark of diagnosis is a prolonged QT interval for heart rate or a QTc interval greater than 440 milliseconds. Unfortunately, there are both false-negative and false-positive QTc intervals. For example, Vincent et al[55] studied 3 families with the same genetic defect and divided them unambiguously into those with the mutation and those without it. Sixteen (14%) of 116 healthy patients had QTc intervals of at least 450 milliseconds, and 5 (6%) of 84 affected patients had QTc intervals of 440 milliseconds or less. Garson et al [117] reported that 6% of 287 patients with the heritable long QT syndrome had normal QT intervals, and in the International Study[114] of the heritable long QT syndrome, 5% of family members with a QTc interval less than 440 milliseconds had a cardiac arrest. Priori et al[137] identified 9 families with 46 members who, unlike the probands, had no evidence for the long QT syndrome. By genetic analysis, they identified 33% of the family members who were gene carriers, for a penetrance of 25%. The percentages of false positives, false negatives, and penetrance may differ in different families.

These conclusions lead to a serious dilemma. Genetic testing is still a research and not a clinical tool, and is available in only a few centers. Because of the number of genes involved and the fact that many different mutations are found for each gene, genetic testing is a major challenge. Even if it were readily available and financially practical, it would solve only part of the dilemma. It would unambiguously show that certain family members did not have the abnormality. On the other hand, we might not know what to do for those who show the gene mutation but have a normal QTc interval and have had no cardiac symptoms. There is agreement that those with a long QTc interval, especially if greater than 500 milliseconds, or those with symptoms should be treated, but no agreement about those with neither abnormality (see below).

Perturbations that provoke cardiac events may differ according to the underlying genetic defect. Thus, swimming seems to be a potent cause of sudden death in those with LQT1,[138,139] auditory or emotional stimuli predominate in those with LQT2,[127,138,139] and those with LTQ3 are more likely to have cardiac episodes at rest or during sleep,[127] perhaps associated with their unusually low heart rates at these times.

In the absence of genetic testing, what else can be done? Schwartz et al[140] have provided a useful scoring system (Table 2). Other more complicated diagnostic schemas have been developed.[141]

TABLE 2.
Diagnostic Criteria for the Long QT Syndrome

Findings	Points
ECG findings	
A. QTc	
≥480 ms	3
460-470 ms	2
450 (males)	1
B. Torsades de pointes*	2
C. T-wave alternans	1
D. Notched T waves in at least 3 leads	0.5
Clinical findings	
A. Syncope*	
With stress	2
Without stress	1
B. Congenital deafness	0.5
Family history	
A. Definite long QT syndrome	1
B. Unexplained sudden cardiac death < 30 years of age	0.5

Note: If the score is ≤ 1, the probability of the long QT syndrome is low. If the score is 2 or 3, the probability is intermediate, and if it is ≥ 4, then the probability of the disease is high.
*Mutually exclusive.
Reproduced with permission from Schwartz PJ, Moss AJ, Vincent GM, et al: Diagnostic criteria for the long QT syndrome. An update. *Circulation* 88:782-784, 1993.

Careful inspection of the T waves may help.[142] Different gene mutations may produce different changes in the ST segment and the T waves. For example, LQT3 caused by a mutation in the sodium channel lengthens the QT interval by prolonging phase 2 but, because potassium channels are normal, does not affect the T waves that are inscribed during phase 3; therefore, there is a long ST segment but a normal T wave. On the other hand, the potassium channel abnormalities distort and widen the T wave or produce wide-based, double-humped but low-amplitude T waves. There is, however, overlap between T wave changes and channel abnormalities, so that a particular ST-T change cannot be unambiguously ascribed to a particular chromosomal abnormality.

What might be of more importance is to calculate the dispersion of QTc intervals. In healthy patients, these vary over a short range, but vary much more widely in those with the long QT syndrome: the dispersion of QT intervals in control patients versus those with the long QT syndrome in 3 studies was 50 ± 20 versus 108 ± 30 milliseconds,[68] 28 ± 14 versus 81 ± 70 milliseconds,[57] and 70 versus 130 milliseconds.[85] Unfortunately, there are no reports of dispersion in a large group of asymptomatic carriers with normal QTc intervals; all of the above studies were done on those with typical long QT syndrome.

Another possible approach is to explore changes in the QT interval with various perturbations such as exercise, pacing, or isoproterenol infusion.[143] With exercise, the QT interval does not shorten appropriately so that the QTc interval lengthens, even if it was normal before.[48,144] Furthermore, although the QT interval does shorten as the heart rate increases, it does not continue to shorten as the heart rate increases further.[48] In practice, most authorities look for QTc prolongation 1 minute after the end of exercise. A similar prolongation of the QTc interval occurs with atrial pacing or isoproterenol infusion.[144]

TREATMENT

Symptomatic Patients

Ventricular fibrillation is treated with electrical defibrillation. Torsades de pointes is treated with intravenous magnesium,[145,146] correction of metabolic abnormalities, and removal of any potential offending medications. Lidocaine should be avoided. Temporary pacing and intravenous β-blockers have also been used.

Those with the long QT syndrome and symptoms (syncope, torsades de pointes, ventricular fibrillation) need to be treated to prevent sudden death. Current therapies start with β-adrenergic blockade and, if this fails, proceed to either left cardiac sympathectomy or else implantation of a pacemaker or an automatic defibrillator. It is important to take a careful history to uncover episodes of brief syncope or light-headedness that did not appear in a routine history; such a history is associated with a greatly increased risk of a future serious cardiac event.[113]

The involvement of the sympathetic nervous system in cardiac events in those with a long QT syndrome has been clear for many years, both from animal experiments[39] and the association of these events with emotional stresses in patients. This led to early therapeutic use of propranolol or sympathectomy.[92,97] β-Adrenergic blockade with propranolol was shown by Schwartz et al[95] to decrease mortality from 73% to 6%. In the study by Garson et al,[117] β-adrenergic blockade (the specific blocker did not appear to matter) was 76% effective in abolishing symptoms and 67% effective in abolishing arrhythmias. Priori et al[85] showed that those who responded to β-adrenergic blockade had reduced dispersion of QT intervals, whereas those who failed treatment had no such reduction. This measurement might therefore be a method of selecting those who are more or less likely to respond to β-adrenergic blockade.

Schwartz recommends starting with propranolol, 2 mg/kg per day, and if this fails to control symptoms, increasing the dose to 3 or even 4 mg/kg per day. Unfortunately, some patients cannot tolerate β-adrenergic blockade (excessive fatigue, bradycardia, asthma), about 25% of patients fail to respond to this therapy,[147] and despite therapy there is still a 10% chance of sudden death within 5 years.[148] Some authorities use nadolol, which has the advantage of needing to be given only once daily so that missing a dose may not be catastrophic.

Failure of propranolol treatment is treated in some centers by left cardiac sympathetic denervation and in others by pacemaker implantation. Sympathectomy is very effective,[149-151] with a 5-year survival of 94%. Schwartz et al[151] have pointed out that the exact type of surgery done influences the results. For example, in Milan, where great care is taken to eliminate all the sympathetic nerves to the left ventricle, the 5-year survival has been 100%. They remove the lower part of the left stellate ganglion and the second to fourth left thoracic ganglia. The surgery does not take long, and the patient ambulates the next day. By avoiding the upper part of the stellate ganglion, Horner syndrome is usually avoided.

Pacemaker implantation is the second choice of others.[152,153] The assumed mechanism of action is that by increasing heart rate and preventing pauses, pause-dependent torsades de pointes can be prevented. Sometimes the pacemakers have a fixed rate, or they can be programmed to make specific changes in response to a pause or a premature beat. Others have used implantable defibrillators, usually in combination with β-adrenergic blockade. Pacemakers of both types markedly reduce the mortality rate but do not completely prevent the occasional death. The role of pacemakers in patients without documented ventricular fibrillation is undecided.[154]

Other promising modalities have been considered, although none have had extensive clinical trials. Because LQT3 is caused by a gain-of-function mutation in the sodium channel, the sodium channel blocker mexiletine has been used. In guinea pig ventricular myocytes, anthopleurin inhibits I_{Na} inactivation and so mimics LQT3.[155,156] Dofetilide is a selective blocker of HERG-related I_{Kr}

and thus mimics LQT2. Mexiletine, isoproterenol, and rapid pacing shortened the action potential in the LQT3-like cells, but either did not shorten the action potential or actually lengthened it in LQT2-like cells. Equivalent findings have been verified in a small number of patients with LQT2 and LQT3 syndromes.[127] Patients with LQT2 syndrome caused by loss of function in the HERG-related I_{Kr} potassium channels, however, respond to an increase of potassium. When potassium concentrations were increased by 1.5 mEq/L secondary to spironolactone, intravenous potassium chloride, or oral potassium chloride,[157] the QTc interval was reduced and T-wave notching disappeared.

In rabbits, clofilium (a class III antiarrhythmic agent) blocks I_{Ks}, the current associated with KvLQT1 and minK protein subunits.[158] It thus simulates LQT1 and produces delayed repolarization, early afterdepolarizations, and torsades de pointes. These changes can be blocked by pinacidil, a potassium channel opener. The human counterpart of this was a 17-year-old boy whose early afterdepolarizations were reduced and whose weekly syncopal episodes were abolished by nicorandil.[159]

Finally, because it is likely that torsades de pointes in LQT3 is eventually set off by excess calcium influx through $I_{Ca(L)}$ channels,[76] preventing arrhythmias with calcium-blocking agents such as verapamil has been considered. Shimizu et al[78] observed patients with long QT syndrome who developed ectopic beats, afterdepolarizations, and even torsades de pointes when given epinephrine. These changes were largely prevented by giving verapamil or propranolol, which also reduced the QT interval and its dispersion.

Asymptomatic Patients

If the patients have a prolonged QTc interval, they should avoid competitive sports and swimming. Because they already have defective ion channels, they should avoid agents known to prolong the QT interval that might well further prolong the interval and produce serious and even fatal arrhythmias.[160]

Opinions are divided about prophylactic treatment in these patients. Some decisions may be based on the likelihood of a serious cardiac event, as shown in Box 2. No schema, however, unequivocally separates those who are at risk of a serious arrhythmia from those who are not. Torsades de pointes has occurred in 50-year-old men who have never had any previous symptoms. What makes the decision more difficult is that in about 9% of patients, the first episode is fatal.[117]

BOX 2.
Risk of Serious Cardiac Events in Long QT Syndrome

A longer QTc interval; the risk is about 10-fold higher for a QTc interval > 0.50 s than for a QTc interval ≤ 0.45 s.[113,139]
Greater dispersion of the QTc interval, abnormal T waves, and T-wave alternans.[201]
If close relatives have had a history of serious cardiac events. The risk is more for first-degree relatives of the proband who share half the gene pool than for second-degree relatives who share only one quarter of the gene pool.
Resting heart rates below 60 and above 100 beats/min.
Younger age—childhood and adolescence. Asymptomatic adults are less likely to have a serious cardiac event.
Females are more likely to have arrhythmias, in part related to their longer QTc intervals and their relatively faster heart rates.

Data from Moss AJ: Long QT syndrome: Clinical approach to the asymptomatic patient. *ACC Curr J Rev* July-August: 41-43, 1994.

Moss[160] recommends 24-hour ambulatory Holter monitoring and exercise testing because they may uncover short runs of ventricular tachycardia, T-wave alternans, excessive QT interval prolongation, or giant U waves, all of which increase the likelihood that these patients will have a malignant arrhythmia.[161]

RELATIONSHIP OF LONG QT INTERVAL TO SIDS

SIDS is the most common cause of death between the ages of 1 month and 1 year in the Western world; it accounts for about 0.5 to 2 deaths per 1000 live births.[162-165] One of its hallmarks is that "a thorough postmortem examination fails to demonstrate an adequate cause of death";[166-169] abnormal signs are subtle, and will be discussed below. A similar lack of physical abnormalities on autopsy also characterizes those who die of an arrhythmia, so the question about whether SIDS is caused by an arrhythmia has long been posed.[170,171]

In a review of the subject written in 1976, Schwartz[7] considered that SIDS might be caused by a form of long QT syndrome associated with decreased activity or a delay in development of the right sympathetic cardiac nerves. In support of this notion, patients with the long QT syndrome often have bradycardia that could be caused by right cardiac sympathetic nerve deficiency.[95] Maron et al[5] investigated 42 sets of parents of infants who had died of SIDS and found that in at least 1 member of 11 sets of parents (26%), the QT interval was prolonged. In addition, 39% of the surviving siblings also had a prolonged QT interval. In these abnormal patients, however, the QTc interval varied from 0.42 to 0.47 seconds; only 5 were greater than 0.44 seconds. Although carriers of the LQT genes may have QTc intervals in this range,[55] the relatively minor changes in the QTc interval do not provide a compelling reason to think that SIDS and the long QT syndrome are closely related. Other investigations of the so-called "near miss" or "aborted SIDS" (now also know as acute life-threatening events, or ALTEs) found no differences in the QTc interval between these patients and controls[172,173]; the relationship between ALTEs and SIDS, however, is unclear.

A slightly different result was obtained by Sadeh et al[6] who found no difference between the QTc intervals in infants who subsequently died of SIDS and a control group, but noted that 5 of 10 infants who later died of SIDS had an impaired ability to shorten the QT interval as heart rate increased. This feature occurs in patients with the long QT syndrome.[48] There the matter rested until the dramatic publication in 1998 by Schwartz et al.[8] They took electrocardiograms on the third or fourth day after birth in 34,442 neonates, of whom 33,034 were followed up for the next year. (They had very few premature infants who were known to have the highest incidence of SIDS.) There were 34 deaths, 24 of them from SIDS. The QTc interval exceeded 0.44 seconds in 12 (50%) of 24 SIDS victims (2 were > 0.50 milliseconds) as compared with 825 (2.5%) of 33,010 of the survivors or those who died of other causes. It is possible that at the time of death the QTc intervals were even longer, because Schwartz et al[174] have shown that normally the QTc interval lengthens in the second month, sometimes by as much as 40 milliseconds, and then returns to control values by about 6 months of age. Interestingly, none of the parents of the infants who died of SIDS had prolonged QT intervals.

The 1998 study had sufficient power to show that a prolonged QTc interval is significantly more common in those who died of SIDS than in others, and the findings need to be addressed. The important questions are whether the long QT interval caused death, and if so whether the long QT was caused by the genetic ion channel abnormalities found in the long QT syndrome.

At present, most investigators believe that most deaths from SIDS are not caused by an arrhythmia, although all the evidence is certainly not in. Torsades de pointes is a dramatic arrhythmia that is unlikely to be overlooked, and yet it has not been reported in those dying of SIDS and only once[175] in those with near miss-SIDS (ALTE). However, in older people, torsades de pointes presents with weakness or syncope, but these would be hard to detect in a supine infant. Furthermore, because death from ventricular fibrillation is rapid and undetectable without an electrocardiogram, failure to document it in SIDS is not a compelling argument. Some studies show that infants dying of SIDS while being monitored had bradycardia leading to apnea just before death,[176,177] and other studies show hypoxemia preceding apnea and bradycardia in other infants.[178] These studies do not support death from the long QT syndrome in these infants, but these were mostly preterm infants being monitored for apnea of prematurity or bronchopulmonary dysplasia. They may therefore represent a subgroup of SIDS infants who were more likely to die of respiratory than cardiac causes, and do not give us much information about other SIDS victims. These arguments thus do not mean that the long QT syndrome cannot cause SIDS, and there are occasional reports of infant deaths that were probably caused by the long QT syndrome.[3,179] Indeed, Guntheroth and Spiers[180] have suggested that the 2 children with the longest QTc intervals in the study by Schwartz et al[8] might indeed have had the long QT syndrome. Given an incidence of the long QT syndrome in the order of 1 per 10,000 births, 2 deaths from it in 34,000 children would not be unreasonable.

Another objection to the long QT syndrome being an important cause of SIDS is that a history of other sudden unexplained cardiac deaths in the families of infants who have died of SIDS has not been reported. Considering the intense focus on SIDS in the last 20 years, the absence of such a history argues against the long QT syndrome being the cause of most deaths from SIDS, although there is doubt whether this history has been carefully sought in the reported studies. There is also one recent report to be considered. Schwartz et al[175] described an infant who was resuscitated from ventricular fibrillation and found to have torsades de pointes. Subsequent investigations showed that this infant had the typical genetic abnormality of LQT3 but that both parents were normal. In other words, this was a new mutation that would explain the absence of a significant family history. Since these new mutations may occur in 15% to 30% of patients with the long QT syndrome,[113,116] then absence in SIDS victims of a family history compatible with the long QT syndrome does not exclude it as a cause of SIDS.

By contrast, the weight of evidence for a central or obstructive apnea as the main mechanism of death is strong.[162,163,165,169] Frequently, petechiae are present in the thymus, pleura, and epicardium. The lungs are congested and edematous, and have small foci of recent alveolar hemorrhage. There are also abnormal microscopic findings in the brain. Naeye[181,182] described brain-stem gliosis in SIDS, a finding confirmed by many subsequent studies. He thought that the gliosis represented the response to many subclinical episodes of hypoxia. More recently, Kinney et al[183-185] described absence or abnormalities of the arcuate nucleus, one of the medullary nuclei associated with respiratory control. They also described decreased kainate receptor binding in the arcuate nucleus of infants dying of SIDS but not from other diseases. These neuropathologic findings seem to fit with one of the important cofactors in increasing the incidence of SIDS, namely, smoking tobacco. Nicotine affects many aspects of fetal brain development.[186-188] Slotkin et al[189] showed that nicotine given to pregnant mice caused loss of neonatal tolerance to hypoxia in their offspring, the clinical counterpart of which was demonstrated by Lewis and Bosque.[190]

All of these findings, both the negative ones concerning cardiac causes of death and positive ones indicating a respiratory cause, suggest that the long QT syndrome is not a common cause of SIDS. It is possible to set rough limits on the proportion of SIDS deaths caused by the long QT syndrome. Based on current information, the incidence of SIDS is 0.64 per 1000 live births in the United States in 1998.[191] If the incidence of long QT syndrome is 1 per 10,000 live births, and 15% of these infants die in infancy, then for each million live births, there will be 640 deaths from SIDS and 100 patients with the long QT syndrome, 15 of whom will die in infancy. Therefore, the long QT syndrome would account for only 2.3% of all deaths ascribed to SIDS. If, on the other hand, the long QT syndrome has an incidence of 1 per 2000 live births, and 25% of these patients die in infancy (both very high figures based on existing information), then for each million live births, there will be 640 deaths from SIDS and 500 patients with the long QT syndrome, 125 of whom will die in infancy. This sets an upper limit to the proportion of SIDS deaths from the long QT syndrome of 19.5%. The exact proportion will become clear when large numbers of SIDS victims and their families are evaluated for the genetic defects of the long QT syndrome.

If most SIDS is not caused by the long QT syndrome, why then do many of the SIDS patients have a long QTc interval? In all probability, the long QT interval represents an abnormality of the sympathetic nervous system, as postulated by Schwartz, and this fits in with the neuropathologic studies that show brain-stem abnormalities in SIDS. If this is true, then the long QTc interval is a marker for the neuroabnormality rather than a mechanism of death in most of the SIDS victims. More research is needed to evaluate the role of the long QT syndrome in SIDS.

SCREENING ISSUES

The seminal publication by Schwartz et al[8] suggested that screening of newborn infants by electrocardiography might help to prevent some deaths from SIDS. This drew many dissenting comments, including one from Lister and me,[192] but further reflection suggests that it is time to revisit the conclusions, at least as far as the long QT syndrome is concerned. The value of a screening test is a function of several factors: the prevalence and severity of the disease, the availability of treatment for it, the costs of the screening test, the frequency of false-negative and false-positive tests (ie, the sensitivity and specificity of the tests), the follow-up costs for confirming or ruling out the diagnosis, side effects associated with the treatment, and the psychological effect on the families. These issues are no different for screening in the long QT syndrome.

Factors in favor of early screening are that the long QT syndrome, if untreated, has a high and early death rate, and that there is effective even if not perfect treatment. The side effects of the various treatment modalities are not negligible but are tolerable. The costs of screening electrocardiography in the United States are relatively high for a neonatal screening test, but for those with very long QT intervals, no confirmatory tests are needed. On the other hand, for those with borderline QT prolongation and those with normal QT intervals but with the genetic mutations (false negatives), molecular testing is still not generally available, and even when available is likely to be expensive. In part, the argument for screening will depend on the incidence of the syndrome. A recent study of the likely costs of universal screening of neonates in the United States[193] based on an incidence of the long QT syndrome of 1 per 10,000 births and a cost of $85 per screen was that the incremental costs (above those incurred by routine care) would average $309,527 per year of lives saved. That cost would increase if many expensive follow-up studies were needed, but could be lower because in a disease with a mortality rate of 50% by 30 years of age, many lives would be saved beyond infancy, and because other affected family members would be identified. Furthermore, if the incidence of the syndrome was higher—for example, 3 per 10,000 live births—then the incremental cost would decrease to about $100,000 per year of lives saved. Whether such screening would have a substantial impact on SIDS deaths would depend on how frequently the long QT syndrome causes neonatal death.

It is instructive to compare the total cost and costs per diagnosis for several types of diseases in which neonatal screening can be done (Table 3). From the extensive literature on this subject, several examples were selected for comparison: congenital dysplasia of the hip,[194] congenital deafness,[195] phenylketonuria,[196-198] congenital hypothyroidism,[197-199] adrenal hyperplasia,[200] galactosemia,[201] and maple syrup urine disease.[197]

Favorable cost-benefit ratios have been found for screening for phenylketonuria,[196-198] congenital hypothyroidism,[196-199] and congenital dysplasia of the hip.[194] The benefits of early detection and treatment of congenital adrenal hyperplasia, congenital deafness, galactosemia, and maple syrup urine disease have not been evaluated, but for at least the first of these may well exceed the costs. Many factors enter into producing favorable cost-benefit ratios. Several of the inborn errors of metabolism can be detected in the same blood sample with one of the modern analytic methods (eg, tandem mass spectrometry), so that the cost of finding each affected patient is shared by many diseases. Some of the diseases produce long-term disability with resultant high costs of medical, surgical, or custodial care: for example, phenylketonuria, congenital hypothyroidism, galactosemia, and congenital dysplasia of the hip. Minimizing these costs by early or noninvasive treatment produces the favorable cost-benefit ratio. Some diseases, however, such as maple syrup urine disease and the long QT syndrome, cause either early death or relatively little medically treatable morbidity. For these, the major benefit is less economic than the prevention of premature death and disability. (Note that converting pound sterling into US dollars ignores the relative standard of living and therefore costs in each country. However, the cost-benefit ratios are less affected because the benefits are also related to living standards.)

The reason why screening for the long QT syndrome is so much more expensive is because the testing itself has the highest cost of all those cited. If the cost of electrocardiographic screening were $10, as it appears to be in Europe, then the cost per diagnosis would be similar to those of other standard screening tests (Table 3).

TABLE 3.
Screening Comparisons

Disease	Incidence in Live Births	Incidence/ Million Live Births	Screen Cost ($US)	Total Cost per Million Live Births ($US × 10^6)	Cost/Diagnosis ($US)
Congenital deafness	~1/500[195]	2000	10-25	10-25	5000-12,500
Congenital hypothyroidism	1/3300[201]	303	5.3[197]	5.3	17,492
Congenital hip dysplasia	1/6000[194]	167	10	10	59,880
Long QT	1/10,000[111]	100	85[193]	85	850,000
Phenylketonuria	1/14,000[201]	71	5.2[197]; 15[196]	5.2; 15	73,329-211,267
Congenital adrenal hyperplasia	1/20,000[201]	83	5.52[200] (2 screens)	5.52	66,506
Galactosemia	1/59,000[201]	17	–*		
Maple syrup urine disease	1/100,000[202]	10	–*		

Assumed total annual birth rate in the United States of 3.8 million.
*By-product of phenylketonuria screen.[197]

Whether indeed neonatal electrocardiographic screening is warranted will be decided when we have better data on the incidence of the long QT syndrome and on the actual costs involved. In the end, decisions will have to be made whether the money is better spent in saving these lives or on other causes.

ACKNOWLEDGMENT

I thank Drs George van Hare and James D. Bristow for their help with this review.

REFERENCES

1. Jervell A, Lange-Nielsen F: Congenital deaf-mutism, functional heart disease with prolongation of the Q-T interval and sudden death. *Am Heart J* 54:59-68, 1957.
2. Levine SA, Woodworth CR: Congenital deaf-mutism, prolonged QT interval, syncopal attacks and sudden death. *N Engl J Med* 259:412-417, 1958.
3. Romano C, Gemme G, Pongiglione R: Aritmie cardiache rare dell'eta'pediatrica: II. Accessi sincopali per fibrillazione ventricolare parossistica. *Clin Pediatr* 45:656-661, 1963.
4. Ward OC: New familial cardiac syndrome in children. *J Irish Med Soc* 54:103-106, 1964.
5. Maron BJ, Clark CE, Goldstein RE, et al: Potential role of QT interval prolongation in sudden infant death syndrome. *Circulation* 54:423-430, 1976.
6. Sadeh D, Shannon DC, Abboud S, et al: Altered cardiac repolarization in some victims of sudden infant death syndrome. *N Engl J Med* 317:1501-1505, 1987.
7. Schwartz PJ: Cardiac sympathetic innervation and the sudden infant death syndrome: A possible pathogenetic link. *Am J Med* 60:167-172, 1976.
8. Schwartz PJ, Stramba-Badiale M, Segantini A, et al: Prolongation of the QT interval and the sudden infant death syndrome. *N Engl J Med* 338:1709-1714, 1998.
9. Sanguinetti MC, Keating MT: Role of delayed rectifier potassium channel in cardiac repolarization and arrhythmias. *News in Physiological Sciences* 12:152-157, 1997.
10. Abbott GW, Sesti F, Splawski I, et al: MiRP1 forms IKr potassium channels with HERG and is associated with cardiac arrhythmia. *Cell* 97:175-187, 1999.
11. Chiang CE, Roden DM: The long QT syndromes: Genetic basis and clinical implications. *J Am Coll Cardiol* 36:1-12, 2000.
12. Viswanathan PC, Shaw RM, Rudy Y: Effects of IKr and IKs heterogeneity on action potential duration and its rate dependence: A simulation study. *Circulation* 99:2466-2474, 1999.

13. Surawicz B: Relationship between electrocardiogram and electrolytes. *Am Heart J* 73:814-834, 1967.
14. Kay GN, Plumb VJ, Arciniegas JG, et al: Torsades de pointes: The long-short initiating sequence and other clinical features: Observations in 32 patients. *Circulation* 2:806-817, 1983.
15. Sagie A, Larson MG, Goldberg RJ, et al: An improved method for adjusting the QT interval for heart rate (the Framingham Heart Study). *J Am Coll Cardiol* 70:797-801, 1992.
16. Boudoulas H, Geleris P, Lewis RP, et al: Linear relationship between electrical systole, mechanical systole, and heart rate. *Chest* 80:613-617, 1981.
17. Lepeschkin E, Surawicz B: The duration of the QU interval and its components in the electrocardiograms of normal persons. *Am Heart J* 46:9-20, 1953.
18. Schlamowitz I: An analysis of the time relations within the cardiac cycle in electrocardiograms of normal men: IV. The effect of position change on the relationships of the Q-T and T-P intervals respectively to the cycle length (R-R interval). *Am Heart J* 34:702-708, 1947.
19. Davignon A, Rautaharju P, Boiselle E, et al: Normal ECG standards for infants and children. *Pediatr Cardiol* 1:121-152, 1980.
20. Bazett HC: An analysis of the time relations of electrocardiograms. *Heart* 7:353-370, 1920.
21. Fridericia LS: Die Systolendauer im Elektrokardiogramm bei normalen Menchen und bei Herzkranken. *Acta Med Scand* 53:469-486, 1920.
22. Karjalainen J, Viitasalo M, Mänttäri M, et al: Relation between QT intervals and heart rates from 40 to 120 beats/min in rest electrocardiograms of men and a simple method to adjust QT interval values. *Circulation* 23:1547-1553, 1994.
23. Funck-Brentano C, Jaillon P: Rate-corrected QT interval: Techniques and limitations. *Am J Cardiol* 72:17B-22B, 1993.
24. Kovács SJ Jr: The duration of the QT interval as a function of heart rate: A derivation based on physical principles and a comparison to measured values. *Am Heart J* 110:872-878, 1985.
25. Lecocq B, Lecocq V, Jaillon P: Physiologic relation between cardiac cycle and QT duration in healthy volunteers. *Am J Cardiol* 64:481-486, 1989.
26. Molnar J, Weiss J, Zhang F, et al: Evaluation of five QT correction formulas using a software-assisted method of continuous QT measurement from 24-hour Holter recordings. *Am J Cardiol* 78:920-926, 1996.
27. Puddu PE, Jouve R, Mariotti S, et al: Evaluation of 10 QT prediction formulas in 881 middle-aged men from the seven countries study: Emphasis on the cubic root of Fridericia's equation. *J Electrocardiol* 21:219-229, 1988.
28. Rautaharju PM, Warren JW, Calhoun HP: Estimation of QT prolongation: A persistent, avoidable error in computer electrocardiography. *J Electrocardiol* 23:111S-117S, 1990.
29. Sarma JS, Sarma RJ, Bilitch M, et al: An exponential formula for heart

rate dependence of QT interval during exercise and cardiac pacing in humans: Reevaluation of Bazett's formula. *Am J Cardiol* 54:103-108, 1984.
30. Lombard WP, Cope OM: Effect of pulse rate on the length of the systoles and diastoles of the normal human heart in the standing position. *Am J Physiol* 49:139-140, 1919.
31. Ashman R: The normal duration of the QT interval. *Am Heart J* 23:522-534, 1942.
32. Rautaharju PM, Zhou SH, Wong S, et al: Sex differences in the evolution of the electrocardiographic QT interval with age. *Can J Cardiol* 8:690-695, 1992.
33. Locati EH, Zareba W, Moss AJ, et al: Age- and sex-related differences in clinical manifestations in patients with congenital long-QT syndrome: Findings from the International LQTS Registry. *Circulation* 97:2237-2244, 1998.
34. Lehmann MH, Timothy KW, Frankovich D, et al: Age-gender influence on the rate-corrected QT interval and the QT-heart rate relation in families with genotypically characterized long QT syndrome. *Circulation* 29:93-99, 1997.
35. Ahnve S, Vallin H: Influence of heart rate and inhibition of autonomic tone on the QT interval. *Circulation* 65:435-439, 1982
36. Browne KF, Prystowsky E, Heger JJ, et al: Modulation of the Q-T interval by the autonomic nervous system. *Pacing Clin Electrophysiol* 6:1050-1056, 1983.
37. Staniforth DH: The QT interval and cycle length: The influence of atropine, hyoscine and exercise. *Br J Clin Pharmacol* 16:615-621, 1983.
38. Davidowski TA, Wolf S: The QT interval during reflex cardiovascular adaptation. *Circulation* 69:22-25, 1984.
39. Schwartz PJ: Sympathetic imbalance and cardiac arrhythmias, in Randall WC (ed): *Nervous Control of Cardiovascular Function.* New York, Oxford University Press, 1984, pp 225-252.
40. Yanowitz F, Preston JB, Abildskov JA: Functional distribution of right and left stellate innervation to the ventricles: Production of neurogenic electrocardiographic changes by unilateral alteration of sympathetic tone. *Circ Res* 18:416-428, 1966.
41. Abildskov JA: Adrenergic effects of the QT interval of the electrocardiogram. *Am Heart J* 92:210-216, 1976.
42. Schwartz PJ, Stone HL, Brown AM: Effects of unilateral stellate ganglion blockade on the arrhythmias associated with coronary occlusion. *Am Heart J* 92:589-599, 1976.
43. Schwartz PJ, Verrier RL, Lown B: Effect of stellectomy and vagotomy on ventricular refractoriness in dogs. *Circ Res* 40:536-540, 1977.
44. Schwartz PJ, Stone HL: Effects of unilateral stellectomy upon cardiac performance during exercise in dogs. *Circ Res* 44:637-645, 1979.
45. Stramba-Badiale M, Lazzarotti M, Schwartz PJ: Development of cardiac innervation, ventricular fibrillation, and sudden infant death syndrome. *Am J Physiol* 263 H1514-1522, 1992.

46. Schwartz PJ, Stone HL: The role of the autonomic nervous system in sudden coronary death. *Ann N Y Acad Sci* 382:162-180, 1982.
47. Austoni P, Rosati R, Gregorini L, et al: Stellectomy and exercise in man. *Am J Cardiol* 43:399A, 1979.
48. Vincent GM, Jaiswal D, Timothy KW: Effects of exercise on heart rate, QT, QTc and QT/QS2 in the Romano-Ward inherited long QT syndrome. *Am J Cardiol* 68:498-503, 1991.
49. Fananapazir L, Bennett DH, Faragher EB: Contribution of heart rate to QT interval shortening during exercise. *Eur Heart J* 4:265-271, 1983.
50. Milne JR, Camm AJ, Ward DE, et al: Effect of intravenous propranolol on QT interval: A new method of assessment. *Br Heart J* 43:1-6, 1980.
51. Rickards AF, Norman J: Relation between QT interval and heart rate: New design of physiologically adaptive cardiac pacemaker. *Br Heart J* 45:56-61, 1981.
52. Susmano A, Graettinger JS, Carleton RA: The relationship between Q-T interval and heart rate. *J Electrocardiol* 2:269-273, 1969.
53. Manion CV, Whitsett TL, Wilson MF: Applicability of correcting the QT interval for heart rate (letter). *Am Heart J* 99:678, 1980.
54. Boyett MR, Jewell BR: A study of the factors responsible for rate-dependent shortening of the action potential in mammalian ventricular muscle. *J Physiol (Lond)* 285:359-380, 1978.
55. Vincent GM, Timothy KW, Leppert M, et al: The spectrum of symptoms and QT intervals in carriers of the gene for the long-QT syndrome. *N Engl J Med* 327:846-852, 1992.
56. Berul CI, Sweeten TL, Dubin AM, et al: Use of the rate-corrected JT interval for prediction of repolarization abnormalities in children. *Am J Cardiol* 74:1254-1257, 1994.
57. Shah MJ, Wieand TS, Rhodes LA, et al: QT and JT dispersion in children with long QT syndrome. *J Cardiovasc Electrophysiol* 8:642-648, 1997.
58. Spodick DH: Reduction of QT-interval imprecision and variance by measuring the JT interval (editorial). *Am J Cardiol* 70:103, 1992.
59. Spodick DH: The long-QT syndrome (letter). *N Engl J Med* 328:287, 1993.
60. Spodick DH, Rifkin RD, Rajasingh MC: Effect of self-correlation on the relation between QT interval and cardiac cycle length. *Am Heart J* 120:157-160, 1990.
61. Morganroth J, Brozovich FV, McDonald JT, et al: Variability of the QT measurement in healthy men, with implications for selection of an abnormal QT value to predict drug toxicity and proarrhythmia. *Am J Cardiol* 67:774-776, 1991.
62. Browne KF, Prystowsky E, Heger JJ, et al: Prolongation of the Q-T interval in man during sleep. *Am J Cardiol* 52:55-59, 1983.
63. Sarma JS, Venkataraman K, Nicod P, et al: Circadian rhythmicity of rate-normalized QT interval in hypothyroidism and its significance for development of class III antiarrhythmic agents. *Am J Cardiol* 66:959-963, 1990.

64. Bexton RS, Vallin HO, Camm AJ: Diurnal variation of the QT interval: Influence of the autonomic nervous system. *Br Heart J* 55:253-258, 1986.
65. Abildskov JA: The prolonged QT interval. *Annu Rev Med* 30:171-179, 1979.
66. De Ambroggi L, Bertoni T, Locati E, et al: Mapping of body surface potentials in patients with the idiopathic long QT syndrome. *Circulation* 74:1334-1345, 1986.
67. De Ambroggi L, Negroni MS, Monza E, et al: Dispersion of ventricular repolarization in the long QT syndrome. *Am J Cardiol* 68:614-620, 1991.
68. Linker NJ, Colonna P, Kekwick CA, et al: Assessment of QT dispersion in symptomatic patients with congenital long QT syndromes. *Am J Cardiol* 69:634-638, 1992.
69. Antzelevitch C, Shimizu W, Yan GX, et al: Cellular basis for QT dispersion. *J Electrocardiol* 30:168S-175S, 1998.
70. Bonatti V, Rolli A, Botti G: Recording of monophasic action potentials of the right ventricle in long QT syndromes complicated by severe ventricular arrhythmias. *Eur Heart J* 4:168-179, 1983.
71. Cowan JC, Hilton CJ, Griffiths CJ, et al: Sequence of epicardial repolarisation and configuration of the T wave. *Br Heart J* 60:424-433, 1988.
72. Nador F, Beria G, De Ferrari GM, et al: Unsuspected echocardiographic abnormality in the long QT syndrome: Diagnostic, prognostic, and pathogenetic implications. *Circulation* 84:1530-1542, 1991.
73. Moore EN: Mechanisms and models to predict a Qtc effect. *Am J Cardiol* 72:4B-9B, 1993.
74. Shimizu W, Ohe T, Kurita T, et al: Early afterdepolarizations induced by isoproterenol in patients with congenital long QT syndrome. *Circulation* 84:1915-1923, 1991.
75. Zhou JT, Zheng LR, Liu WY: Role of early afterdepolarization in familial long QTU syndrome and torsades de pointes. *Pacing Clin Electrophysiol* 15:2164-2168, 1992.
76. Viswanathan PC, Rudy Y: Pause induced early afterdepolarizations in the long QT syndrome: A simulation study. *Cardiovasc Res* 42:530-542, 1999.
77. Shimizu W, Ohe T, Kurita T, et al: Epinephrine-induced ventricular premature complexes due to early afterdepolarizations and effects of verapamil and propranolol in a patient with congenital long QT syndrome. *J Cardiovasc Electrophysiol* 5:438-444, 1994.
78. Shimizu W, Ohe T, Kurita T, et al: Effects of verapamil and propranolol on early afterdepolarizations and ventricular arrhythmias induced by epinephrine in congenital long QT syndrome. *Circulation* 26:1299-1309, 1995.
79. Ben-David J, Zipes DP: Differential response to right and left ansae subclaviae stimulation of early afterdepolarizations and ventricular tachycardia induced by cesium in dogs. *Circulation* 78:1241-1250, 1988.
80. Priori SG, Mantica M, Schwartz PJ: Delayed afterdepolarizations elicit-

ed in vivo by left stellate ganglion stimulation. *Circulation* 78:178-185, 1988.

81. Viskin S, Alla SR, Barron HV, et al: Mode of onset of torsades de pointes in congenital long QT syndrome. *Circulation* 28:1262-1268, 1996.
82. Gilmour RF Jr, Riccio ML, Locati EH, et al: Time- and rate-dependent alterations of the QT interval precede the onset of torsade de pointes in patients with acquired QT prolongation. *J Am Coll Cardiol* 30:209-217, 1997.
83. Schwartz PJ: Idiopathic long QT syndrome: Progress and questions. *Am Heart J* 109:399-411, 1985.
84. Day CP, McComb JM, Campbell RW: QT dispersion: An indication of arrhythmia risk in patients with long QT intervals. *Br Heart J* 63:342-344, 1990.
85. Priori SG, Napolitano C, Diehl L, et al: Dispersion of the QT interval: A marker of therapeutic efficacy in the idiopathic long QT syndrome. *Circulation* 89:1681-1689, 1994.
86. Antzelevitch C, Sun ZQ, Zhang ZQ, et al: Cellular and ionic mechanisms underlying erythromycin-induced long QT intervals and torsades de pointes. *Circulation* 28:1836-1848, 1996.
87. Piquette RK: Torsades de pointes induced by cisapride/clarithromycin interaction. *Ann Pharmacother* 33:22-26, 1999.
88. Tonini M, De Ponti F, Di Nucci A, et al: Review article: Cardiac adverse effects of gastrointestinal prokinetics. *Aliment Pharmacol Ther* 13:1585-1591, 1999.
89. Vitola J, Vukanovic J, Roden DM: Cisapride-induced torsades de pointes [see comments]. *J Cardiovasc Electrophysiol* 9:1109-1113, 1998.
90. Walker BD, Singleton CB, Bursill JA, et al: Inhibition of the human ether-a-go-go-related gene (HERG) potassium channel by cisapride: Affinity for open and inactivated states. *Br J Pharmacol* 128:444-450, 1999.
91. Ward RM, Lemons JA, Molteni RA: Cisapride: A survey of the frequency of use and adverse events in premature newborns. *Pediatrics* 103:469-472, 1999.
92. Crampton RS: Another link between the left stellate ganglion and the long Q-T syndrome. *Am Heart J* 96:130-132, 1978.
93. Moss AJ, Schwartz PJ: Sudden death and the idiopathic long Q-T syndrome (editorial). *Am J Med* 66:6-7, 1979.
94. Schwartz PJ, Malliani A: Electrical alternation of the T-wave: Clinical and experimental evidence of its relationship with the sympathetic nervous system and with the long Q-T syndrome. *Am Heart J* 89:45-50, 1975.
95. Schwartz PJ, Periti M, Malliani A: The long Q-T syndrome. *Am Heart J* 89:378-390, 1975.
96. Park MK, Guntheroth WG: Long Q-T syndrome: A preventable form of sudden death. *J Fam Pract* 7:945-948, 1978.
97. Moss AJ, McDonald J: Unilateral cervicothoracic sympathetic ganglionectomy for the treatment of long QT interval syndrome. *N Engl J Med* 285:903-904, 1971.

98. Moss AJ, Schwartz PJ, Crampton RS, et al: The long QT syndrome: A prospective international study. *Circulation* 71:17-21, 1985.
99. Schwartz PJ: Prevention of arrhythmias in the long QT syndrome, in Kulbertus HE (ed): *Medical Management of Cardiac Arrhythmias.* Edinburgh, Scotland, Churchill Livingstone, 1986, pp 153-161.
100. Moss AJ: Prolonged QT-interval syndromes [published erratum appears in *JAMA* 257:487, 1987]. *JAMA* 256:2985-2987, 1986.
101. Curran ME, Splawski I, Timothy KW, et al: A molecular basis for cardiac arrhythmia: HERG mutations cause long QT syndrome. *Cell* 80:795-803, 1995.
102. Keating MT: Molecular genetics of long QT syndrome. *Soc Gen Physiol Ser* 50:53-60, 1995.
103. Keating MT, Sanguinetti MC: Pathophysiology of ion channel mutations. *Curr Opin Genet Dev* 6:326-333, 1996.
104. Keating MT, Sanguinetti MC: Molecular genetic insights into cardiovascular disease. *Science* 272:681-685, 1996.
105. Keating MT: The long QT syndrome: A review of recent molecular genetic and physiologic discoveries. *Medicine (Baltimore)* 75:1-5, 1996.
106. Sanguinetti MC, Spector PS: Potassium channelopathies. *Neuropharmacology* 36:755-762, 1997.
107. Splawski I, Tristani-Firouzi M, Lehmann MH, et al: Mutations in the hminK gene cause long QT syndrome and suppress IKs function. *Nat Genet* 17:338-340, 1997.
108. Splawski I, Timothy KW, Vincent GM, et al: Molecular basis of the long-QT syndrome associated with deafness. *N Engl J Med* 336:1562-1567, 1997.
109. Splawski I, Shen J, Timothy KW, et al: Genomic structure of three long QT syndrome genes: KVLQT1, HERG, and KCNE1. *Genomics* 51:86-97, 1998.
110. Vincent GM, Timothy K, Fox J, et al: The inherited long QT syndrome: From ion channel to bedside. *Cardiol Rev* 7:44-55, 1999.
111. Ackerman MJ: The long QT syndrome: Ion channel diseases of the heart. *Mayo Clin Proc* 73:250-269, 1998.
112. Schwartz PJ: The long QT syndrome. *Curr Probl Cardiol* 22:297-351, 1997.
113. Moss AJ, Schwartz PJ, Crampton RS, et al: The long QT syndrome: Prospective longitudinal study of 328 families. *Circulation* 84:1136-1144, 1991.
114. Schwartz PJ, Zaza A, Locati E, et al: Stress and sudden death: The case of the long QT syndrome. *Circulation* 83:II71-80, 1991.
115. Rashba EJ, Zareba W, Moss AJ, et al: Influence of pregnancy on the risk for cardiac events in patients with hereditary long QT syndrome: LQTS Investigators. *Circulation* 97:451-456, 1998.
116. Priori SG, Napolitano C, Ronchetti E: Characterization of the prevalence of mink polymorphism and mutations in 140 long QT syndrome families. *PACE* 21:39, 1998.
117. Garson A Jr, Dick MD, Fournier A, et al: The long QT syndrome in

children: An international study of 287 patients. *Circulation* 87:1866-1872, 1993.

118. Ackerman MJ: The long QT syndrome. *Pediatr Rev* 19:232-238, 1998.
119. Ackerman MJ, Tester DJ, Porter CJ, et al: Molecular diagnosis of the inherited long-QT syndrome in a woman who died after near-drowning. *N Engl J Med* 341:1121-1125, 1999.
120. Chen Q, Zhang D, Gingell RL, et al: Homozygous deletion in KVLQT1 associated with Jervell and Lange-Nielsen syndrome. *Circulation* 99:1344-1347, 1999.
121. Dumaine R, Wang Q, Keating MT, et al: Multiple mechanisms of Na+ channel–linked long-QT syndrome. *Circ Res* 78:916-924, 1996.
122. Franqueza L, Lin M, Splawski I, et al: Long QT syndrome-associated mutations in the S4-S5 linker of KvLQT1 potassium channels modify gating and interaction with minK subunits. *J Biol Chem* 274:21063-21070, 1999.
123. Li H, Chen Q, Moss AJ, et al: New mutations in the KVLQT1 potassium channel that cause long-QT syndrome. *Circulation* 97:1264-1269, 1998.
124. Sanguinetti MC, Jiang C, Curran ME, et al: A mechanistic link between an inherited and an acquired cardiac arrhythmia: HERG encodes the IKr potassium channel. *Cell* 81:299-307, 1995.
125. Sanguinetti MC, Curran ME, Spector PS, et al: Spectrum of HERG K+-channel dysfunction in an inherited cardiac arrhythmia [published erratum appears in *Proc Natl Acad Sci U S A* 93:8796, 1996]. *Proc Natl Acad Sci U S A* 93:2208-2212, 1996.
126. Sanguinetti MC, Zou A: Molecular physiology of cardiac delayed rectifier K+ channels. *Heart Vessels* 12:170-172, 1997.
127. Schwartz PJ, Priori SG, Locati EH, et al: Long QT syndrome patients with mutations of the SCN5A and HERG genes have differential responses to Na+ channel blockade and to increases in heart rate: Implications for gene-specific therapy. *Circulation* 92:3381-3386, 1995.
128. Vincent GM: Heterogeneity in the inherited long QT syndrome. *J Cardiovasc Electrophysiol* 6:137-146, 1995.
129. Vincent GM: The molecular genetics of the long QT syndrome: genes causing fainting and sudden death. *Annu Rev Med* 49:263-274, 1998.
130. Wang Z, Tristani-Firouzi M, Xu Q, et al: Functional effects of mutations in KvLQT1 that cause long QT syndrome. *J Cardiovasc Electrophysiol* 10:817-826, 1999.
131. Neyroud N, Tesson F, Denjoy I, et al: A novel mutation in the potassium channel gene KVLQT1 causes the Jervell and Lange-Nielsen cardioauditory syndrome. *Nat Genet* 15:186-189, 1997.
132. Priori SG, Schwartz PJ, Napolitano C, et al: A recessive variant of the Romano-Ward long-QT syndrome? *Circulation* 97:2420-2425, 1998.
133. Donger C, Denjoy I, Berthet M, et al: KVLQT1 C-terminal missense mutation causes a forme fruste long-QT syndrome. *Circulation* 96:2778-2781, 1997.
134. Mohammad-Panah R, Demolombe S, Neyroud N, et al: Mutations in a

dominant-negative isoform correlate with phenotype in inherited cardiac arrhythmias. *Am J Hum Genet* 64:1015-1023, 1999.
135. Neyroud N, Denjoy I, Donger C, et al: Heterozygous mutation in the pore of potassium channel gene KvLQT1 causes an apparently normal phenotype in long QT syndrome. *Eur J Hum Genet* 6:129-133, 1998.
136. Zareba W, Moss AJ, Schwartz PJ, et al: Influence of genotype on the clinical course of the long-QT syndrome: International Long-QT Syndrome Registry Research Group. *N Engl J Med* 339:960-965, 1998.
137. Priori SG, Napolitano C, Schwartz PJ: Low penetrance in the long-QT syndrome: Clinical impact. *Circulation* 99:529-533, 1999.
138. Ackerman MJ, Tester DJ, Porter CJ: Swimming, a gene-specific arrhythmogenic trigger for inherited long QT syndrome. *Mayo Clin Proc* 74:1088-1094, 1999.
139. Moss AJ, Robinson JL, Gessman L, et al: Comparison of clinical and genetic variables of cardiac events associated with loud noise versus swimming among subjects with the long QT syndrome. *Am J Cardiol* 84:876-879, 1999.
140. Schwartz PJ, Moss AJ, Vincent GM, et al: Diagnostic criteria for the long QT syndrome: An update. *Circulation* 88:782-784, 1993.
141. Benhorin J, Merri M, Alberti M, et al: Long QT syndrome: New electrocardiographic characteristics. *Circulation* 82:521-527, 1990.
142. Moss AJ, Zareba W, Benhorin J, et al: ECG T-wave patterns in genetically distinct forms of the hereditary long QT syndrome. *Circulation* 92:2929-2934, 1995.
143. Berul CI, Sweeten TL, Hill SL, et al: Provocative testing in children with suspect congenital long QT syndrome. *Ann Noninvasive Electrocardiol* 3:3-11, 1998.
144. Vetter VL, Berul CI, Sweeten TL: Response of corrected QT interval to exercise, pacing and isoproterenol. *Cardiol Young* 3:63, 1993.
145. Bailie DS, Inoue H, Kaseda S, et al: Magnesium suppression of early afterdepolarizations and ventricular tachyarrhythmias induced by cesium in dogs. *Circulation* 77:1395-1402, 1988.
146. Ben-David J, Zipes DP: Torsades de pointes and proarrhythmia. *Lancet* 341:1578-1582, 1993.
147. Schwartz PJ: Long Q-T syndrome, in Horowitz LN (ed): *Current Management of Arrhythmias.* Philadelphia, BC Decker, 1991, pp 194-198.
148. Eldar M, Griffin JC, Van Hare GF, et al: Combined use of beta-adrenergic blocking agents and long-term cardiac pacing for patients with the long QT syndrome. *J Am Coll Cardiol* 20:830-837, 1992.
149. Epstein AE, Rosner MJ, Hageman GR, et al: Posterior left thoracic cardiac sympathectomy by surgical division of the sympathetic chain: An alternative approach to treatment of the long QT syndrome. *Pacing Clin Electrophysiol* 19:1095-1104, 1996.
150. Ouriel K, Moss AJ: Long QT syndrome: An indication for cervicothoracic sympathectomy. *Cardiovasc Surg* 3:475-478, 1995.
151. Schwartz PJ, Locati EH, Moss AJ, et al: Left cardiac sympathetic den-

ervation in the therapy of congenital long QT syndrome: A worldwide report. *Circulation* 84:503-511, 1991.
152. Moss AJ, Liu JE, Gottlieb S, et al: Efficacy of permanent pacing in the management of high-risk patients with long QT syndrome. *Circulation* 84:1524-1529, 1991.
153. Viskin S, Fish R, Roth A, et al: Prevention of torsades de pointes in the congenital long QT syndrome: Use of a pause prevention pacing algorithm. *Heart* 79:417-419, 1998.
154. Schwartz PJ, Priori SG, Napolitano C: The long QT syndrome, in Jalife J, Zipes DP (eds): *Cardiac Electrophysiology. From Cell to Bedside.* Philadelphia, WB Saunders, 2000, pp 597-615.
155. Priori SG, Napolitano C, Cantù F, et al: Differential response to Na+ channel blockade, beta-adrenergic stimulation, and rapid pacing in a cellular model mimicking the SCN5A and HERG defects present in the long-QT syndrome. *Circ Res* 78:1009-1015, 1996.
156. Priori SG, Napolitano C, Paganini V, et al: Molecular biology of the long QT syndrome: Impact on management. *Pacing Clin Electrophysiol* 20:2052-2057, 1997.
157. Compton SJ, Lux RL, Ramsey MR, et al: Genetically defined therapy of inherited long-QT syndrome: Correction of abnormal repolarization by potassium. *Circulation* 94:1018-1022, 1996.
158. Carlsson L, Abrahamsson C, Drews L, et al: Antiarrhythmic effects of potassium channel openers in rhythm abnormalities related to delayed repolarization. *Circulation* 85:1491-1500, 1992.
159. Sato T, Hata Y, Yamamoto M, et al: Early afterdepolarization abolished by potassium channel opener in a patient with idiopathic long QT syndrome. *J Cardiovasc Electrophysiol* 6:279-282, 1995.
160. Moss AJ: Long QT syndrome: Clinical approach to the asymptomatic patient. *ACC Curr J Rev* July-August: 41-43, 1994.
161. Weintraub RG, Gow RM, Wilkinson JL: The congenital long QT syndromes in childhood. *Circulation* 16:674-680, 1990.
162. Shannon DC, Kelly DH: SIDS and near-SIDS (first of two parts). *N Engl J Med* 306:959-965, 1982.
163. Shannon DC, Kelly DH: SIDS and near-SIDS (second of two parts). *N Engl J Med* 306:1022-1028, 1982.
164. Dwyer T, Ponsonby A-L: SIDS epidemiology and incidence. *Pediatr Ann* 24:350-356, 1995.
165. Ariagno RL, Glotzbach SF: Sudden infant death syndrome, in Rudolph AM, Hoffman JIE, Rudolph CD (eds): *Rudolph's Pediatrics.* Stanford, Conn, Appleton & Lange, 1996, 868-878.
166. Bergman AB: Unexplained sudden infant death. *N Engl J Med* 287:254-255, 1972.
167. Bergman AB, Ray CG, Pomeroy MA, et al: Studies of the sudden infant death syndrome in King County, Washington: 3. Epidemiology. *Pediatrics* 49:860-870, 1972.
168. Bergman AB: Sudden infant death syndrome. *Postgrad Med* 51:156-157, 1972.

169. Valdes-Dapena M: The postmortem examination. *Pediatr Ann* 24:365-372, 1995.
170. Froggatt P, James TN: Sudden unexpected death in infants: Evidence on a lethal cardiac arrhythmia. *Ulster Med J* 42:136-152, 1973.
171. James TN: Sudden death in babies: New observations in the heart. *Am J Cardiol* 22:479-506, 1968.
172. Kelly DH, Shannon DC, Liberthson RR: The role of the QT interval in the sudden infant death syndrome. *Circulation* 55:633-635, 1977.
173. Southall DP, Arrowsmith WA, Stebbens V, et al: QT interval measurements before sudden infant death syndrome. *Arch Dis Child* 61:327-333, 1986.
174. Schwartz PJ, Montemerlo M, Facchini M, et al: The QT interval throughout the first 6 months of life: A prospective study. *Circulation* 66:496-501, 1982.
175. Schwartz PJ, Priori SG, Dumaine R, et al: A molecular link between the sudden infant death syndrome and the long-QT syndrome. *N Engl J Med* 343:262-267, 2000.
176. Meny RG, Carroll JL, Carbone MT, et al: Cardiorespiratory recordings from infants dying suddenly and unexpectedly at home. *Pediatrics* 93:44-49, 1994.
177. Poets CF, Meny RG, Chobanian MR, et al: Gasping and other cardiorespiratory patterns during sudden infant deaths. *Pediatr Res* 45:350-354, 1999.
178. Poets CF, Samuels MP, Noyes JP, et al: Home monitoring of transcutaneous oxygen tension in the early detection of hypoxaemia in infants and young children. *Arch Dis Child* 66:676-682, 1991.
179. Southall DP, Arrowsmith WA, Oakley JR, et al: Prolonged QT interval and cardiac arrhythmias in two neonates: Sudden infant death syndrome in one case. *Arch Dis Child* 54:776-779, 1979.
180. Guntheroth WG, Spiers PS: Prolongation of the QT interval and the sudden infant death syndrome. *Pediatrics* 103:813-814, 1999.
181. Naeye RL: The sudden infant death syndrome. *Monogr Pathol* 19:262-270, 1978.
182. Naeye RL: Sudden infant death. *Sci Am* 242:56-62, 1980.
183. Filiano JJ, Kinney HC: Sudden infant death syndrome and brainstem research. *Pediatr Ann* 24:379-383, 1995.
184. Kinney HC, Filiano JJ, Harper RM: The neuropathology of the sudden infant death syndrome: A review. *J Neuropathol Exp Neurol* 51:115-126, 1992.
185. Panigrahy A, Filiano JJ, Sleeper LA, et al: Decreased kainate receptor binding in the arcuate nucleus of the sudden infant death syndrome. *J Neuropathol Exp Neurol* 56:1253-1261, 1997.
186. Slotkin TA, McCook EC, Seidler FJ: Cryptic brain cell injury caused by fetal nicotine exposure is associated with persistent elevations of c-fos protooncogene expression. *Brain Res* 750:180-188, 1997.
187. Slotkin TA: Fetal nicotine or cocaine exposure: Which one is worse? *J Pharmacol Exp Ther* 285:931-945, 1998.

188. Trauth JA, Seidler FJ, McCook EC, et al: Persistent c- fos induction by nicotine in developing rat brain regions: Interaction with hypoxia. *Pediatr Res* 45:38-45, 1999.
189. Slotkin TA, Lappi SE, McCook EC, et al: Loss of neonatal hypoxia tolerance after prenatal nicotine exposure: Implications for sudden infant death syndrome. *Brain Res Bull* 38:69-75, 1995.
190. Lewis KW, Bosque EM: Deficient hypoxia awakening response in infants of smoking mothers: Possible relationship to sudden infant death syndrome. *J Pediatr* 127:691-699, 1995.
191. Guyer B, Hoyert DL, Martin JA, et al: Annual summary of vital statistics—1998. *Pediatrics* 104:1229-1246, 1999.
192. Hoffman JI, Lister G: The implications of a relationship between prolonged QT interval and the sudden infant death syndrome. *Pediatrics* 103:815-817, 1999.
193. Zupancic JAF, Triedman JK, Alexander M, et al: Cost-effectiveness and implications of newborn screening for prolongation of QT interval for the prevention of sudden infant death syndrome. *J Pediatr* 136:481-489, 2000.
194. Clegg J, Bache CE, Raut VV: Financial justification for routine ultrasound screening of the neonatal hip. *J Bone Joint Surg Br* 81:852-857, 1999.
195. Kemper AR, Downs SM: A cost-effectiveness analysis of newborn hearing screening strategies. *Arch Pediatr Adolesc Med* 154:484-488, 2000.
196. Lord J, Thomason MJ, Littlejohns P, et al: Secondary analysis of economic data: A review of cost-benefit studies of neonatal screening for phenylketonuria. *J Epidemiol Community Health* 53:179-186, 1999.
197. Pollitt RJ, Green A, McCabe CJ, et al: Neonatal screening for inborn errors of metabolism: Cost, yield and outcome. *Health Technol Assess* 1:i-iv, 1-202, 1997.
198. Simonsen H, Brandt NJ, Nørgaard-Pedersen B: [Neonatal screening in Denmark: Status and future perspectives]. *Ugeskr Laeger* 160:5777-5782, 1998.
199. Hisashige A: Technology assessment of the neonatal mass screening programs in Japan. *Annual Meeting and International Society of Technology Assessment in Health Care* 11:93A, 1995.
200. Brosnan CA, Brosnan P, Therrell BL, et al: A comparative cost analysis of newborn screening for classic congenital adrenal hyperplasia in Texas. *Public Health Rep* 113:170-178, 1998.
201. Kwon C, Farrell PM: The magnitude and challenge of false-positive newborn screening test results. *Arch Pediatr Adolesc Med* 154:714-718, 2000.
202. Elsias LJ III: Newborn screening, in Rudolph AM, Hoffman JIE, Rudolph CD (eds): *Rudolph's Pediatrics.* Stamford, Conn, Appleton & Lange, 1996, pp 282-288.

CHAPTER 5

Kawasaki Disease

Jane C. Burns, MD
Professor and Chief, Division of Allergy and Immunology, Department of Pediatrics, UCSD School of Medicine, La Jolla, Calif

ABSTRACT

Kawasaki disease is an acute self-limited vasculitis of infancy and early childhood that is now the leading cause of acquired heart disease in children in the United States and Japan. An infectious cause is suspected, although the etiology remains unknown. Children typically are seen with the acute onset of fever followed by signs of mucosal inflammation and vasodilatation that evolve over the first week of the illness. Laboratory tests reveal a marked systemic inflammatory response. If untreated, 1 in 4 children will develop permanent damage to the coronary arteries. Intravenous γ globulin in conjunction with aspirin is effective in reducing the inflammation and preventing coronary artery abnormalities if administered within the first 10 days of illness. This poses a difficult situation for the pediatric care provider who must distinguish Kawasaki disease from other rash/fever syndromes in a timely manner so that appropriate therapy can be initiated.

Kawasaki disease (KD) is a self-limited vasculitis of unknown etiology that predominantly affects children younger than 5 years.[1] It is now the most common cause of acquired heart disease in children in the United States and Japan.[2,3] This chapter reviews the history, epidemiology, clinical features, treatment, pathology, and prognosis for patients with KD.

NEW DISEASE/OLD DISEASE

The sign/symptom complex that we recognize today as KD was first described as a distinct clinical entity by the pediatrician Tomisaku Kawasaki of the Red Cross Hospital in Tokyo, Japan.[4] Kawasaki[5] saw his first patient in 1961. By 1967, he had gathered a series of 50 patients who shared similar clinical signs and symptoms. His meticulous description of the evolution of the illness and laboratory parameters (recently translated into English) is a masterpiece of clinical descriptive writing.[6] In this first publication, Kawasaki described "mucocutaneous lymph node syndrome" (now KD) as a benign self-limited illness that was newly emerging in Japan. The benign nature of KD would be challenged by the pathologist Noburu Tanaka,[7] who was among the first to suspect that KD could affect the coronary arteries and have a fatal outcome. It was not until the epidemiologic survey conducted by the Japanese Ministry of Health in 1970 that KD was clearly linked to coronary arteritis.[8,9] As a result of that survey, more than 3000 clinical cases were identified, including 10 fatal cases. But was KD truly a new disease in Japan? In their investigation into the history of KD, Kushner et al[10] argued that although the disease may have been new to postwar Japan, it was likely present in the West as far back as the 19th century, but was concealed in other disease categories.

Two young pediatricians at the University of Hawaii independently recognized a newly emerging syndrome in Japanese-American children residing in Hawaii during the early 1970s. Marian Melish and Raquel Hicks[11] saw patients with a curious syndrome characterized by high fever, rash, nonexudative conjunctival injection, oral mucosal erythema, urethritis, and arthritis. An autopsy of a fatal case was performed by the pathologist Eunice Larson,[12] who discovered coronary artery aneurysms with thrombosis that was indistinguishable from the pathologic lesions of infantile polyarteritis nodosa (IPN). In 1977, Larson with her mentor, the late Benjamin Landing,[13] reviewed a series of autopsies of KD and IPN and concluded that these 2 entities were pathologically indistinguishable. Thus, Kawasaki in Japan and Melish and Hicks in Hawaii might well have been witnessing the new emergence of an old disease. History may indeed inform the present, and future historical investigation may lead to new testable hypotheses regarding the etiology of KD.

EPIDEMIOLOGY

KD has now been reported from every continent, and it seems clear that where there are children, there is KD.[14] The pattern of disease in Japan has been documented in 14 nationwide surveys.[3,15-18] From this enormous database, we have learned that (1) KD occurred initially in nationwide epidemics (1979, 1982, and 1986), but now occurs only in limited regional epidemics; (2) there are approximately 5000 to 6000 new cases per year in Japan; (3) cur-

TABLE 1.
Diagnostic Criteria for Kawasaki Disease

Fever ≥ 5 days
Bilateral conjunctival injection
Changes of the mucous membranes of the upper respiratory tract: injected pharynx; injected, fissured lips; strawberry tongue
Changes of the peripheral extremities: peripheral edema, peripheral erythema, periungual desquamation
Polymorphous rash
Cervical adenopathy

The diagnosis of KD is considered confirmed by the presence of fever and 4 of the remaining 5 criteria and if the illness cannot be explained by some other known disease process.
(Adapted from Morens DM, O'Brien RJ: Kawasaki disease in the United States. *J Infect Dis* 137:91-93, 1978.)

rent estimates of incidence rates vary between 120 and 150 cases per 100,000 children younger than 5 years; (4) the disease is 1.5 times more common in boys than girls, and 85% of children with KD are younger than 5 years; (5) the recurrence rate is low (4%); and (6) the attack rate in siblings (1%) is 10-fold higher than in the general population.

In the United States, a case definition was adopted by the Centers for Disease Control and Prevention (CDC) (Table 1) and was based on Kawasaki's original clinical criteria, but added the caveat that the illness not be explained by some other known disease process.[19] Regional and statewide investigations in the continental United States suggest an annual endemic incidence of 4 to 18.8 cases per 100,000 children younger than 5 years.[20-26] These widely different estimates may reflect differences in study methods, regional differences in the distribution of ethnic groups who have different susceptibilities to KD, or true regional and temporal differences in KD prevalence. The most accurate estimates are likely to be from studies that used surveillance based on the discharge diagnosis code for KD (446.1) according to the *International Classification of Diseases, Ninth Revision, Clinical Modification (ICD-9-CM)*.[24-26] Although KD has been reported in most ethnic groups, the disease is overrepresented among Asian-American populations.[20,21,24,27-29] In Hawaii, the annual hospitalization rate for all ethnic groups averaged during a 4-year period (1994-1997) was 47.7 per 100,000 children younger than 5 years.[26] However, that rate for Japanese-American residents of Hawaii is estimated at

135 per 100,000 children younger than 5 years,[30] a figure almost identical to current attack rates in Japan.[3] These data suggest an influence of genetic factors on disease susceptibility, with a higher incidence among Japanese regardless of their country of residence.

As in Japan, approximately 85% of US patients are younger than 5 years, the disease is more common in boys, and regional epidemics have been observed.[20-29] However, a major difference in the epidemiology between the 2 countries that remains unexplained is that the mean and median ages of patients with KD in Japan are consistently younger (6-12 months) than in the United States (2-3 years).

Several lines of evidence point to a role for humidity, rainfall, or exposure to water as a risk factor for developing KD. The first piece of evidence was generated by the CDC in an investigation of an outbreak of KD in Denver, Colo, in 1982.[31] Children with KD were more likely to have been exposed to a freshly shampooed carpet in the preceding 30 days before the onset of disease as compared with age-matched "best friend" or census tract control subjects. In addition, the onset of disease was clustered between 2 and 3 weeks after exposure to carpet cleaning, suggesting perhaps an incubation period for an infectious agent. The second water-related association with KD was another investigation by the CDC in which residence near a body of water appeared as a potential risk factor for KD.[21,32] A third association described increased humidifier use among patients with KD during a recent outbreak, again in Denver.[33] Finally, a detailed analysis of regional weather parameters showed a striking relationship between the number of KD cases and the average monthly rainfall in San Diego, Calif.[24] Taken together, these studies suggest a possible precipitating role for humidity or moisture in triggering the onset of KD. If these observations are truly clues to solving the KD mystery, perhaps further attention should be given to water-borne pathogens as possible etiologic agents.

ETIOLOGY

The following observations are usually invoked to argue that KD is an infectious disease: (1) the clinical syndrome resembles other acute self-limited infectious diseases, including adenovirus and enterovirus infection and streptococcal and staphylococcal toxin-mediated diseases; (2) there is a seasonal occurrence with a winter/spring predominance; (3) KD is rare in children younger than 6 months and in adolescents or adults, which may suggest a protective role for transplacental maternal antibody and acquired immunity from asymptomatic infection in older individuals; and (4) recurrences are rare, which also suggests acquired immunity after primary infection. An appealing hypothesis is that KD is caused by a newly emerged single agent that is common in the environment and that is immunogenically similar to another common agent to which most adults are immune. This cross-protective immunity would explain the absence of observed adult cases, even in the 1950s and 1960s, when the disease may have been newly emerging in Japan. It might also help to explain the efficacy of intravenous immunoglobulin (IVIG) in the treatment of KD. The answer to the question of whether KD is a new or old disease would help in the formulation of hypotheses about the etiologic agent or agents.

Many candidate infectious agents have been sought, but no convincing evidence implicates any one of them as the culprit in this disease. Debates continue on the possible role of superantigens in the genesis of the immune activation in KD. Data supporting a role for a bacterial superantigen have been presented by some investigators,[34-36] whereas other studies have found no link to either a superantigen or toxin-secreting bacteria.[37-39] Intriguing data suggesting an IgA response to a conventional antigen have recently been presented and await further confirmation.[40] Suffice it to say that after more than 30 years of searching, the etiology of KD remains unknown.

CLINICAL FEATURES

A central dilemma for the pediatric practitioner is that there is no definitive diagnostic test for KD, but there is effective treatment and potentially dire consequences if the diagnosis is missed and therapy not administered early in the course of the illness. Given this situation, it would seem prudent to increase one's index of suspicion of KD and lower one's threshold for instituting potentially lifesaving therapy. One could argue that the risks of unnecessary treatment with IVIG are small compared with the very real risks of coronary artery aneurysms.[41-43] KD should be considered in the differential diagnosis of every young infant or child with fever, rash, and red eyes (Table 2). History and physical examination should seek supporting or refuting evidence for this diagnosis (Table 3). The possibility of KD should be strongly considered in any patient with prolonged, unexplained fever and any of the associated cutaneous features. This becomes even more important when the patient is younger than 6 months because many patients

TABLE 2.
Differential Diagnosis of a Red Eye in the Pediatric Patient With Rash and Prolonged Fever

Kawasaki syndrome*
Streptococcal and staphylococcal toxin-mediated disease (eg, scarlet fever, toxic shock syndrome)
Adenovirus and other viral infections (enterovirus, measles*)
Drug reaction or Stevens-Johnson syndrome*
Leptospirosis*
Yersinia pseudotuberculosis infection
Rickettsial infection
Reiter syndrome*
Inflammatory bowel disease*
Postinfectious immune complex disease* (eg, postmeningococcemia)
Sarcoidosis*
Systemic lupus erythematosus*
Behçet disease*

*May be associated with anterior uveitis by slit-lamp examination.
(Adapted from Smith LS, Newburger JW, Burns JC: Kawasaki disease and the eye. *Pediatr Infect Dis J* 8:116-118, 1989. Used by permission.)

in this age group allegedly lack the other supporting clinical criteria.[44,45] Whether this is a failure to note a subtle rash or conjunctival injection in these very young patients or whether the associated clinical features are truly less pronounced or even absent in this patient population is unclear. What is clear is that the diagnosis in these infants is frequently delayed and is established only after aneurysms are detected by echocardiography. In recognition of this fact, the American Heart Association created a new disease category called "atypical KD" that includes patients who meet only 4 of the 6 clinical criteria but have coronary artery abnormalities documented by echocardiogram.[46]

To aid the practitioner in the recognition of KD, each of the clinical features (Table 1) will be considered and discussed separately.

1. Fever. KD usually presents with the abrupt onset of high fevers (>39.0°C) that wax and wane. Common antipyretics are often ineffective in controlling the fever. Although the CDC case definition, which was created for epidemiologic, not clinical applications,[19] specified that the fever must have persisted for 5 or

TABLE 3.
Clinical Pearls

Taking the history

1. Refusal to walk: This may be a consequence of swelling of the feet or arthralgia/arthritis.
2. Crying with diaper changes: This may indicate pain with internal rotation of the hip and be a sign of axial arthropathy.
3. Hoarseness: The genesis of this symptom in acute Kawasaki disease (KD) is unclear but may be related to lymph node swelling that affects vocal cord function.

Physical examination

1. Perilimbal sparing: The conjunctival injection of KD is not usually associated with conjunctival edema, and thus the limbus (avascular region around the cornea) is plainly seen and appears as a white halo around the iris.[53]
2. Erythema of the urethral meatus: This is most easily detected in circumcised males and is associated with the urethritis of acute KD.
3. Generalized lymphadenopathy as manifested by bilateral axillary nodes, splenomegaly, exudative pharyngitis, exudative conjunctivitis, and discrete intraoral lesions are specifically not associated with KD and should prompt a search for an alternative diagnosis.[47]
4. A slit-lamp examination by a pediatric ophthalmologist may detect mild anterior uveitis in greater than 80% of patients examined during the first week of illness.[52]
5. Tachycardia out of proportion to anemia and fever is often present.

Laboratory investigation

1. The infection most commonly confused with KD is adenovirus infection. Detection of adenoviral antigens by direct immunofluorescence of nasal scrapings may be helpful to differentiate the 2 diseases.[65]
2. A rising erythrocyte sedimentation rate (ESR) in the face of clinical improvement and defervescence is very characteristic of KD and is distinctly different from most viral and bacterial infections, in which the patient and ESR improve together. The ESR and quantitative C-reactive protein (CRP) do not correlate well in this disease.[6] Sometimes, the CRP is high early in the disease while the ESR is elevated later.
3. Sterile pyuria in KD is associated with mononuclear cells in the urine, not neutrophils. Voided urine specimens are preferred over catheterized specimens since the inflammation is in the urethra distal to the bladder.[12] Making a cytospin preparation of the urine sediment and staining as for a blood smear (Wright-Giemsa stain) will reveal mononuclear cells with bizarre intracytoplasmic inclusions. The leukocyte esterase test on the urine dipstick is usually negative.
4. The serum γ-glutamyltransferase (GGT) is elevated in two thirds of patients with acute KD.[58]

more days, the diagnosis of KD can be established earlier in the course of the illness if other supporting clinical features are present.

2. Rash. Most patients with KD (92.9% in one series[47]) have some kind of rash during the course of their illness. The rash may take many forms but is never frankly bullous or purpuric. A true erythroderma (sunburned appearance) is also not consistent with KD. Petechiae can be present, and a peculiar micropustular rash may be noted (1-mm pustules) on extensor surfaces and intertriginous areas.[48,49] The micropustular rash was noted in 4 (5.3%) of 75 patients in one Japanese series.[48] The rash is accentuated in the groin in approximately half of the patients[47,50] and is often misdiagnosed as a diaper dermatitis in young infants. The rash of KD is frequently mistaken for an allergic reaction to medications, usually antibiotics, that have been prescribed for various suspected infections, usually otitis media. KD may be associated with tympanic membrane erythema, perhaps similar to the vasodilation in the conjunctiva. However, this erythema is usually not associated with an effusion in the middle ear. The polymorphous rash of KD may be misdiagnosed as urticaria, erythema multiforme (both major and minor), or a benign viral exanthem. Skin biopsy is only helpful in ruling in one of these alternative diagnoses, which, unlike KD, may have a characteristic histopathology.
3. Red eyes. The conjunctival injection in KD is specifically not an inflammatory process in that conjunctival biopsy specimens reveal no cellular infiltrate or vasculitis.[51] Perilimbal sparing is characteristic of KD and may help to differentiate the red eye of KD from other infections or allergic reactions in which edema and swelling of the conjunctiva are common. A slit-lamp examination will reveal anterior uveitis in as many as 80% of patients examined within the first week of illness and before administration of IVIG.[52] The red eyes of patients with KD are not associated with tearing or exudate, and these signs should prompt the search for an alternative diagnosis.[47] Similarly, extensive keratitis and marked photophobia are uncommon.[53]
4. Oropharyngeal changes. The red cracked lips of patients with KD are often mistaken for chapping associated with dehydration. The strawberry tongue appears the same in KD and in bacterial toxin-mediated illnesses, including scarlet fever and staphylococcal toxic shock syndrome. The oropharynx may be diffusely red in KD patients, but discrete intraoral lesions and tonsillar exudate are not seen.[47]

5. Cervical lymphadenopathy. Some patients with KD present solely with high fever and a unilateral mass of cervical nodes.[54,55] Only later during the first week of illness do the other clinical features appear. Often, the rash is thought to be an allergic reaction to antibiotics administered for treatment of presumed bacterial lymphadenitis. The enlarged nodes may be in the anterior or posterior cervical chains, although a unilateral anterior cervical mass of nodes is the most common presentation. Generalized lymphadenopathy is not associated with KD.[47]
6. Extremity changes. The nonpitting edema of the dorsa of the hands and feet may be difficult to distinguish from the normal pudgy extremities of some infants and toddlers. Parents can usually identify abnormal puffiness in the extremities of their child. Inability to put on shoes because of swelling, refusal to walk, and requesting that the soles and palms be rubbed are frequent among patients with KD. The erythema of the palms and soles, like the other features of KD, may wax and wane over short intervals, and frequent repeated observations of patients for the stigmata of KD are often helpful. Periungual desquamation of the fingers and toes is usually a late finding and does not appear until the second to third week of the illness.[1]

Clinical features that are not part of the case definition but can be associated with acute KD include the following:

1. Cardiac: tachycardia and gallop rhythm associated with myocarditis, pericarditis with effusion, murmur associated with valvulitis, congestive heart failure caused by myocarditis, ischemia, or both, myocardial infarction caused by thrombosis of aneurysms, and sudden death caused by arrhythmia or rupture of coronary artery aneurysm.[56]
2. Gastrointestinal: hydrops of the gallbladder associated with vomiting and right upper quadrant pain,[57] biochemical evidence of hepatobiliary and hepatocellular damage,[58] and diarrhea.
3. Musculoskeletal: arthritis and arthralgia of weight-bearing joints (35% of patients) or small joints (15% of patients).[49]
4. Neurologic: irritability with slowing on electroencephalogram (EEG), meningeal signs with cerebrospinal fluid (CSF) pleocytosis,[59] sensorineural hearing loss,[60] and cranial nerve palsies.[61]
5. Genitourinary: urethritis with sterile pyuria.[12]

CARDIAC COMPLICATIONS

The most significant complication of the vasculitis of acute KD is the development of ectasia or aneurysms in the coronary arteries and other medium-sized, extraparenchymal muscular arteries.[56,62] Dilatation of the coronary arteries (>2 SDs above the mean based on body surface area)[63] as measured by echocardiogram is common during acute KD. In a retrospective review of echocardiograms performed during a 1-year period, we found that 12 (33.3%) of 36 patients had dilated coronary arteries according to these criteria (JCB, unpublished data). This dilatation disappeared after IVIG therapy in all but 2 patients, who developed aneurysms. The long-term significance of this transient dilatation is currently unknown. More permanent structural damage to the coronary arteries as reflected by ectasia or aneurysm formation may be clinically silent for years to decades and may ultimately present as sudden death in a young adult.[64]

LABORATORY EVALUATION

No single laboratory test establishes the diagnosis of KD. Although no laboratory tests are included in the current case definition, clinicians certainly use the laboratory to seek evidence of marked systemic inflammation or to establish alternative diagnoses (Table 3). Laboratory testing should include a complete blood cell count with differential, erythrocyte sedimentation rate, platelet count, C-reactive protein, liver transaminases, γ-glutamyltransferase (GGT), and a urinalysis. Cultures of blood, urine, and CSF for bacteria, throat culture for streptococcus, streptococcal serology, nasal secretions for indirect immunofluorescent testing for adenovirus,[65] and serology for Epstein-Barr virus and measles virus may be helpful in selected patients to establish an alternative diagnosis.

TREATMENT OF ACUTE KD

The goal of therapy in KD is to rapidly reduce inflammation and thus the potential for damage to the arterial wall. Initially, patients with KD were treated with a variety of antibiotics, steroids, and aspirin in an attempt to modify the clinical course.[6,66] Despite these therapies, 1 in 4 patients developed coronary artery abnormalities.

IVIG THERAPY

Influenced by reports of high-dose IVIG for the treatment of idiopathic thrombocytopenic purpura,[67] Furusho et al[68] in Japan attempted therapy with IVIG for patients with KD in the early 1980s and reported beneficial effects. These findings were subsequently confirmed by other groups both in Japan and North America.[69-71] The US Multicenter KD Study Group reported that treatment with IVIG (1.6-2 g/kg), in conjunction with high doses of aspirin (80-100 mg/kg per day), was effective in abolishing fever and clinical signs of inflammation in 85% of patients and reduced the prevalence of coronary artery abnormalities to 3% to 5%.[69,70] There is much speculation, but little data, on the mechanism of action of IVIG in acute KD. Possible mechanisms include Fc receptor blockade, specific antiagent antibody, anti-idiotype antibodies, antitoxin antibodies, and anticytokine antibodies. Current recommended therapy is 2 g/kg of IVIG as a single infusion over 10 to 12 hours.[46,72] The optimal management of patients (approximately 15%) who are refractory to the first dose of IVIG has not been prospectively studied. Retrospective studies suggest that most of these patients will become afebrile after a second infusion of 2 g/kg of IVIG.[73,74]

ASPIRIN

Aspirin is used in patients with KD at different doses to achieve different therapeutic goals: high-dose aspirin (80-100 mg/kg per day) is used for its anti-inflammatory effect, medium-dose aspirin (30 mg/kg per day) is used for its antipyretic effect, and low-dose aspirin (3-5 mg/kg per day) is used for its antiplatelet effect. No prospective randomized trial has established that aspirin at any dose is useful in the treatment of acute KD. The US Multicenter KD Study Group used high-dose aspirin through the 14th day of illness, followed by 3 to 5 mg/kg per day of aspirin for an additional 2 months or until the erythrocyte sedimentation rate and platelet count returned to normal. Many centers have reduced the total number of days of high-dose aspirin therapy by switching to low-dose therapy after the patient has remained afebrile for 48 hours. In Japan, the maximum dose is 30 mg/kg per day because of intolerance to higher doses and the development of drug-induced hepatitis in some patients. Complications of high-dose aspirin therapy in US patients with KD have been rarely reported and include gastrointestinal hemorrhage and Reye syndrome.[75,76] A trial conducted in the United States that compared initial low-dose (3-5 mg/kg per day) versus high-dose (80-100 mg/kg per day) aspirin therapy combined with IVIG found that patients who received low-dose aspirin had more fever after IVIG administration, more frequently required re-treatment with IVIG, and had prolonged hospital stays as a consequence.[77] Therefore, low-dose aspirin as initial therapy is not advised. The use of nonsteroidal drugs as antipyretic and anti-inflammatory agents in KD has not been prospectively studied.

OTHER THERAPIES

Methylprednisolone (30 mg/kg per dose) has been successfully used to treat refractory patients with persistent fever despite re-treatment with IVIG.[78] The appropriate role of steroids in the treatment of KD has not been defined and deserves further study. Other immune modulators such as competitive inhibitors of tumor necrosis factor-α (TNF-α)[79,80] and TNF-α messenger RNA synthesis inhibitors (eg, pentoxifylline)[81] have not been systematically studied in patients with KD.

PATHOLOGY

The pathologic changes associated with acute KD have been gleaned from autopsy reports of children dying of cardiovascular complications of the vasculitis[82] and from biopsy material collected from skin,[6,83] conjunctiva,[51] lymph nodes,[6,84,85] liver,[86] gallbladder,[87] small bowel,[88] and right ventricle.[89] Biopsy material from superficial sites has been surprisingly unhelpful in that the small vessels in these specimens are minimally affected by the inflammatory process in this disease. Skin biopsy specimens have revealed only nonspecific changes including edema and dilatation of small blood vessels in the dermal papilla with mild mononuclear cell infiltration.[6,83] Electron microscopy revealed some degenerative changes in endothelial cells.[83] Biopsy of the pustular eruption seen in approximately 5% of patients revealed intraepidermal spongiform pustules with numerous neutrophils.[48]

Tissue sampling from deeper sites from living patients has documented a number of histologic abnormalities that suggest a diffuse inflammatory process. Lymph node biopsy specimens have shown abnormal hyperplasia of the endothelium of the postcapillary venule with associated reticulocyte hyperplasia.[6] Other studies have described multiple foci of necrosis and fibrin thrombi in the microvasculature associated with endothelial cell swelling.[84,85] Liver biopsy specimens have demonstrated portal infiltrates with neutrophils and degeneration or swelling of bile duct epithelial cells.[86] Gallbladder histology on surgical specimens has revealed periarteriolar infiltrates, edema, and hemorrhage in the gallbladder wall and fibrinous exudate on the serosal surface.[87] Small-bowel biopsy specimens showed minimally increased cellularity by routine histology, but an increase in activated epithelial cells and infiltrating CD4+ cells was demonstrated by immunologic staining.[88]

A study of right ventricular biopsy specimens performed 2 months to 11 years after acute KD in more than 200 patients revealed myocardial abnormalities, including fibrosis, disorganization of myocytes with abnormal branching, and hypertrophy of myocytes.[89] The extent of myocardial damage was not predicted by severity of the acute illness or the development of coronary artery abnormalities.

Histologic examination of medium-sized, extraparenchymal muscular arteries such as the coronary, renal, hepatic, splanchnic, internal iliac, and brachial arteries obtained at autopsy has shown marked changes throughout the length of the vessel.[13,62,90] The histologic progression of the vascular lesion in KD has been characterized as beginning in both the adventitial and intimal surfaces and proceeding towards the media. Early intimal changes include a mononuclear cell accumulation with intimal thickening. This is followed by lymphocyte infiltration of the luminal side of the intima and can progress to intimal fibrinoid necrosis. In the adventitia, there is a mixed inflammatory cell infiltration that progresses toward the intima, creating medial disruption and edema. Finally, luminal thrombosis and aneurysmal dilatation may occur. Lesions in all different stages of progression are seen even within a single vessel. Characterization of the cellular infiltrate in these vessels has been pursued in hopes of finding clues to the antigens that may be inciting the inflammatory response. The role of IgA-secreting plasma cells seen in some autopsy tissues is currently under investigation.[40]

PROGNOSIS

PATIENTS WITH NO DETECTABLE CORONARY ARTERY LESIONS

Little data are available to guide physicians in counseling parents of a child whose echocardiograms have remained normal after KD. Kato et al[91] followed the status of 258 Japanese patients with normal angiograms after KD and found no cardiac symptoms or abnormalities during the follow-up period that ranged from 10 to 21 years. Although these data are reassuring, other data provide evidence of long-term endothelial cell dysfunction after KD. Two studies that used provocative tests of endothelial cell-mediated vasodilatation have shown abnormal results years after KD even in the patients with normal echocardiograms during their acute illness.[92,93] The clinical or prognostic significance of these findings in asymptomatic patients is unknown.

An autopsy study by Tanaka et al[94] described 5 children who died of unrelated causes 2 months to 2 years after acute KD. All cases showed varying degrees of intimal thickening and fibrosis. Unfortunately, the antemortem status of their coronary arteries was unknown. A second autopsy study by Fujiwara et al[95] described 4 children who died 9 to 22 days after disease onset and who had no abnormalities of the coronary arteries detected by echocardiogram. All of these children had histologic evidence of coronary arteritis. However, it is impossible to know whether these children would have gone on to develop aneurysms had they lived longer. An additional 2 patients were reported who died later after KD. One had normal echocardiograms during his acute and convalescent period and died 46 days after KD of staphylococcal pneumonia. The coronary arteries were normal at autopsy. A second patient had dilatation of the coronary arteries by echocardiogram during acute KD that resolved during convalescence. This patient died 2 years later from a myocardial infarction that occurred at the time of cardiac catheterization. At autopsy, he had only one focal area of fibrous intimal thickening in the coronary arteries, which were otherwise normal.

In an attempt to address questions about long-term prognosis for this group of patients with KD, the Japanese Ministry of Health has organized a prospective study of a cohort of approximately 6500 Japanese patients with KD. After 10 years, no excess mortality has been detected among these individuals.[96] However, questions regarding long-term outcome will require another 2 to 3 decades of observation. Unfortunately, no similar longitudinal follow-up study of Western children has been organized. Thus, in a population with a higher a priori risk of atherosclerosis, no information is being systematically gathered on potential long-term affects of KD on the health and function of the coronary arteries.

PATIENTS WITH CORONARY ARTERY LESIONS

Damage to the coronary arteries after KD is a dynamic process, and approximately half of the patients with aneurysms will remodel the vessel wall and fill in the aneurysms in the first year after their acute KD.[91,97] Many studies have documented, however, that these vessels remain functionally abnormal and are unable to dilate normally in response to increased myocardial oxygen demand.[98] Thus, the terms “healing” and “resolution” may be misleading when applied to coronary artery aneurysms.

The management of children with coronary artery abnormalities after acute KD is individualized based on the type and location of lesions. Stenosis of aneurysms that have healed in patients with myointimal proliferation is a potentially lethal complication. Pediatric cardiologists in Japan and the United States generally recommend long-term antiplatelet therapy (eg, aspirin, dipyridamole). Newer antiplatelet agents such as clopidogrel (inhibitor of adenosine diphosphate [ADP]-mediated platelet activation)[99] have not yet been systematically studied in this patient population. Systemic anticoagulation with warfarin (Coumadin) may be desirable in patients with turbulent flow through the abnormal vessel segment. Invasive approaches including angioplasty, stenting, coronary bypass grafting, and cardiac transplantation may be necessary.[100]

SUMMARY

KD is a self-limited pediatric vasculitis that must be treated promptly to avoid potentially lethal coronary artery damage. A high index of suspicion coupled with a low threshold for treating patients for KD who have prolonged fever without other explanation is appropriate. More directed therapy and specific diagnostic tests must await elucidation of the causative agent.

REFERENCES

1. Kawasaki T, Kosaki F, Okawa S, et al: A new infantile acute febrile mucocutaneous lymph node syndrome (MCLS) prevailing in Japan. *Pediatrics* 54:271-276, 1974.
2. Taubert KA, Rowley AH, Shulman ST: A nationwide survey of Kawasaki disease and acute rheumatic fever. *J Pediatr* 119:279-282, 1991.
3. Yanagawa H, Nakamura Y, Ojima T, et al: Changes in epidemic patterns of Kawasaki disease in Japan. *Pediatr Infect Dis J* 18:64-66, 1999.
4. Burns JC, Kushner HI, Bastian JF, et al: Kawasaki disease: A brief history. *Pediatrics* [online] 106:http://www.pediatrics.org/cgi/content /full/106/2/e27, 2000.
5. Kawasaki T: Pediatric acute mucocutaneous lymph node syndrome: Clinical observation of 50 cases [in Japanese]. *Arerugi (Jpn J Allergy)* 16:178-222, 1967.
6. Shike H, Shimizu C, Burns JC: English translation of Kawasaki T. Pediatric acute mucocutaneous lymph node syndrome: Clinical observation of 50 cases, submitted for publication.
7. Tanaka N, Seikimoto K, Naoe S: Kawasaki disease: Relationship with infantile polyarteritis nodosa. *Arch Pathol Lab Med* 100:81-86, 1976.
8. Shigematsu I: Epidemiology of mucocutaneous lymph node syndrome [in Japanese]. *Nippon Shonika Gakkai Zasshi (J Jpn Pediatr Soc)* 76:695-696, 1972.
9. Kosaki F, Kawasaki T, Okawa S, et al: Clinicopathological conference on 10 fatal cases with acute febrile mucocutaneous lymph node syndrome [in Japanese]. *Shonika Rinsho (Jpn J Pediatr)* 24:2545-2559, 1971.
10. Kushner HI, Turner CL, Bastian JF, et al: Kawasaki disease before Kawasaki, submitted for publication.
11. Melish ME, Hicks RM, Larson E: Mucocutaneous lymph node syndrome in the U.S. *Pediatr Res* 8:427A, 1974.

12. Melish ME, Hicks RM, Larson EJ: Mucocutaneous lymph node syndrome in the United States. *Am J Dis Child* 130:599-607, 1976.
13. Landing BH, Larson EJ: Are periarteritis nodosa with coronary artery involvement and fatal mucocutaneous lymph node syndrome the same? Comparison of 20 patients from North America with patients from Hawaii and Japan. *Pediatrics* 59:651-662, 1976.
14. Taubert KA: Epidemiology of Kawasaki disease in the United States and worldwide. *Prog Pediatr Cardiol* 6:181-185, 1997.
15. Yanagawa H, Yashiro M, Nakamura Y, et al: Results of 12 nationwide epidemiological incidence surveys of Kawasaki disease in Japan. *Arch Pediatr Adolesc Med* 149:779-783, 1995.
16. Yanagawa H, Yashiro M, Nakamura Y, et al: Epidemiologic pictures of Kawasaki disease in Japan: From the nationwide incidence survey in 1991 and 1992. *Pediatrics* 95:475-479, 1995.
17. Yanagawa H, Nakamura Y, Yashiro M, et al: Update of the epidemiology of Kawasaki disease in Japan: From the results of 1993-94 nationwide survey. *J Epidemiol* 6:148-157, 1996.
18. Yanagawa Y, Nakamura Y, Yashiro M, et al: Results of the nationwide epidemiologic survey of Kawasaki disease in 1995 and 1996 in Japan. *Pediatrics* [online] 102:http://www.pediatrics.org/cgi/content/full/102/6/e65, 1998.
19. Morens DM, O'Brien RJ: Kawasaki disease in the United States. *J Infect Dis* 137:91-93, 1978.
20. Shulman ST, McCauley JB, Pachman LM, et al: Risk of coronary abnormalities due to Kawasaki disease in urban area with small Asian population. *Am J Dis Child* 141:420-425, 1987.
21. Rausch AM, Kaplan SL, Nihill MR, et al: Kawasaki syndrome clusters in Harris Country, Texas, and eastern North Carolina: A high endemic rate and a new environmental risk factor. *Am J Dis Child* 142:441-444, 1988.
22. Taubert KA, Rowley AH, Shulman ST: Seven-year national survey of Kawasaki disease and acute rheumatic fever. *Pediatr Infect Dis J* 13:704-708, 1994.
23. Davis RL, Waller PL, Mueller BA, et al: Kawasaki syndrome in Washington State: Race-specific incidence rates and residential proximity to water. *Arch Pediatr Adolesc Med* 149:66-69, 1995.
24. Bronstein DE, Dille AN, Austin JP, et al: Relationship of climate, ethnicity, and socioeconomic status to Kawasaki Disease in San Diego County, 1994-1998. *Pediatr Infect Dis J* 19:1087-1091, 2000.
25. Holman RC, Belay ED, Clarke MJ, et al: Kawasaki syndrome among American Indian and Alaska native children, 1980-1995. *Pediatr Infect Dis J* 18:451-455, 1999.
26. Holman RC, Shahriari A, Effler PV, et al: Kawasaki syndrome hospitalizations among children in Hawaii and Connecticut. *Arch Pediatr Adolesc Med* 154:804-808, 2000.
27. Morens DM, Anderson LJ, Hurwitz ES: National surveillance of Kawasaki disease. *Pediatrics* 65:21-25, 1980.

28. Bell DM, Brink EW, Nitzkin JL, et al: Kawasaki syndrome: Description of two outbreaks in the United States. *N Engl J Med* 304:1568-1575, 1981.
29. Dean AG, Melish ME, Hicks R, et al: An epidemic of Kawasaki syndrome in Hawaii. *J Pediatr* 100:552-557, 1982.
30. Marian Melish, personal communication, November 17, 1999.
31. Patriarca PA, Rogers MF, Morens DM, et al: Kawasaki syndrome: Association with the application of rug shampoo. *Lancet* 2:578-580, 1982.
32. Rausch AM: Kawasaki syndrome: Review of new epidemiologic and laboratory developments. *Pediatr Infect Dis J* 6:1016-1021, 1987.
33. Treadwell TA, Shahrian A, Belay ED, et al: Kawasaki syndrome in Colorado, November 1997-April 1998. *Pediatr Res* 47:559A, 2000.
34. Abe J, Kotzin BL, Jujo K, et al: Selective expansion of T cells expressing T-cell receptor variable regions V beta 2 and V beta 8 in Kawasaki disease. *Proc Natl Acad Sci U S A* 89:4066-4070, 1992.
35. Yamashiro Y, Nagata S, Oguchi S, et al: Selective increase of VB2+ T cells in the small intestinal mucosa in Kawasaki Disease. *Pediatr Res* 39:264-266, 1996.
36. Leung DYM, Giorno RC, Kazemi LV, et al: Evidence for superantigen involvement in cardiovascular injury due to Kawasaki syndrome. *J Immunol* 155:5018-5021, 1995.
37. Pietra BA, De IJ, Giannini EH, et al: TCR V beta family repertoire and T cell activation markers in Kawasaki disease. *J Immunol* 153:1881-1888, 1994.
38. Choi IH, Chwae YJ, Shim WS, et al: Clonal expression of CD8+ T cells in Kawasaki Disease. *J Immunol* 159:481-486, 1997.
39. Jason J, Montana E, Donald F, et al: Kawasaki disease and the T-cell antigen receptor. *Hum Immunol* 59:29-38, 1998.
40. Rowley AH, Eckerley CA, Jack HM et al: IgA plasma cells in vascular tissue of patients with Kawasaki syndrome. *J Immunol* 159:5946-5955, 1997.
41. Klassen TP, Rowe PC, Gafni A: Economic evaluation of intravenous immune globulin therapy for Kawasaki syndrome. *J Pediatr* 122:538-542, 1993.
42. Witt MR, Minich L, Bohnsack JF, et al: Kawasaki disease: More patients are being diagnosed who do not meet American Heart Association criteria. *Pediatrics* [online] 104:http://www.pediatrics.org/cgi/content/full/104/1/e10, 1999.
43. Stapp J, Marshall GS: Fulfillment of diagnostic criteria in Kawasaki disease. *South Med J* 93:44-47, 2000.
44. Burns JC, Wiggins JW Jr, Toews WH, et al: Clinical spectrum of Kawasaki disease in infants younger than 6 months of age. *J Pediatr* 109:759-763, 1986.
45. Rosenfeld EA, Corydon KE, Shulman ST: Kawasaki disease in infants less than one year of age. *J Pediatr* 126:524-529, 1995.
46. Dajani AS, Taubert KA, Gerber MA, et al: Diagnosis and therapy of Kawasaki disease in children. *Circulation* 87:1776-1780, 1993.

47. Burns JC, Mason WH, Glode MP, et al: Clinical and epidemiologic characteristics of patients referred for evaluation of possible Kawasaki disease. *J Pediatr* 118:680-686, 1991.
48. Kimura T, Miyazawa H, Watanabe K, et al: Small pustules in Kawasaki disease. *Am J Dermatopathol* 10:218-223, 1988.
49. Hicks RV, Melish ME: Kawasaki Syndrome. *Pediatr Clin North Am* 33:1151-1175, 1986.
50. Urbach AH, McGregor RS, Malatack JJ, et al: Kawasaki disease and perineal rash. *Am J Dis Child* 142:1174-1176, 1988.
51. Burns JC, Wright JD, Newburger JW, et al: Conjunctival biopsy in patients with Kawasaki Disease. *Pediatr Pathol* 15:547-553, 1995.
52. Burns JC, Joffe L, Sargent RA, et al: Anterior uveitis associated with Kawasaki syndrome. *Pediatr Infect Dis J* 4:258-261, 1985.
53. Smith LS, Newburger JW, Burns JC: Kawasaki disease and the eye. *Pediatr Infect Dis J* 8:116-118, 1989.
54. April MM, Burns JC, Newburger JW, et al: Kawasaki disease and cervical adenopathy: An update for the otolaryngologist. *Arch Otolaryngol* 115:512-514, 1989.
55. Park AH, Batchra N, Rowley A, et al: Patterns of Kawasaki syndrome presentation. *Int J Pediatr Otorhinolaryngol* 40:41-50, 1997.
56. Kato H, Koike S, Yamamoto M, et al: Coronary aneurysms in infants and young children with acute febrile mucocutaneous lymph node syndrome. *J Pediatr* 86:892-898, 1975.
57. Suddelson EA, Reid B, Woolley MM, et al: Hydrops of the gallbladder associated with Kawasaki syndrome. *J Pediatr Surg* 22:956-959, 1987.
58. Ting EC, Capparelli EV, Billman GF, et al: Elevated gamma-glutamyltransferase concentrations in patients with acute Kawasaki disease. *Pediatr Infect Dis J* 17:431-432, 1998.
59. Dengler LD, Capparelli EV, Bastian JF, et al: Cerebrospinal fluid profile in patients with acute Kawasaki disease. *Pediatr Infect Dis J* 17:478-481, 1998.
60. Sundel RP, Newburger JW, McGill T, et al: Sensorineural hearing loss associated with Kawasaki disease. *J Pediatr* 117:371-377, 1990.
61. Hattori T, Tokugawa K, Fukushige J, et al: Facial palsy in Kawasaki disease. *Eur J Pediatr* 146:601-602, 1987.
62. Tanaka N, Naoe S, Masuda H, et al: Pathological study of sequella of Kawasaki disease (MCLS): With special reference to the heart and coronary arterial lesions. *Acta Pathol Jpn* 36:1513-1527, 1986.
63. de Zori A, Clan SD, Gauvreau K, et al: Coronary artery dimensions may be misclassified as normal in Kawasaki disease. *J Pediatr* 133:254-258, 1998.
64. Burns JC, Shike H, Gordon JB, et al: Sequella of Kawasaki disease in adolescents and young adults. *J Am Coll Cardiol* 28:253-257, 1996.
65. Barone SR, Pontrelli LR, Krilov LR: The differentiation of classic Kawasaki disease, atypical Kawasaki disease, and acute adenoviral infection: Use of clinical findings and rapid direct fluorescent antigen test. *Arch Pediatr Adolesc Med* 54:453-456, 200.

66. Kato H, Koike S, Yokoyama T: Kawasaki disease: Effect of treatment on coronary artery. *Pediatrics* 63:175-179, 1979.
67. Imbach P, Barandun S, d'Apuzzo V, et al: High-dose intravenous gamma globulin for idiopathic thrombocytopenic purpura in childhood. *Lancet* 1:1228-1230, 1981.
68. Furusho K, Kamiya T, Nakano H et al: High-dose intravenous gamma globulin for Kawasaki disease. *Lancet* 2:1055-1058, 1984.
69. Newburger JW, Takahashi M, Burns JC, et al: Treatment of Kawasaki syndrome with intravenous gamma globulin. *N Engl J Med* 315:341-347, 1986.
70. Newburger JW, Takahashi M, Beiser AS, et al: Single infusion of intravenous gamma globulin compared to four daily doses in the treatment of acute Kawasaki Syndrome. *N Engl J Med* 324:1633-1639, 1991.
71. Morikawa Y, Ohashi Y, Harada K, et al: A multicenter, randomized controlled trial of intravenous gamma globulin therapy in children with acute Kawasaki disease. *Acta Paediatr Jpn* 36:347-354, 1994.
72. American Academy of Pediatrics: Kawasaki disease, in Pickering LK (ed): *2000 Red Book: Report of the Committee on Infectious Diseases*, ed 25. Elk Grove Village, Ill, American Academy of Pediatrics, 2000, pp 360-363.
73. Burns JC, Capparelli EV, Brown JA, et al: Intravenous gamma globulin treatment and retreatment in Kawasaki disease. *Pediatr Inf Dis J* 17:1144-1148, 1998.
74. Han RK, Silverman ED, Newman A, et al: Management and outcome of persistent or recurrent fever after initial intravenous gamma globulin therapy in acute Kawasaki disease. *Arch Pediatr Adolesc Med* 154:694-699, 2000.
75. Matsubara T, Mason W, Kashani IA, et al: Gastrointestinal hemorrhage complicating aspirin therapy in acute Kawasaki disease. *J Pediatr* 128:701-703, 1996.
76. Takahashi M, Mason W, Thomas D, et al: Reye syndrome following Kawasaki syndrome confirmed by liver histopathology, in Kato H (ed): *Kawasaki Disease. Proceedings of the 5th International Kawasaki Disease Symposium, Fukuoka, Japan.* Amsterdam, The Netherlands, Elsevier Science, 1995, pp 436-444.
77. Melish ME, Takahashi M, Shulman ST, et al: Comparison of low dose aspirin vs. high dose aspirin as an adjunct to intravenous gamma globulin in the treatment of Kawasaki syndrome. *Pediatr Rcs* 31:170A, 1992.
78. Wright DA, Newburger JW, Baker A, et al:. Treatment of immune globulin-resistant Kawasaki disease with pulsed doses of corticosteroids. *J Pediatr* 128:146-149, 1996.
79. Maini R, St Clair EW, Breedveld F, et al: Infliximab (chimeric anti-tumor necrosis factor alpha monoclonal antibody) versus placebo in rheumatoid arthritis patients receiving concomitant methotrexate: A randomized phase III trial. *Lancet* 354:1932-1939, 1999.

80. Lowell DJ, Giannini EH, Reiff A, et al: Etanercept in children with polyarticular juvenile rheumatoid arthritis. *N Engl J Med* 342:763-769, 2000.
81. Furukawa S, Matsubara T, Umezawa Y, et al: Pentoxifylline and intravenous gamma globulin combination therapy for acute Kawasaki disease. *Eur J Pediatr* 153:663-667, 1994.
82. Fujiwara H, Hamashima Y: Pathology of the heart in Kawasaki disease. *Pediatrics* 61:100-107, 1978.
83. Hirose S, Hamashima Y: Morphological observation on the vasculitis in the mucocutaneous lymph node syndrome: A skin biopsy study of 27 patients. *Eur J Pediatr* 129:17-27, 1978.
84. Giesdker DW, Pastuszak WT, Forouhar FA, et al: Lymph node biopsy for early diagnosis in Kawasaki disease. *Am J Surg Pathol* 6:493-501, 1982.
85. Tanaka N: Kawasaki disease in Japan: Relationship with infantile periarteritis nodosa. *Pathol Microbiol* 43:204-218, 1975.
86. Bader-Meunier B, Hadchouel M, Fabre M, et al: Intrahepatic bile duct damage in children with Kawasaki disease. *J Pediatr* 120:750-752, 1992.
87. Dinulos J, Mitchell DK, Egerton J, et al: Hydrops of the gallbladder associated with Epstein-Barr virus infection: A report of two cases and review of the literature. *Pediatr Infect Dis J* 13:924-949, 1994.
88. Nagata S, Yamashiro Y, Maeda M, et al: Immunohistochemical studies on small intestinal mucosa in Kawasaki disease. *Pediatr Res* 33:557-563, 1993.
89. Yutani C, Go S, Kamiya T, et al: Cardiac biopsy of Kawasaki disease. *Arch Pathol Lab Med* 105:470-473, 1981.
90. Naoe S, Takahashi K, Masuda H, et al: Kawasaki disease with particular emphasis on arterial lesions. *Acta Pathol Jpn* 41:785-797, 1991.
91. Kato H, Sugimura T, Akagi T, et al: Long-term consequences of Kawasaki disease: A 10-21-year follow-up study of 594 patients. *Circulation* 94:1379-1385, 1996.
92. Mitani Y, Okuda Y, Shimpo H, et al: Impaired endothelial function in epicardial coronary arteries after Kawasaki disease. *Circulation* 96:454-461, 1997.
93. Dhillon R, Clarkson P, Donald AE, et al: Endothelial dysfunction late after Kawasaki disease. *Circulation* 94:2103-2106, 1996.
94. Tanaka N, Naoe S, Masuda H, et al: Pathological study of sequella of Kawasaki disease with special reference to the heart and coronary arterial lesions. *Acta Pathol Jpn* 36:1513-1527, 1986.
95. Fujiwara T, Fujiwara H, Nakano H: Pathological features of coronary arteries in children with Kawasaki disease in which coronary arterial aneurysm was absent at autopsy. *Circulation* 78:345-350, 1988.
96. Nakamura Y, Yanagawa H, Kato H, et al: Mortality among patients with a history of Kawasaki disease: The third look. *Acta Paediatr Jpn* 40:419-423, 1998.
97. Suzuki A, Kamiya T, Kuwahara N, et al: Coronary arterial lesions of Kawasaki disease: Cardiac catheterization findings of 1,100 cases. *Pediatr Cardiol* 7:3-9, 1986.

98. Paridon SM, Galioto FM, Vincent JA, et al: Exercise capacity and incidence of myocardial perfusion defects after Kawasaki disease in children and adolescents. *J Am Coll Cardiol* 25:1420-1424, 1995.
99. CAPRIE Steering Committee: A randomized, blinded trial of clopidogrel versus aspirin in patients at risk of ischemic events. *Lancet* 348:61-66, 1996.
100. Newburger JW, Burns JC: Kawasaki disease. *Vasc Med* 4:187-202, 1999.

CHAPTER 6

Treating Obesity in Youth: Should Dietary Glycemic Load Be a Consideration?

Cara B. Ebbeling, PhD
Instructor in Pediatrics, Harvard Medical School, Research Associate, Division of Endocrinology, Children's Hospital, Boston, Mass

David S. Ludwig, MD, PhD
Assistant Professor in Pediatrics, Harvard Medical School, Director, Obesity Program, Division of Endocrinology, Children's Hospital, Boston, Mass

ABSTRACT

Although the adverse effects of excess adiposity on health outcomes are widely recognized, there is no consensus regarding the most appropriate dietary strategies for managing obesity in youth. Recently, a novel dietary variable termed glycemic load has been postulated to influence hunger and body weight regulation. Glycemic load, a measure of the effects of a meal on blood glucose levels, is determined by the type and the amount of carbohydrate consumed. According to a hypothetical model, ingestion of high–glycemic load meals induces a sequence of hormonal changes that alter partitioning of metabolic fuels, exacerbate hunger, and over the long-term, promote weight gain. This chapter provides an overview of the available evidence suggesting that dietary glycemic load, and its related factor, the glycemic index, should be taken into consideration in the design of weight loss interventions.

The increasing prevalence of obesity[1,2] in youth is of major concern because excess adiposity elevates risk for physiologic and psychosocial morbidities across the lifespan.[3,4] Although dietary intervention constitutes an important component of most pediatric obesity treatment programs,[5] opinions vary regarding the optimal macronutrient composition of pediatric diets, irrespective of obesity status.[6-12] According to public health guidelines[13,14] conveyed in the Food Guide Pyramid[13] and recommendations for medical nutrition therapy,[15-17] a diet containing no more than 30% of total energy from fat is advocated for preventing and treating obesity and associated comorbidities. These guidelines and recommendations are based, in part, on the potential for excess dietary fat to increase caloric density, promoting positive energy balance and weight gain,[13] and the link between saturated fat intake and cardiovascular disease (CVD).[18] However, observational studies do not show a consistent relationship between dietary fat and adiposity in children and young adults.[19-22] Those who question current guidelines argue that data are lacking to substantiate a causal relationship between fat in pediatric diets and either development of atherosclerosis or risk for adult disease.[7,8] Furthermore, as the prevalence of obesity has continued to rise over the last 3 decades, a decrease in the contribution of fat to total energy intake has been associated with a compensatory and concomitant increase in carbohydrate.[6,23,24] Advocates of current dietary recommendations acknowledge the need to consider other factors in addition to dietary fat, such as the consumption of refined carbohydrates (including fruit juice), when treating obesity in youth.[10,12,25]

Traditionally, carbohydrates have been classified as simple (monosaccharides, disaccharides) or complex (polysaccharides, starches), based on chemical structure (degree of polymerization).[26,27] However, there is considerable overlap in the postprandial glycemic response to foods containing simple versus complex carbohydrates.[28] Beginning 20 years ago,[29-31] the traditional classification scheme has been increasingly recognized as an oversimplification with respect to the physiologic effects of carbohydrate. The glycemic index (GI), a concept first proposed by Jenkins et al,[29] represents an alternative method for characterizing carbohydrate type based on postprandial blood glucose responses to ingestion of carbohydrate-containing foods. The GI of a food is defined as the area under the glycemic response curve (AUC) 2 hours after consumption of a portion of food containing 50 g of carbohydrate divided by the AUC for a reference substance (ie, either glucose or white bread) containing the same absolute amount of carbohydrate.

$$\text{GI} = \frac{\text{AUC for test food}}{\text{AUC for reference}} \times 100$$

Foods listed among the most popular sources of energy in pediatric and adolescent diets (eg, breads, ready-to-eat cereals, potatoes, soft drinks, cakes, cookies)[32] have a high GI.[28] By contrast, intakes of nonstarchy vegetables and fruits, typically characterized by a low GI,[28] are insufficient relative to current public health guidelines.[33]

Because the GI does not consider carbohydrate amount,[34] a glycemic load variable has recently been used in epidemiologic data analyses[35-38] to fully characterize the effects of dietary patterns on postprandial glycemia. This chapter provides a systematic overview of the available evidence suggesting that glycemic load (ie, arithmetic product of carbohydrate amount and type) is an important consideration when treating obesity in youth, with emphasis directed towards the role of GI in modulating postprandial physiology and thereby influencing body weight. Data are reviewed using the framework of the hypothetical model presented in Fig 1. This model was developed based on findings from human studies focusing on acute responses to feeding, short-term intervention studies, animal research, and epidemiologic investigations.

DETERMINANTS OF GLYCEMIC LOAD

GLYCEMIC INDEX (CARBOHYDRATE TYPE)

Glycemic load can be effectively modulated at constant macronutrient intakes by selecting foods with the use of the GI concept.[39] For practical purposes, the GI of foods can be simply categorized as low (nonstarchy vegetables and fruits, legumes, nuts, milk, and the sugars fructose and lactose) (Table 1), moderate (unprocessed grain products, pasta, and the sugar sucrose), and high (refined grain products such as breads and ready-to-eat cereals, potatoes, and the sugar glucose).[28] Differences in GI among foods may be attributed to several factors affecting rates of digestion and absorption. These factors can be broadly classified relative to the chemical structure of carbohydrates per se[40-42] and properties of carbohydrate-containing foods.[42] With regard to chemical structure, the monomeric subunits of disaccharides and the glycosidic linkages in starch molecules influence rates of digestion and absorption. Food properties that influence GI include soluble fiber, food structure, and acidity (see below).

Comparisons among sugars with different chemical structures indicate that both sucrose (disaccharide: 1 glucose, 1 fructose; table sugar) and lactose (disaccharide: 1 glucose, 1 galactose; milk sugar) have lower GIs than many foods containing starch (glucose polymer).[28] Each monosaccharide is absorbed into the portal circulation. However, while a large portion of ingested glucose passes through the liver and enters the systemic circulation,[43] the liver is the primary site of fructose and galactose metabolism.[44] These

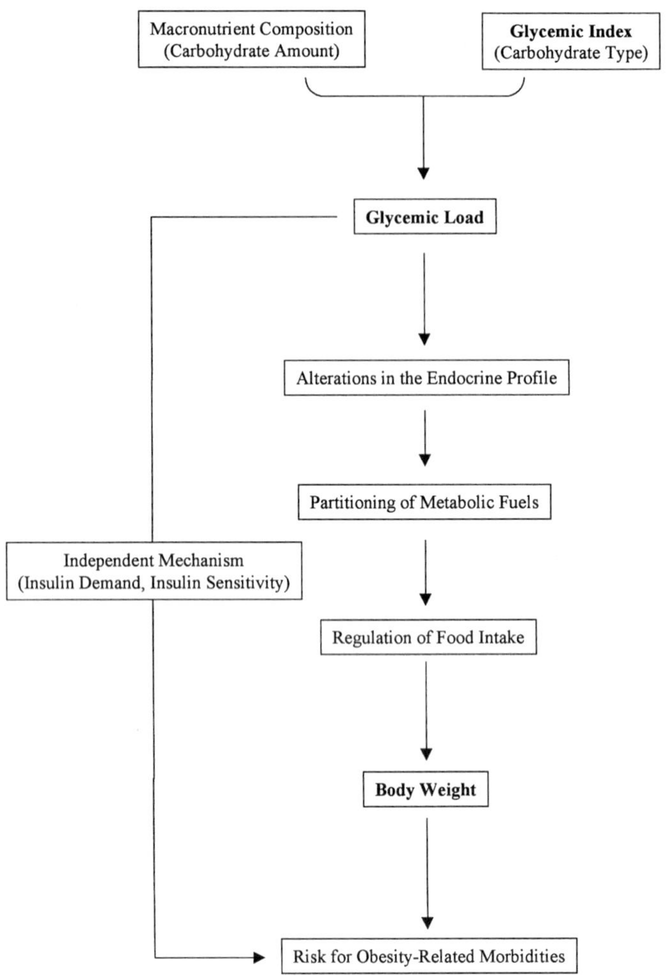

FIGURE 1.
Proposed model linking dietary glycemic index and load to body weight and obesity-related morbidities. Repeated ingestion of meals containing a high glycemic load (determined by amount and type of carbohydrate) elicits acute responses (ie, abrupt increase in blood glucose and rapid insulin response, followed by a period of reactive hypoglycemia and elevated levels of counterregulatory hormones) that direct partitioning of metabolic fuels towards storage. Diets designed to lower glycemic load may attenuate the postprandial insulin response, improve access to stored fuels, decrease hunger, and ultimately facilitate weight loss. A low–glycemic load diet also may reduce insulin demand and increase insulin sensitivity via a weight-independent mechanism, reducing risk for obesity-related morbidities such as type 2 diabetes.

TABLE 1.
Examples of Low Glycemic Index Foods

Nonstarchy Vegetables			
Alfalfa sprouts	Cabbage	Kohlrabi	Snow peas
Artichoke	Cauliflower	Leeks	Sauerkraut
Asparagus	Celery	Lettuce	Spinach
Bamboo shoots	Cucumber	Mushrooms	Summer squash
Beans (green, wax)	Eggplant	Okra	Swiss chard
	Green onions	Onions	Tomatoes
Bean sprouts	Greens (collard, endive, escarole, kale, mustard, turnip)	Peppers	Turnip
Bok choy		Radishes	Water chestnuts
Broccoli		Salsa	Zucchini
Brussels sprouts		Scallions	
Fresh Fruit			
Apples	Clementines	Lemon	Pears
Apricot	Grapefruit	Lime	Plums
Berries	Grapes	Nectarines	Tangelos
Cantaloupe	Honeydew	Oranges	Tangerines
Cherries	Kiwi	Peaches	
Legumes			
Black beans	Chickpeas (Garbanzo beans)	Lentils	Split peas
Black-eyed peas		Navy beans	Lima beans
	Hummus	Pinto beans	White (navy) beans
Butter beans	Kidney beans	Soy beans	
Nuts			
Almonds	Cashews	Peanut butter (natural)	Pistachios
Almond butter (natural)	Hazelnuts		Soy nuts
	Macadamia nuts	Pecans	Walnuts
Brazil nuts	Peanuts	Pine nuts	
Dairy			
Milk	Yogurt (plain, sugar-free flavored)		

monosaccharides are substrates for several metabolic pathways including glycolysis, glycogenesis, and gluconeogenesis.[44] Differences in hepatic metabolism likely account, in part, for the attenuated glycemic effects of foods containing sucrose and lactose in comparison with popular sources of energy derived from starch (eg, refined grain products, potatoes).

The GI of starch-containing foods depends, in part, on the chemical structure of the starch molecule. Two forms of starch are amylose and amylopectin. The amylose molecule is a linear structure in which the glucose residues are linked through α-1,4 glycosidic bonds. In contrast, amylopectin contains not only α-1,4 but also α-1,6 glycosidic bonds creating branch points. Consumption of amylose-rich rice,[45,46] crackers,[47] and muffins[48] induces blunted glycemic responses compared with analogous foods containing a relatively low amylose:amylopectin (Am:Ap) ratio. The branched structure of amylopectin may increase the surface area vulnerable to enzymatic attack by preventing the hydrogen bonding that stabilizes the linear structure of amylose.[47] With alterations in crystalline structure consequent to processing (eg, exposure to high temperatures, cooling, storage), amylose becomes more resistant to digestion compared with amylopectin.[49,50] However, although Am:Ap is among the factors affecting GI, the amylose and amylopectin contents of commercial and agricultural products have not been documented extensively.

Soluble fiber (guar gum, psyllium, β-glucan, pectin, an arabinoxylan) attenuates blood glucose responses to carbohydrate loads[51-56] by increasing the viscosity of partially digested food in the small intestine. Increased viscosity effectively enhances the thickness of the unstirred water layer, preventing rapid absorption of carbohydrate into the circulation.[57] Also, gastric emptying may be prolonged by soluble fiber,[56,58] although findings are inconsistent.[52,53] Irrespective of mechanism, soluble fiber thus has the potential to exert a beneficial effect on postprandial glycemia, whether provided as a natural component of food[54] or in extracted form as a supplement, enriched product, or recipe ingredient.[51-56]

Compared with soluble fiber, purified insoluble fiber has minimal effect on GI.[57] Nevertheless, the integrity of insoluble fiber (ie, structure of intact foods) is an important consideration.[39,59-62] Ingestion of fruit purée or juice, compared with intact fruit, causes exaggerated insulin responses and greater postabsorptive drops in blood glucose.[59,60] Likewise, progressive processing of grains (eg, whole grains to cracked grains to coarsely milled flour to finely milled flour) yields increasingly greater and less sustained glycemic and insulinemic responses.[39,61-64] Several mechanisms have been proposed to explain the effects of food structure on postprandial glycemia and insulinemia. For instance, undisrupted fiber may decrease accessibility of starch to digestive enzymes.[62] Foods with increased solidity require more chewing during ingestion,[59,61] and solidity may decrease the rate of gastric emptying.[61]

Acetic acid presented in the form of a salad dressing containing vinegar[65] or lactic acid in sourdough bread[66] is sufficient to attenuate the postprandial glycemic response to a carbohydrate load. However, the mechanism by which acid exerts a beneficial effect has not been fully elucidated. Although the provision of organic acids in relatively high concentrations reduces gastric emptying,[67] amounts of acid that can be easily obtained by adherence to simple dietary recommendations (ie, using oil and vinegar salad dressing, eating sourdough bread rather than white bread) apparently do not have a significant effect on the rate of carbohydrate delivery to the duodenum.[65,66]

CARBOHYDRATE AMOUNT AND MACRONUTRIENT COMPOSITION

When carbohydrate type (ie, GI) is held constant, glycemic load is affected by the absolute amount of carbohydrate ingested and compensatory changes in consumption of other macronutrients that independently modulate postprandial glycemia.[39,68] Reducing the contribution of carbohydrate to total energy intake, by increasing the contributions of fat and protein, attenuates glucose and insulin responses.[39] Furthermore, coingestion of fat and protein may attenuate GI, diminishing glycemic load at a given absolute level of dietary carbohydrate by altering physiologic responses to feeding.[69,70]

Fat slows gastric emptying and, thus, reduces the rate at which carbohydrate enters the small intestine and is absorbed into the circulation.[71,72] However, data are inconsistent with regard to the effect of fat coingestion on the insulin response to carbohydrate.[71,73-75] Collier et al[73,74] observed no change in the insulin response with addition of saturated fat (consumed in the form of butter) to a fixed amount of carbohydrate (consumed in the form of either potatoes or lentils). In contrast, Welch et al[71] noted a reduced insulin response when corn oil (a source of polyunsaturated fat) was added to a potato meal. Inconsistency among studies may be caused, in part, by differences in type of fat.

Protein may attenuate glycemic responses to carbohydrate ingestion given that it is an insulin secretagogue[69,76] and also stimulates release of glucagon.[77,78] Ingesting protein in combination with carbohydrate may help prevent relative hyperinsulinemia and hypoglucagonemia, maintaining availability of metabolic fuels and attenuating appetite.[39] Among the macronutrients, protein has the most pronounced effect on satiety and suppression of spontaneous energy intake.[79] Skov et al[80] noted that an ad libitum diet prescription containing 25% of energy as protein (45% carbohydrate, 30% fat) elicited greater weight loss in obese adults during a 6-month intervention period compared with a high-carbohydrate prescription (58% carbohydrate, 12% protein, 30% fat). Although this finding is consistent with the model presented in Fig 1, the investigators did not assess endocrine parameters or voluntary energy intake. The precise mechanism for the satiating effect of protein remains elusive and likely involves multiple variables (eg, amino acid profiles of specific proteins; effects of particular amino acids on digestion, insulin and glucagon kinetics, and the central nervous system).[81-83] There is no well-defined tolerable upper limit for dietary protein in obese but otherwise healthy patients, and the human body can adapt to a wide range of protein intakes.[84] Nevertheless, given the potentially adverse effects of excess protein on mineral homeostasis and kidney function,[85-87] prescription of dietary protein must depend on overall health status and existing comorbidities.

ACUTE RESPONSES TO INGESTION OF CARBOHYDRATE

ALTERATIONS IN THE ENDOCRINE PROFILE

The glycemic load of a meal markedly affects postprandial hormonal and metabolic responses, and these responses may mediate, in part, the influence of diet composition on body weight regulation. After ingestion of glucose (eg, in an oral glucose tolerance test), blood glucose and serum insulin levels initially increase rapidly, followed by a period of reactive hypoglycemia.[88-90] High GI foods induce similar patterns of change in blood glucose and insulin.[29,39,62,91] Many,[39,92-94] but not all,[95-97] studies have shown that the GI concept is relevant to mixed meals. Apparent discrepancies may reflect, in part, methodologic differences among studies. When the postprandial glycemic response is defined as the incremental rather than absolute AUC, the glycemic responses to mixed meals can be accurately ranked based on information regarding the GI values of component foods.[92]

Focusing specifically on obese adolescents, Ludwig et al[39] recently reported differential effects of mixed meals varying in carbohydrate amount and type. Patients consumed 3 different breakfasts on separate occasions. Two of the breakfasts were identical with respect to the contribution of macronutrients to total energy (64% carbohydrate, 16% protein, 20% fat) but varied in carbohydrate type (ie, steel-cut oats in which the structural integrity of the kernel is preserved in one meal versus high-GI instant oatmeal in the other meal). The third breakfast contained a vegetable omelet and was lower in the amount of carbohydrate (40% carbohydrate, 30% protein, 30% fat) and, consequently, glycemic load. Results are summarized in Fig 2. When the macronutrient composition was held constant, glycemic and insulinemic responses were reduced after the breakfast containing the low-GI steel-cut oats, as opposed to the high-GI instant oatmeal. Altering macronutrient composition by replacing carbohydrate with protein and fat, further attenuated responses beyond what could be achieved by altering only carbohydrate type. Blood glucose nadir was lowest for the instant oatmeal breakfast compared with the 2 other meals (a difference of 10 mg/dL). Plasma glucagon was suppressed after both high-carbohydrate breakfasts, presumably because of the inhibitory effects of hyperglycemia on glucagon secretion and the lower

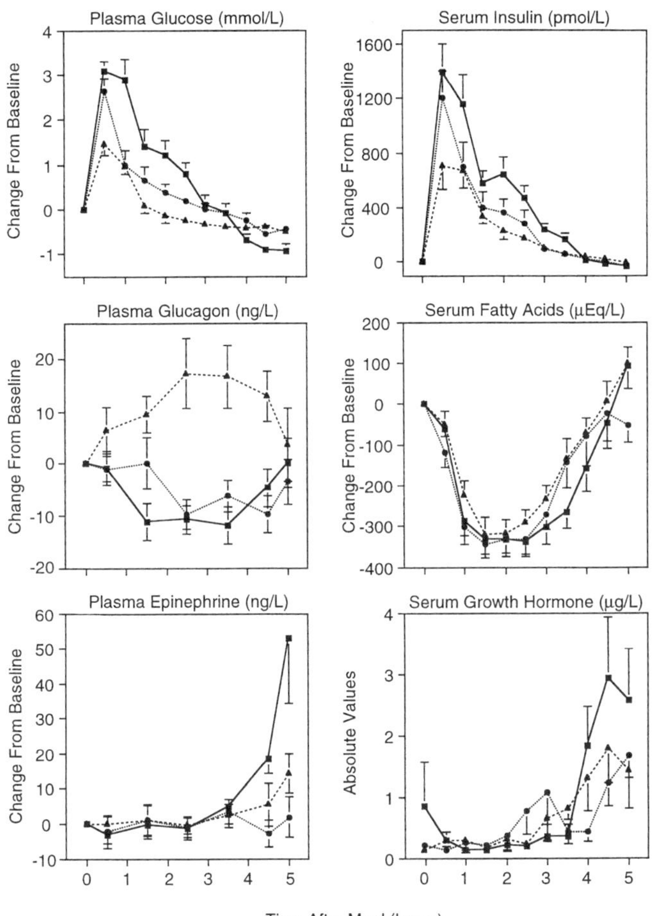

FIGURE 2.
Hormonal and metabolic changes in adolescent boys after consumption of test breakfasts. Plot symbols: *square,* instant oatmeal; *circle,* steel-cut oats; *triangle,* omelet. (Courtesy of Ludwig DS, Majzoub JA, Al-Zahrani A, et al: High glycemic index foods, overeating, and obesity. Reproduced by permission of *Pediatrics* 103:http://www.pediatrics.org/cgi/content/full/103/3/e26, copyright, 1999.)

protein content of these meals. By contrast, glucagon levels increased above baseline after consumption of the vegetable omelet. The concentration of circulating free fatty acids was suppressed to the greatest extent after the instant oatmeal breakfast. The counterregulatory hormones epinephrine and growth hormone increased markedly in the postabsorptive period after the instant oatmeal breakfast, but not after the other 2 meals, even though all meals had identical calorie content. Hunger ratings and voluntary food intake during the 5-hour postprandial period were highest after consumption of instant oatmeal and most attenuated after the vegetable omelet (data not shown). These findings suggest that high–glycemic load meals induce a sequence of hormonal changes that limit access to the 2 major metabolic fuels (glucose and fatty acids) in the postabsorptive period and may promote positive energy balance.

PARTITIONING OF METABOLIC FUELS

Data derived from animal research provide a mechanism relating glycemic load to energy metabolism. Specifically, the high insulin levels associated with consumption of high–glycemic load diets may favor partitioning of metabolic fuels from oxidation to storage. Cusin et al[98] found that insulin administration caused hypoglycemia, hyperphagia, and weight gain in rats. Moreover, insulin-treated rats compared with control rats showed increased insulin sensitivity in adipose tissue, but decreased insulin sensitivity in muscle tissue, during euglycemic-hyperinsulinemic clamps. In 2 studies conducted by Kabir et al,[99,100] rats were fed diets varying in GI for 3 weeks. Animals receiving high-GI (cornstarch, high amylopectin) compared with low-GI (mung bean starch, high amylose) starch demonstrated decreased insulin-stimulated glucose oxidation and increased incorporation of glucose into lipid, based on ^{14}C-glucose tracer studies.[99] Furthermore, consumption of the high-GI starch resulted in higher fatty acid synthase activity in adipose tissue and lower phosphoenolpyruvate carboxykinase mRNA in liver,[100] two key insulin-regulated lipogenic and gluconeogenic enzymes, respectively. In a human study, an energy-restricted diet with a low (vs high) glycemic load had beneficial effects on resting energy expenditure and nitrogen balance, possibly because of improved access to metabolic fuels during the active phase of weight loss.[101]

REGULATION OF FOOD INTAKE

Given that obesity is a disease of energy imbalance (ie, excess energy consumption relative to expenditure), the effects of endocrine-regulated partitioning of metabolic fuels on voluntary food intake is a critical component of the model linking glycemic load to weight control. With transient declines in blood glucose caused by elevated insulin levels, hunger increases as the body attempts to restore energy homeostasis.[102] Hypoglycemia or glucoprivation may preferentially stimulate consumption of high-GI foods,[103] leading to cycles of hypoglycemia and hyperphagia. Considering that hyperphagia may persist for an extended period after attainment of normal blood glucose levels,[104] such cycles may provide a plausible physiologic basis for generally poor long-term outcomes with conventional diet therapy often characterized by a high glycemic load.[105]

As summarized in Table 2, several studies have examined hunger, voluntary energy intake, and satiety in response to manipulation of dietary factors that affect GI. The vast majority of these studies suggest that GI is important in regulating acute food intake, thus lending support to the model presented in Fig 1. However, conclusions from investigations focusing specifically on glycosidic linkages (Table 2) are less consistent compared with those examining other factors influencing GI. Apparent inconsistencies may be attributed to differences in the Am:Ap range between high- and low-amylose meals, variable macronutrient compositions, and differences in food structure among investigations. Nevertheless, food structure and soluble fiber are arguably more critical considerations than the chemical structure of starch molecules when prescribing diets for weight loss. Results of several studies indicate that botanic and physical structure and soluble fiber (Table 2) influence satiety, hunger, and voluntary energy intake through effects on glycemic and insulinemic responses to test meals.

OUTCOMES OF SHORT-TERM INTERVENTION STUDIES

In several short-term intervention studies, glycemic load has been manipulated by altering carbohydrate type (ie, GI), with a focus on promoting weight loss and reducing risk for obesity-related morbidities (eg, type 2 diabetes, CVD) (Fig 1). An overview of the methods and outcomes of these studies is presented in Table 3 and discussed below.

BODY WEIGHT

Three studies have documented changes in body weight or composition with dietary interventions focusing on selection of low-GI foods. Participants in two of these studies were adults,[123,124] and one of the studies used data obtained from children who were treated for

Text continued on p. 201

TABLE 2.
Effects of Nutrient and Food Factors Influencing Glycemic Index on Hunger, Voluntary Energy Intake, and Satiety

Factor Influencing GI Reference	Relevant Dietary Comparison	Study Design	Effect of GI on Hunger, Voluntary Energy Intake, and Satiety
Monomeric Subunits	*Both sucrose (disaccharide: 1 glucose, 1 fructose; table sugar) and lactose (disaccharide: 1 glucose, 1 galactose; milk sugar) have a lower GI than many foods containing starch (glucose polymer).*		
Spitzer and Rodin[106]	Preload: 50 g glucose or 50 g fructose dissolved in 500 mL water	Random group assignment; Buffet at 2.25 hours after preload	Lower voluntary energy intake after fructose compared with glucose
Rodin et al[107]	Preload: 50 g glucose or 50 g fructose dissolved in 500 mL water	Random group assignment, with obese and lean subjects in each group; Buffet at 2.25 hours after preload	Lower voluntary energy intake after fructose compared with glucose; Reduced insulin secretion predictive of lower energy intake in obese subjects
Rodin[108]	Preload: 50 g glucose or 50 g fructose dissolved in 500 mL water	Within-subject design; Obese and lean subjects; Buffet at 38 minutes after preload	Lower voluntary energy intake after fructose compared with glucose; Relationship between plasma insulin levels and energy intake after glucose, but not fructose, for obese and lean subjects

Rodin[109]	Preload: 50 g glucose, 50 g fructose, or 50 g fructose + 15 g starch ingested in the form of pudding	Within-subject design; Buffet at 2.25 hours after preload	Lower voluntary energy intake after fructose compared with glucose; Attenuated effects of fructose on energy intake with addition of starch to preload; Glucose and fructose + starch elicited similar insulin responses
Kong et al[110]	Preload: 75 g glucose or 75 g fructose dissolved in 300 mL water	Within-subject design; Buffet at 2 hours after preload	No difference in voluntary energy intake after fructose compared with glucose
Glycosidic Linkages	*Glycemic potential is inversely related to the amylose:amylopectin ratio.*		
vanAmelsvoort and Weststrate[111]	Test meals with different Am:Ap (0.10 or 0.82); 62% (of energy) carbohydrate, 12% protein, 26% fat	Within-subject design; Hunger and satiety assessed for 6 hours after test meal	Greater satiety and less hunger at 4-6 hours after high amylose (Am:Ap = 0.82) meals
Weststrate and vanAmelsvoort[112]	Test meals with different Am:Ap (Breakfast: 0.06 or 0.63; Lunch: 0.29 or 0.59); Breakfast: 47% carbohydrate, 15% protein, 39% fat; Lunch: 53% carbohydrate, 12% protein, 34% fat	Within-subject design; Hunger and satiety assessed for 4 to 6 hours after test meals	No differences in satiety and hunger ratings attributed to amylose content of test meals
Granfeldt et al[113]	Test meals containing 50 g carbohydrate from barley varying in Am:Ap	Within-subject design; Satiety assessed for 3 hours after test meals	No differences in satiety among kernels varying in amylose; Higher amylose barley flour induced greater satiety
Holt and Brand Miller[114]	High- or low-amylose puffed rice cakes (50 g available carbohydrate)	Within-subject design; Satiety assessed for 2 hours after test meals	Greater satiety after consumption of high- compared with low-amylose rice cakes

(continued)

TABLE 2. (continued)

Factor Influencing GI Reference	Relevant Dietary Comparison	Study Design	Effect of GI on Hunger, Voluntary Energy Intake, and Satiety
Botanic and Physical Structure	*Disruption of plant structure with processing (eg, milling, puréeing) elicits products with higher GIs compared with intact foods.*		
Haber et al[59]	Whole apple, apple purée, or apple juice (60 g available carbohydrate)	Within-subject design; Satiety assessed for 3 hours after fruit, purée, or juice consumption	Whole fruit more satisfying than purée; Purée more satisfying than juice; Greater satiety for up to 2 hours for whole fruit and purée compared with juice
Bolton et al[60]	Grapes or grape juice (30 g glucose, 30 g fructose) Orange or orange juice (12 g glucose, 15 g fructose, 23 g sucrose)	Within-subject design; Satiety/hunger assessed for 3 hours after fruit or juice consumption	Greater satiety for up to 2 hours after consumption of whole fruit compared with juice
Leathwood and Pollet[115]	Test meals containing potato (32.9 g carbohydrate) or bean (24.5 g carbohydrate) purée	Within-subject design; Hunger assessed for 4 hours after test meals	Delayed return of hunger after test meals containing bean, compared with potato, purée
Holt and Brand Miller[61]	Test meals containing differentially processed wheat: whole grain, cracked grain, course flour, fine flour	Within-subject design; Satiety assessed for 2 hours after test meals	Trend for smaller particle sizes to reduce satiety; Satiety correlated with insulin response
Gustafsson et al[116]	Test meals containing raw or cooked carrots	Within-subject design; Satiety assessed for 3.5 hours after test meals	Greater satiety for up to 3 hours after consumption of raw compared with cooked carrots

Gustafsson et al[117]	Isocaloric test meals in which potato powder was partially substituted with spinach (equivalent amounts of digestible carbohydrate)	Within subject design; Satiety assessed for 3.5 hours after test meals	Greater satiety with spinach compared with potato powder; Similar results whether spinach was cut or minced
Holt and Brand Miller[114]	Ordinary or quick-cooking rice (50 g available carbohydrate)	Within-subject design; Satiety assessed for 2 hours after test meals	Greater satiety after consumption of ordinary, compared with quick-cooking rice
Benini et al[118]	Test meals in which physical structure was disrupted by removal of fiber (high-fiber vs low-fiber meals)	Within-subject design; Hunger and satiety assessed for 5 hours after test meals	Delayed return of hunger with high-fiber meal; No difference in satiety ratings between meals
Holt et al[119]	Test meals (breakfasts) containing corn flakes or All-Bran	Within-subject design; Voluntary energy intake assessed by weighed food diaries throughout the day	Less voluntary energy intake at lunch after All-Bran breakfast
Ludwig et al[39]	Test meals containing instant oatmeal or steel-cut oats (identical meal fed for breakfast and then lunch on same day)	Within-subject design; Hunger assessed for 5 hours after breakfast (with simultaneous evaluation of glycemic response); Voluntary energy intake measured for 5 hours after lunch	Less hunger and voluntary energy intake after consumption of steel-cut oats; Glycemic response predicted energy intake
Soluble Fiber	*Viscosity of soluble fiber modulates GI by preventing rapid absorption of carbohydrate into the circulation.*		
Krotkiewski[120]	Guar gum or wheat bran, 10 g, twice daily (before lunch and dinner)	Within-subject design; Treatment alternated weekly for approximately 6 weeks; Each fiber consumed for approximately 3 weeks; Hunger ratings obtained before breakfast, lunch, dinner, and evening snack	Guar gum reduced hunger ratings compared with wheat bran

(continued)

TABLE 2. (continued)

Factor Influencing GI Reference	Relevant Dietary Comparison	Study Design	Effect of GI on Hunger, Voluntary Energy Intake, and Satiety
DiLorenzo et al[58]	Pectin or methylcellulose, 15 g, added to an egg sandwich meal	Within-subject design; Satiety assessed for approximately 2 hours after consumption of the fiber preload; Documentation of time to next meal	Greater satiety and prolonged time to the next meal after consumption of pectin versus methylcellulose
Lavin and Read[52]	Preload: 300-kcal glucose drink with or without 5 g guar gum	Within-subject design; Hunger and satiety assessed for 3 hours after preload; Preselected meal at 3.5 hours after preload	Greater satiety and less hunger after consumption of guar gum; No difference in voluntary energy intake during test meal; Guar gum decreased postprandial glycemia and insulinemia
Rigaud et al[53]	Psyllium (7.4 g) or placebo given 15 minutes before a test meal (450 kcal) provided at approximately noon	Within-subject design; Hunger assessed for 6 hours after test meal; Voluntary energy intake recorded during the interval between test meal and bedtime	Psyllium reduced hunger and voluntary energy intake, associated with attenuated postprandial glycemia and insulinemia

Acidity	*Organic acids attenuate postprandial glycemia via a mechanism that has not been fully elucidated.*		
Liljeberg and Bjorck[66]	Meals containing whole meal bread (reference), bread with lactic acid (similar to amount formed during sourdough fermentation), bread with sodium propionate (acid load, on a molar basis, 3 times higher than lactic acid)	Within-subject design; Satiety assessed for 3 hours after consumption of test meals	No difference in satiety after consumption of lactic acid compared with reference bread; Greater satiety after consumption of sodium propionate compared with reference bread
Multiple Factors			
Holt et al[121]	Test meals containing different breakfast cereals (35.8 g available carbohydrate)	Within-subject design; Satiety assessed for 3 hours after test meals	Inverse relationship between satiety score and both glycemic index and insulin response
Holt et al[122]	Preload: 1 of 38 test foods representing 6 food categories (bakery products, snacks and confectionery, breakfast cereals, carbohydrate-rich foods, protein-rich foods, fruits), isoenergetic portions containing variable amounts of carbohydrate	Separate groups of subjects for each food category; Satiety assessed for 2 hours after preload; Standard ad libitum meal provided at 2 hours after preload	No relationships between satiety and plasma glucose or insulin responses; Negative association between food intake and insulin response

Abbreviations: GI, Glycemic index; *Am:Ap,* amylose:amylopectin.

TABLE 3.
Potential Benefits of Manipulating Glycemic Index Based on Short-term Intervention Studies

Reference	Subjects	Study Design	Intervention Strategy	Outcomes
Jenkins et al[139]	Patients (3 women, 9 men) with hyperlipidemia; Age (range): 40-72 years; Percent of ideal weight (range): 94-127	Three 1-month sequential study periods (Pretest: lipid clinic diet; Test: low-GI diet; Posttest: lipid clinic diet)	Outpatient dietary counseling with an exchange system; weight-maintaining	Reductions in serum cholesterol (total, LDL) and triglycerides with low-GI diet
Jenkins et al[140]	Patients (8 women, 22 men) with hyperlipidemia; 3 treated with cholestyramine; Middle-aged; Nonobese	Three 1-month sequential study periods (Pretest: lipid clinic diet; Test: low-GI diet; Posttest: lipid clinic diet)	Outpatient dietary counseling with an exchange system; weight-maintaining	Reductions in serum cholesterol (total, LDL) with low-GI diet; Changes most pronounced for patients with hyperlipidemia
Jenkins et al[136]	6 healthy men; Age (mean): approximately 33 years; Percent ideal weight (mean): approximately 104	Randomized cross-over, two 2-week intervention periods (isocaloric high- vs low-GI diets)	Outpatient feeding study; Diet composition held constant (61% carbohydrate, 19% protein, 20%fat); weight-maintaining	Significant decrease in fructosamine and serum cholesterol during low-GI period; Greater decrease in urinary c-peptide and flatter AUC for 12-hour blood glucose during low-GI period
Jenkins et al[141]	Patients (6 women, 2 men) with type 2 diabetes; 6 patients treated with insulin and 2 with oral agents; Age (range): 51 to 70 years; Percent ideal weight (range): 109 to 150	Randomized crossover, two 2-week intervention periods (high- vs low-GI diets)	Outpatient study (provision of preweighed carbohydrate-containing foods and menu plans); Diet composition held relatively constant (53% to 54% carbohydrate, 21% to 22% protein, 24% to 26% fat)	Reduction in body weight, serum cholesterol, and fructosamine over both periods; Decreases in fasting blood glucose and HbA1c over low-GI period only

Collier et al[142]	Children (1 girl, 6 boys) with type 1 diabetes; Age (range): 7 to 17 years; Percent normal weight (range): 92 to 112	Randomized crossover, two 6-week intervention periods (control vs low-GI diets)	Outpatient dietary counseling using an exchange system; diet composition: 47% to 49% carbohydrate, 16% to 18% protein, 33% to 37% fat; Caloric intake similar for both periods	Incremental blood glucose, glycosolated albumin, and cholesterol decreased during low-GI period, no change during control period
Brand et al[143]	Patients (6 women, 10 men) with type 2 diabetes; 10 treated with sulfonylureas; Age (mean ± SD): 62 ± 9 years; BMI (mean ± SD): 25 ± 5 kg/m^2	Randomized crossover, two 12-week intervention periods (isocaloric high- vs low-GI diets)	Outpatient dietary counseling; diet composition: 44% to 46% carbohydrate, 19% to 22% protein, 30% to 31% fat	HbA1c lower after low-GI diet; Lower integrated AUC for plasma glucose on profile days (provision of standard high- or low-GI meals during respective periods) with low-GI diet; No changes in plasma lipids
Wolever et al[144]	Patients (8 women, 7 men) with type 2 diabetes; 4 treated with insulin and 9 with glibenclamide; Age (mean): approximately 67 years; Weight (mean): approximately 70 kg	Randomized crossover, two 2-week intervention periods (high- vs low-GI diets)	Outpatient study (provision of selected foods, patients required to purchase other foods according to specified menu plan); Weight-maintaining energy prescriptions for 9 of the patients; Hypocaloric prescriptions to induce weight loss of 0.5-1 kg/wk for 6 patients who were overweight or obese; Diet composition (58% to 59%carbohydrate, 20% protein, 21% to 22% fat) held constant	Fasting serum fructosamine dropped more with the low-GI diet; Urinary c-peptide and serum cholesterol lower with low-GI diet

(continued)

TABLE 3. (continued)

Reference	Subjects	Study Design	Intervention Strategy	Outcomes
Wolever et al[145]	Patients (3 women, 3 men) with type 2 diabetes; Age (range): 53 to 72 years; BMI (range): 24.5-39.3 kg/m^2	Randomized crossover, two 6-week intervention periods (high- vs low-GI diets)	Outpatient study (provision of selected foods, patients required to purchase other foods according to specified menu plan); Hypocaloric to induce weight loss of 0.5-1 kg/wk; Diet composition (57% carbohydrate, 23% fat, 20% protein) held constant	No difference in weight loss or drop in fasting blood glucose between periods; Decrease in fructosamine and cholesterol on low-GI diet with no change on high-GI diet
Fontvieille et al[146]	Patients with type 1 (2 women, 10 men) or type 2 (4 women, 2 men) diabetes; 6 patients with type 2 diabetes treated with hypoglycemic agents; Age (mean ± SD): 47.2 ± 11.6 years; BMI (mean ± SD): 24.8 ± 2.6 kg/m^2	Randomized crossover, two 5-week intervention periods (isocaloric high- vs low-GI diets)	Outpatient dietary counseling; Nutrient intakes (including total and soluble fiber) held constant; Diet composition: 45% to 46% carbohydrate; 18% to 19% protein; 36% fat	No differences between type 1 and type 2 diabetic patients for measured outcomes; Improvements in fructosamine and serum triglycerides with the low-GI diet; No differences between diets for body weight, HbA1c, and other blood lipids
Frost et al[147]	Patients (15 women, 36 men) with type 2 diabetes; Age (mean): approximately 54 to 56 years; BMI (mean): approximately 29 to 30 kg/m^2	Randomized trial, parallel design; 12-week intervention period (conventional vs low-GI diets)	Outpatient dietary counseling; Prescriptions for energy and diet composition (50% carbohydrate, 35% fat, 15% protein) consistent between groups	Greater reductions in fructosamine and cholesterol with low-GI diet

Slabber et al[123]	30 hyperinsulinemic women; Age (mean): approximately 35 years; BMI (mean): approximately 35 kg/m^2	Randomized trial, parallel design; 12-week intervention period (conventional vs low-GI diets)	Outpatient dietary counseling with energy restriction imposed with exchange lists; Diet composition (50% carbohydrate, 30% fat, 20% protein) consistent between groups	Greater weight loss and drop in fasting serum insulin with low-GI diet
Kiens and Richter[148]	7 healthy lean men; Age (range): 20 to 30 years; Body mass (range): 63 to 83 kg	Randomized crossover, two 30-day intervention periods (isocaloric high- vs low-GI diets)	Outpatient feeding study; Diet composition (46% to 47% carbohydrate, 41% fat, 13% to 14% protein) held constant; Dietary fiber higher for low- compared with high-GI diet	No changes in fasting blood glucose or insulin; Whole-body glucose disposal (euglycemic hyperinsulinemic clamp at end of intervention period): similar across diets at low plasma insulin level, decreased at high insulin level with the low-GI diet
Frost et al[149]	28 healthy women; 16 (of 28) with parental history of premature coronary heart disease; Age (median): 34 to 37 years; BMI (median): 23 to 25 kg/m^2	Randomized trial, parallel design; 3-week intervention period (isocaloric high- vs low-GI diets)	Outpatient dietary counseling	Insulin sensitivity improved with the low-GI vs high-GI diet, irrespective of medical history
Jarvi et al[137]	Patients (5 women, 15 men) with type 2 diabetes; Age (range): 50 to 77 years; BMI (mean ± SD): 25.3 ± 2.7 kg/m^2	Randomized crossover, two 24-day intervention periods (isocaloric high- vs low-GI diets)	Outpatient feeding study (preweighed diets); Diet composition held constant (55% carbohydrate, 28% fat, 16% protein); Weight-maintaining	Incremental AUC for blood glucose and insulin lower for low-GI diet during a profile day; Greater decreases in serum fructosamine and cholesterol (total, LDL) with low-GI diet; PAI-1 decreased with low-GI but remained unchanged with high-GI diet

(continued)

TABLE 3. (continued)

Reference	Subjects	Study Design	Intervention Strategy	Outcomes
Luscombe et al[150]	Patients (7 women, 14 men) with type 2 diabetes; 16 patients treated with oral hypoglycemic agents; Age (mean ± SD): 57.4 ± 13.3 years; BMI (mean ± SD): 30.4 ± 5.0 kg/m^2	Randomized crossover, three 4-week intervention periods (high-carbohydrate, low-GI diet; high-monounsaturated fat, high-GI diet; high-carbohydrate, high-GI diet)	Outpatient study with provision of specific study foods and menus; Relatively constant levels of saturated fat, fiber, and protein; High-monounsaturated fat diet provided slightly more energy than other diets	No difference among diets for fasting plasma glucose, fructosamine, plasma insulin, or urinary c-peptide; HDL-cholesterol higher on high-monounsaturated fat and low-GI diets compared with high-GI diet
Spieth et al[125]	Children (58 girls, 49 boys); Age (mean): approximately 10 years; BMI (mean): approximately 33 kg/m^2	Retrospective cohort study of children attending an outpatient obesity program (reduced-fat vs low-GI diet prescriptions); Average length of follow-up: approximately 4 months	Dietary counseling; Reduced fat (n = 43): –250 to –500 kcal/d, 55% to 60% carbohydrate, 15% to 20% protein, 25% to 30% fat; Ad libitum low-GI (n = 64): 45% to 50% carbohydrate, 20% to 25% protein, 30% to 35% fat	Greater decreases in BMI and body weight with low-GI diet
Bouche et al[124]	11 overweight men	Double-blind crossover, two 5-week intervention periods (high- vs low-GI diets)	Energy and macronutrient intakes consistent between periods	Greater decrease in fat mass (measured by dual x-ray absorptiometry) with low-GI diet
Giacco et al[151]	Patients (33 women, 21 men) with type 1 diabetes; Age (mean): approximately 28 years; BMI (mean): approximately 24 kg/m^2	Randomized trial, parallel design, 24-week intervention period (high- vs low-fiber diets varying in GI)	Outpatient dietary counseling; Diet composition (50% carbohydrate, 30% fat, 20% protein) consistent between groups	Reductions in mean daily blood glucose concentrations, HbA1c, and number of hypoglycemic events with the high-fiber (low-GI) diet

Abbreviations: GI, Glycemic index; *LDL,* low-density lipoprotein; *AUC,* area under curve; *HbAlc,* hemoglobin Alc; *BMI,* body mass index; *PAI-1,* plasminogen activator inhibitor 1; *HDL,* high-density lipoprotein.

obesity in an outpatient hospital-based clinic.[125] Slabber et al[123] prescribed diets containing 50% carbohydrate, 20% protein, and 30% fat to obese, hyperinsulinemic women who were assigned to 1 of 2 treatment groups for 12 weeks. One of the groups was instructed to obtain carbohydrates from relatively low- and moderate-GI foods (eg, lentils, pasta), avoiding high-GI products (eg, white bread). For the other group, carbohydrate-containing foods were not differentiated based on GI. Although postprandial changes in endocrine metabolism were not evaluated, a greater decrease in serum insulin levels under fasting conditions was accompanied by more weight loss (mean ± SD: –9.35 ± 2.49 vs –7.41 ± 4.23 kg) for the group consuming the low-GI foods. In a recent study focusing on overweight men, Bouche et al[124] used a crossover design (5-week intervention periods) to examine the effects of low- versus high-GI diets. Although there were no detectable differences in body weight at the end of the 2 intervention periods, abdominal fat mass, determined by dual-energy x-ray absorptiometry, was significantly lower after the low-GI diet, based on a preliminary report.

A recent retrospective analysis of data from children who received dietary counseling in an outpatient obesity clinic suggests that therapy focusing on reducing glycemic load may be more effective for treating obesity than a conventional low-fat diet.[125] The low–glycemic load prescription focused on selection of low-GI foods and had a targeted macronutrient composition of 45% to 50% carbohydrate, 20% to 25% protein, and 30% to 35% fat. Patients were instructed to eat to satiety and snack when hungry. There was no prescription-imposed caloric restriction. In contrast, the low-fat diet prescription incorporated an energy restriction of 250 to 500 kcal/d compared with usual intake, with a targeted macronutrient intake of 55% to 60% carbohydrate, 15% to 20% protein, and 25% to 30% fat. Patients who were prescribed the low–glycemic load diet had an average decrease in body mass index (BMI) that was significantly greater than those who received the low-fat prescription (–1.53 kg/m^2, 95% confidence interval [CI]: –1.94 to –1.12 vs –0.06 kg/m^2, 95% CI: –0.56 to 0.44). In multivariate models, this difference remained significant after adjustment for potentially confounding variables (ie, age, gender, ethnicity, baseline weight status, referral to behavioral therapy, treatment duration). Although these findings must be considered preliminary because patients were not formally randomly assigned to treatment groups, the data are consistent with the model presented in Figure 1.

GLUCOSE HOMEOSTASIS AND RISK FOR CVD

The emerging type 2 diabetes epidemic in the pediatric population has been attributed, in large part, to the increase in prevalence of obesity.[126,127] Indeed, most children and adolescents who receive a diagnosis of type 2 diabetes are overweight or obese,[128,129] and pediatric populations with the greatest prevalence of obesity also have the highest rates of type 2 diabetes.[127,130] Furthermore, insulin resistance and type 2 diabetes in children are associated with an increased risk for CVD.[127,131] Although weight management typically is recommended for preventing or treating type 2 diabetes and thereby reducing risk for disease,[128] the importance of GI in medical nutrition therapy is a topic of debate.[132-134]

Studies examining the utility of GI for improving glycemic control, reducing CVD risk factors, or both, typically have been designed to prevent changes in body weight, possibly limiting the full benefits of low-GI diets in the context of the model presented in Fig 1. Nevertheless, improvements in glycemic control and reductions in risk for CVD, independent of weight loss (Fig 1), have been documented in several intervention studies with low-GI diets (Table 3). With regard to diabetes prevention through a mechanism independent of weight loss, diets composed of low-GI foods elicit lower insulin levels and less c-peptide secretion compared with high-GI diets when calorie intake is held constant.[135,136] A decrease in insulin demand, accompanied by an increase in insulin sensitivity independent of weight loss,[137] may help prevent β-cell "exhaustion" that precipitates frank type 2 diabetes.[138]

CHRONIC EFFECTS OF DIETARY GLYCEMIC LOAD

Although data from long-term (ie, ≥1 year) intervention studies focusing on dietary glycemic load are presently nonexistent, findings from epidemiologic investigations suggest that glycemic load is an important variable with regard to risk for obesity[22] and related morbidities, including type 2 diabetes[35,36] and CVD.[37,38,152] Concerning obesity, Ludwig et al[22] examined the influence of dietary fiber, a predictor of GI,[153] on weight gain in the Coronary Artery Risk Development in Young Adults (CARDIA) Study. They noted that fiber intake was inversely associated with fasting blood insulin levels and weight gain, speculating that the reduced glycemic response of high-fiber diets was implicated in the underlying mechanism for the observed associations. Data from the Nurses' Health Study[36] and Health Professionals' Follow-up Study[35] indicate significantly higher prevalence rates of diabetes among individuals in the highest quintile of glycemic load compared with those in the lowest quintile, after adjustment for BMI and other potentially confounding variables. With regard to CVD, Frost et al[152] noted an inverse relationship between GI and serum high-density lipoprotein (HDL) cholesterol concentrations in the Survey of British Adults. Consistent with this finding, glycemic load was associated with risk for a coronary event in the Nurses' Health Study.[38]

SUMMARY AND CONCLUSIONS

To answer the question posed in the title of this chapter, available data reviewed in the context of the hypothetical model presented in Fig 1 argue for the importance of considering dietary glycemic load when treating obesity in youth. However, even among those who agree that the utility of low-fat diets for weight loss and prevention of related comorbidities must be scrutinized, opinions vary with regard to appropriate strategies for reducing glycemic load. Some practitioners argue that decreasing the amount of carbohydrate, rather than attempting to alter carbohydrate type, should be a main focus of diet prescriptions, given that application of the GI concept may be too complex for most patients.[133] Nevertheless, the data reviewed herein indicate that modulating carbohydrate type (ie, GI) can have potentially beneficial acute and chronic effects at carbohydrate intakes approximating current public health guidelines and recommendations for medical nutrition therapy. When presented in the context of a modified food pyramid (level 1: vegetables, fruits; level 2: reduced-fat dairy, lean protein, nuts, and legumes; level 3: unrefined grains and pasta; level 4: refined grains, potatoes, sweets),[154] children and adolescents can understand and apply the concept.[125] Because many of the most popular foods consumed by children[32] are located on levels 3 and 4 of this pyramid, there may be great potential for attaining not only clinical but also public health benefits by recommending diets characterized by a low glycemic load. Nevertheless, randomized clinical trials comparing the effectiveness of low glycemic load versus conventional diet prescriptions are a necessary prerequisite to resolving controversy with respect to dietary therapy for treatment of pediatric obesity.

REFERENCES

1. Troiano RP, Flegal KM, Kuczmarski RJ, et al: Overweight prevalence and trends for children and adolescents: The National Health and Nutrition Examination Surveys, 1963 to 1991. *Arch Pediatr Adolesc Med* 149:1085-1091, 1995.

2. Seidell JC: Obesity: A growing problem. *Acta Paediatr Suppl* 428:46-50, 1999.
3. Dietz WH: Health consequences of obesity in youth: Childhood predictors of adult disease. *Pediatrics* 101:518-525, 1998.
4. Must A, Strauss RS: Risks and consequences of childhood and adolescent obesity. *Int J Obes* 23:S2-S11, 1999.
5. Jelalian E, Saelens BE: Empirically supported treatments in pediatric psychology: Pediatric obesity. *J Pediatr Psychol* 24:223-248, 1999.
6. Milner JA, Allison RG: The role of dietary fat in child nutrition and development: Summary of an ASNS workshop. *J Nutr* 129:2094-2105, 1999.
7. Olsen RE: Is it wise to restrict fat in the diets of children? *J Am Diet Assoc* 100:28-32, 2000.
8. Satter E: A moderate view on fat restriction for young children. *J Am Diet Assoc* 100:32-36, 2000.
9. Dwyer J: Should dietary fat recommendations for children be changed? *J Am Diet Assoc* 100:36-37, 2000.
10. Krebs NF, Johnson SL: Guidelines for healthy children: Promoting eating, moving, and common sense. *J Am Diet Assoc* 100:137-139, 2000.
11. Lytle LA: In defense of a low-fat diet for healthy children. *J Am Diet Assoc* 100:39-41, 2000.
12. VanHorn L: Primary prevention of cardiovascular disease starts in childhood. *J Am Diet Assoc* 100:41-42, 2000.
13. US Department of Health and Human Services, US Department of Agriculture: Dietary guidelines for Americans. http://www.usda.gov/cnpp/Pubs/DG2000/Index.htm, 2000.
14. Johnson RK, Nicklas TA: Position of the American Dietetic Association: Dietary guidance for healthy children aged 2 to 11 years. *J Am Diet Assoc* 99:93-101, 1999.
15. Gidding SS, Leibel RL, Daniels S, et al: Understanding obesity in youth. *Circulation* 94:3383-3387, 1996.
16. American Academy of Pediatrics, Committee on Nutrition: Cholesterol in childhood. *Pediatrics* 101:141-147, 1998.
17. American Academy of Pediatrics, Committee on Nutrition: *Pediatric Nutrition Handbook,* ed 4. Elk Grove Village, Ill, American Academy of Pediatrics, 1998.
18. Fisher EA, VanHom L, McGill HC: A statement for healthcare professionals from the nutrition committee, American Heart Association. *Circulation* 95:2332-2333, 1997.
19. Atkin L-M, Davies PSW: Diet composition and body composition in preschool children. *Am J Clin Nutr* 72:15-21, 2000.
20. Gazzaniga JM, Bums TL: Relationship between diet composition and body fatness, with adjustment for resting energy expenditure and physical activity, in preadolescent children. *Am J Clin Nutr* 58:21-28, 1993.
21. Tucker LA, Seljaas GT, Hager RL: Body fat percentage of children varies according to their diet composition. *J Am Diet Assoc* 97:981-986, 1997.

22. Ludwig DS, Pereira MA, Kroenke CH, et al: Dietary fiber, weight gain and cardiovascular disease risk factors in young adults: The CARDIA Study. *JAMA* 282:1539-1546, 1999.
23. Hu FB, Stampfer MJ, Manson JE, et al: Trends in the incidence of coronary heart disease and changes in diet and lifestyle in women. *N Engl J Med* 343:530-537, 2000.
24. Cavadini C, Siega-Riz AM, Popkin BM: US adolescent food intake trends from 1965 to 1996. *Arch Dis Child* 83:18-24, 2000.
25. Barlow SE, Dietz WH: Obesity evaluation and treatment: Expert committee recommendations. *Pediatrics* 102:http://www. pediatrics.org/cgi /content/full/102/3/e29, 1998.
26. Technical Committee on Carbohydrates: Complex carbohydrates: The science and the label. *Nutr Rev* 53:186-193, 1995.
27. Asp N-G: Nutritional classification and analysis of food carbohydrates. *Am J Clin Nutr* 59:679S-681S, 1994.
28. Foster-Powell K, Brand Miller J: International tables of glycemic index. *Am J Clin Nutr* 62:871S-890S, 1995.
29. Jenkins DJA, Wolever TMS, Taylor RH, et al: Glycemic index of foods: A physiological basis for carbohydrate exchange. *Am J Clin Nutr* 34:362-366, 1981.
30. Crapo PA, Olefsky JM: Food fallacies and blood sugar. *N Engl J Med* 309:44-45, 1983.
31. Hollenbeck CB, Coulston AM, Donner CC, et al: The effects of variations in percent of naturally occurring complex and simple carbohydrates on plasma glucose and insulin response in individuals with non-insulin-dependent diabetes mellitus. *Diabetes* 34:151-155, 1985.
32. Subar AF, Krebs-Smith SM, Cook A, et al: Dietary sources of nutrients among US children, 1989-1991. *Pediatrics* 102:913-923, 1998.
33. Krebs-Smith SM, Cook A, Subar AF, et al: Fruit and vegetable intakes of children and adolescents in the United States. *Arch Pediatr Adolesc Med* 150:81-86, 1996.
34. Wolever TMS, Jenkins DJA, Jenkins AL, et al: The glycemic index: Methodology and clinical implications. *Am J Clin Nutr* 54:846-854, 1991.
35. Salmeron J, Ascherio A, Rimm EB, et al: Dietary fiber, glycemic load, and risk of NIDDM in men. *Diabetes Care* 20:545-550, 1997.
36. Salmeron J, Manson JE, Stampfer MJ, et al: Dietary fiber, glycemic load, and risk of non-insulin-dependent diabetes mellitus in women. *JAMA* 277:472-477, 1997.
37. Stampfer MJ, Hu FB, Manson JE, et al: Primary prevention of coronary heart disease in women through diet and lifestyle. *N Engl J Med* 343:16-22, 2000.
38. Liu S, Willett WC, Stampfer MJ, et al: A prospective study of dietary glycemic load, carbohydrate intake, and risk of coronary heart disease in women. *Am J Clin Nutr* 71:1455-1461, 2000.
39. Ludwig DS, Majzoub JA, Al-Zahrani A, et al: High glycemic index

foods, overeating, and obesity. *Pediatrics* 103:http://www.pediatrics.org/cgi/content/full/103/3/e26, 1999.
40. Wolever TMS, Wong GS, Kenshole A, et al: Lactose in the diabetic diet: A comparison with other carbohydrates. *Nutr Res* 5:1335-1345, 1985.
41. Gannon MC, Nuttall FQ, Krezowski PA, et al: The serum insulin and plasma glucose responses to milk and fruit products in type 2 (non-insulin-dependent) diabetic patients. *Diabetologia* 29:784-791, 1986.
42. Bjorck I, Granfeldt Y, Liljeberg H, et al: Food properties affecting the digestion and absorption of carbohydrates. *Am J Clin Nutr* 59:699S-705S, 1994.
43. Jackson RA, Roshania RD, Hawa MI, et al: Impact of glucose ingestion on hepatic and peripheral glucose metabolism in man: An analysis based on simultaneous use of the forearm and double isotope techniques. *J Clin Endocrinol Metab* 63:541-549, 1986.
44. Groff JL, Gropper SS: *Advanced Nutrition and Human Metabolism,* ed 3. Belmont, Calif, Wadsworth, 2000.
45. Goddard MS, Young G, Marcus R: The effect of amylose content on insulin and glucose responses to ingested rice. *Am J Clin Nutr* 39:388-392, 1984.
46. Brand Miller J: Rice: A high or low glycemic index food? *Am J Clin Nutr* 56:1034-1036, 1992.
47. Behall KM: Effect of starch structure on glucose and insulin responses in adults. *Am J Clin Nutr* 47:428-432, 1988.
48. Krezowski PA, Nuttall FQ, Gannon MC, et al: Insulin and glucose responses to various starch-containing foods in type II diabetic subjects. *Diabetes Care* 10:205-212, 1987.
49. Champ MM, Molis C, Flourie B, et al: Small-intestinal digestion of partially resistant cornstarch in healthy subjects. *Am J Clin Nutr* 68:705-710, 1998.
50. Vonk RJ, Hagedoorn RE, deGraaff R, et al: Digestion of so-called resistant starch sources in the human small intestine. *Am J Clin Nutr* 72:432-438, 2000.
51. Jenkins DJA, Wolever TMS, Nineham R, et al: Improved glucose tolerance four hours after taking guar with glucose. *Diabetologia* 19:21-24, 1980.
52. Lavin JH, Read NW: The effect on hunger and satiety of slowing the absorption of glucose: Relationship with gastric emptying and postprandial blood glucose and insulin responses. *Appetite* 25:89-96, 1995.
53. Rigaud D, Paycha F, Meulemans A, et al: Effect of psyllium on gastric emptying, hunger feeling and food intake in normal volunteers: A double blind study. *Eur J Clin Nutr* 52:239-245, 1998.
54. Bourdon I, Yokoyama W, Davis P, et al: Postprandial lipid, glucose, insulin, and cholecystokinin responses in men fed barley pasta enriched with β-glucan. *Am J Clin Nutr* 69:55-63, 1999.
55. Lu ZX, Walker KZ, Muir JG, et al: Arabinoxylan fiber, a byproduct of wheat flour processing, reduces the postprandial glucose response in normoglycemic subjects. *Am J Clin Nutr* 71:1123-1128, 2000.

56. Schwartz SE, Levine RA, Weinstock RS, et al: Sustained pectin ingestion: Effect on gastric emptying and glucose tolerance in non-insulin-dependent diabetic patients. *Am J Clin Nutr* 48:1413-1417, 1988.
57. Jenkins DJA, Jenkins AL: Dietary fiber and the glycemic response. *Proc Soc Exp Biol Med* 180:422-431, 1985.
58. DiLorenzo C, Williams CM, Hajnal F, et al: Pectin delays gastric emptying and increases satiety in obese subjects. *Gastroenterology* 95:1211-1215, 1988.
59. Haber GB, Heaton KW, Murphy D, et al: Depletion and disruption of dietary fibre. Effects on satiety, plasma-glucose, and serum-insulin. *Lancet* 2:679-682, 1977.
60. Bolton RP, Heaton KW, Burroughs LF: The role of dietary fiber in satiety, glucose, and insulin: Studies with fruit and fruit juice. *Am J Clin Nutr* 34:211-217, 1981.
61. Holt SHA, Brand Miller J: Particle size, satiety and the glycaemic response. *Eur J Clin Nutr* 48:496-502, 1994.
62. Granfeldt Y, Hagander B, Bjorck I: Metabolic responses to starch in oat and wheat products. On the importance of food structure, incomplete gelatinization or presence of viscous dietary fibre. *Eur J Clin Nutr* 49:189-199, 1995.
63. Jenkins DJA, Wesson V, Wolever TMS, et al: Wholemeal versus wholegrain breads: Proportion of whole or cracked grain and the glycaemic response. *Br Med J* 297:958-960, 1988.
64. Heaton KW, Marcus SN, Emmett PM, et al: Particle size of wheat, maize, and oat test meals: Effects on plasma glucose and insulin responses and on the rate of starch digestion in vitro. *Am J Clin Nutr* 47:675-682, 1988.
65. Brighenti F, Castellani G, Benini L, et al: Effect of neutralized and native vinegar on blood glucose and acetate responses to a mixed meal in healthy subjects. *Eur J Clin Nutr* 49:242-247, 1995.
66. Liljeberg HGM, Bjorck IME: Delayed gastric emptying rate as a potential mechanism for lowered glycemia after eating sourdough bread: Studies in humans and rats using test products with added organic acids or an organic salt. *Am J Clin Nutr* 64:886-893, 1996.
67. Hunt JN, Knox MT: The slowing of gastric emptying by nine acids. *J Physiol* 201:161-179, 1969.
68. Wolever TMS, Bentum-Williams A, Jenkins DJA: Physiological modulation of plasma free fatty acid concentrations by diet. *Diabetes Care* 18:962-970, 1995.
69. Estrich D, Ravnik A, Schlierf G, et al: Effects of co-ingestion of fat and protein upon carbohydrate-induced hyperglycemia. *Diabetes* 16:232-237, 1967.
70. Jenkins DJA, Wolever TMS, Wong GS, et al: Glycemic responses to foods: Possible differences between insulin-dependent and noninsulin-dependent diabetics. *Am J Clin Nutr* 40:971-981, 1984.
71. Welch IM, Bruce C, Hill SE, et al: Duodenal and ileal lipid suppresses postprandial blood glucose and insulin responses in man: Possible

implications for the dietary management of diabetes mellitus. *Clin Sci* 72:209-216, 1987.
72. Sidery MB, Macdonald IA, Blackshaw PE: Superior mesenteric artery blood flow and gastric emptying in humans and the differential effects of high fat and high carbohydrate meals. *Gut* 35:186-190, 1994.
73. Collier G, O'Dea K: The effect of coingestion of fat on the glucose, insulin, and gastric inhibitory polypeptide responses to carbohydrate and protein. *Am J Clin Nutr* 37:941-944, 1983.
74. Collier G, McLean A, O'Dea K: Effect of co-ingestion of fat on the metabolic responses to slowly and rapidly absorbed carbohydrates. *Diabetologia* 26:50-54, 1984.
75. Gatti E, Noe D, Pazzucconi F, et al: Differential effect of unsaturated oils and butter on blood glucose and insulin response to carbohydrate in normal volunteers. *Eur J Clin Nutr* 46:161-166, 1992.
76. Nuttall FQ, Mooradian AD, Gannon MC, et al: Effect of protein ingestion on the glucose and insulin response to a standardized oral glucose load. *Diabetes Care* 7:465-470, 1984.
77. Rorsman P, Ashcroft RM, Berggren P-O: Regulation of glucagon release from pancreatic A-cells. *Biochem Pharmacol* 41:1783-1790, 1991.
78. Brand-Miller JC, Colagiuri S, Gan ST: Insulin sensitivity predicts glycemia after a protein load. *Metabolism* 49:1-5, 2000.
79. Stubbs RJ: Macronutrient effects on appetite. *Int J Obes* 19:S11-S19, 1995.
80. Skov AR, Toubro S, Ronn B, et al: Randomized trial on protein vs carbohydrate in ad libitum fat reduced diet for the treatment of obesity. *Int J Obes* 23:528-536, 1999.
81. vanLoon LJC, Saris WHM, Verhagen H, et al: Plasma insulin responses after ingestion of different amino acid or protein mixtures with carbohydrate. *Am J Clin Nutr* 72:96-105, 2000.
82. Fruhbeck G: Slow and fast dietary proteins. *Nature* 391:843-844, 1998.
83. Peters JC, Harper AE: Acute effects of dietary protein on food intake, tissue amino acids, and brain serotonin. *Am J Physiol* 252:R902-R914, 1987.
84. Garlick PJ, McNurlan MA, Patlak CS: Adaptation of protein metabolism in relation to limits to high dietary protein intake. *Eur J Clin Nutr* 53:S34-S43, 1999.
85. Kerstetter JE, Mitnick ME, Gundberg CM, et al: Changes in bone turnover in young women consuming different levels of dietary protein. *J Clin Endocrinol Metab* 84:1052-1055, 1999.
86. Anderson JW, Blake JE, Turner J, et al: Effects of soy protein on renal function and proteinuria in patients with type 2 diabetes. *Am J Clin Nutr* 68:1347S-1353S, 1998.
87. Metges CC, Barth CA: Metabolic consequences of a high dietary-protein intake in adulthood: Assessment of the available evidence. *J Nutr* 130:886-889, 2000.
88. Freinkel N, Metzger BE: Oral glucose tolerance curve and hypoglycemias in the fed state. *N Engl J Med* 280:820-828, 1969.

89. Rosenbloom AL, Wheeler L, Bianchi R, et al: Age-adjusted analysis of insulin responses during normal and abnormal glucose tolerance tests in children and adolescents. *Diabetes* 24:820-828, 1975.
90. Lev-Ran A: Nadirs of oral glucose tolerance tests are independent of age and sex. *Diabetes Care* 6:405-408, 1983.
91. Jenkins DJA, Wolever TMS, Jenkins AL, et al: The glycaemic index of foods tested in diabetic patients: A new basis for carbohydrate exchange favouring the use of legumes. *Diabetologia* 24:257-264, 1983.
92. Wolever TMS, Jenkins DJA: The use of glycemic index in predicting the blood glucose response to mixed meals. *Am J Clin Nutr* 43:167-172, 1986.
93. Bornet FRJ, Costagliola D, Rizkalla SW, et al: Insulinemic and glycemic indexes of six starch-rich foods taken alone and in a mixed meal by type 2 diabetics. *Am J Clin Nutr* 45:588-595, 1987.
94. Jarvi AE, Karlstrom BE, Granfeldt YE, et al: The influence of food structure on postprandial metabolism in patients with non-insulin-dependent diabetes mellitus. *Am J Clin Nutr* 61:837-842, 1995.
95. Coulston AM, Hollenbeck CB, Liu GC, et al: Effect of source of dietary carbohydrate on plasma glucose, insulin, and gastric inhibitory polypeptide responses to test meals in subjects with noninsulin-dependent diabetes mellitus. *Am J Clin Nutr* 40:965-970, 1984.
96. Coulston AM, Hollenbeck CB, Swislocki ALM, et al: Effect of source of dietary carbohydrate on plasma glucose and insulin responses to mixed meals in subjects with NIDDM. *Diabetes Care* 10:395-400, 1987.
97. Hollenbeck CB, Coulston AM, Reaven GM: Comparison of plasma glucose and insulin responses to mixed meals of high-, intermediate-, and low-glycemic potential. *Diabetes Care* 11:323-329, 1988.
98. Cusin I, Rohner-Jeanrenaud F, Terrettaz J, et al: Hyperinsulinemia and its impact on obesity and insulin resistance. *Int J Obes* 14:S1-S11, 1992.
99. Kabir M, Rizkalla SW, Champ M, et al: Dietary amylose-amylopectin starch content affects glucose and lipid metabolism in adipocytes of normal and diabetic rats. *J Nutr* 128:35-43, 1998.
100. Kabir M, Rizkalla SW, Quignard-Boulange A, et al: A high glycemic index starch diet affects lipid storage-related enzymes in normal and to a lesser extent in diabetic rats. *J Nutr* 128:1878-1883, 1998.
101. Agus MSD, Swain JF, Larson CL, et al: Dietary composition and physiologic adaptations to energy restriction. *Am J Clin Nutr* 71:901-907, 2000.
102. Campfield LA, Smith FJ, Rosenbaum M, et al: Human eating: Evidence for a physiological basis using a modified paradigm. *Neurosci Biobehav Rev* 20:133-137, 1996.
103. Thompson DA, Campbell RG: Hunger in humans induced by 2-deoxy-D-glucose: Glucoprivic control of taste preference and food intake. *Science* 198:1065-1068, 1977.
104. Friedman MI, Granneman J: Food intake and peripheral factors after

recovery from insulin-induced hypoglycemia. *Am J Physiol* 244:R374-R382, 1983.
105. NIH Technology Assessment Conference Panel: Methods for voluntary weight loss and control. *Ann Intern Med* 119:764-770, 1993.
106. Spitzer L, Rodin J: Effects of fructose and glucose preloads on subsequent food intake. *Appetite* 8:135-145, 1987.
107. Rodin J, Reed D, Jamner L: Metabolic effects of fructose and glucose: Implications for food intake. *Am J Clin Nutr* 47:683-689, 1988.
108. Rodin J: Comparative effects of fructose, aspartame, glucose, and water preloads on calorie and macronutrient intake. *Am J Clin Nutr* 51:428-435, 1990.
109. Rodin J: Effects of pure sugar vs. mixed starch fructose loads on food intake. *Appetite* 17:213-219, 1991.
110. Kong M-F, Chapman I, Goble E, et al: Effects of oral fructose and glucose on plasma GLP-1 and appetite in normal subjects. *Peptides* 20:545-551, 1999.
111. vanAmelsvoort JM, Weststrate JA: Amylose-amylopectin ratio in a meal affects postprandial variables in male volunteers. *Am J Clin Nutr* 55:712-718, 1992.
112. Weststrate JA, vanAmelsvoort JM: Effects of the amylose content of breakfast and lunch on postprandial variables in male volunteers. *Am J Clin Nutr* 58:180-186, 1993.
113. Granfeldt Y, Liljeberg H, Drews A, et al: Glucose and insulin responses to barley products: influence of food structure and amylose-amylopectin ratio. *Am J Clin Nutr* 59:1075-1082, 1994.
114. Holt SHA, Brand Miller J: Increased insulin responses to ingested foods are associated with lessened satiety. *Appetite* 24:43-54, 1995.
115. Leathwood P, Pollet P: Effects of slow release carbohydrates in the form of bean flakes on the evolution of hunger and satiety in man. *Appetite* 10:1-11, 1988.
116. Gustafsson K, Asp NG, Hagander B, et al: Influence of processing and cooking of carrots in mixed meals on satiety, glucose and hormonal response. *Int J Food Sci Nutr* 46:3-12, 1995.
117. Gustafsson K, Asp NG, Hagander B, et al: Satiety effects of spinach in mixed meals: Comparison with other vegetables. *Int J Food Sci Nutr* 46:327-334, 1995.
118. Benini L, Castellani G, Brighenti F, et al: Gastric emptying of a solid meal is accelerated by the removal of dietary fibre naturally present in food. *Gut* 36:825-830, 1995.
119. Holt SHA, Delargy HJ, Lawton CL, et al: The effects of high-carbohydrate vs high-fat breakfasts on feelings of fullness and alertness, and subsequent food intake. *Int J Food Sci Nutr* 50:13-28, 1999.
120. Krotkiewski M: Effect of guar gum on body-weight, hunger ratings and metabolism in obese subjects. *Br J Nutr* 52:97-105, 1984.
121. Holt S, Brand J, Soveny C, et al: Relationship of satiety to postprandial glycaemic, insulin and cholecystokinin responses. *Appetite* 18:129-141, 1992.

122. Holt SH, Brand Miller JC, Petocz P: Interrelationships among postprandial satiety, glucose and insulin responses and changes in subsequent food intake. *Eur J Clin Nutr* 50:788-797, 1996.
123. Slabber M, Bamard HC, Kuyl IM, et al: Effects of a low-insulin-response, energy-restricted diet on weight loss and plasma insulin concentrations in hyperinsulinemic obese females. *Am J Clin Nutr* 60:48-53, 1994.
124. Bouche C, Rizkalla SW, Luo J, et al: Regulation of lipid metabolism and fat mass distribution by chronic low glycemic index diet in non diabetic subjects. *Diabetes* 49:A40-A41, 2000.
125. Spieth LE, Hamish JD, Lenders CM, et al: A low glycemic index diet in the treatment of pediatric obesity. *Arch Pediatr Adolesc Med* 154:947-951, 2000.
126. Rosenbloom AL, Joe JR, Young RS, et al: Emerging epidemic of type 2 diabetes in youth. *Diabetes Care* 22:345-354, 1999.
127. Dabelea D, Pettitt DJ, Jones KL, et al: Type 2 diabetes mellitus in minority children and adolescents: An emerging problem. *Endocrinol Metab Clin North Am* 28:709-729, 1999.
128. American Diabetes Association: Type 2 diabetes in children and adolescents. *Diabetes Care* 22:381-389, 2000.
129. Libman I, Arslanian SA: Type II diabetes mellitus: No longer just adults. *Pediatr Ann* 28:589-593, 1999.
130. Young TK, Dean HJ, Flett B, et al: Childhood obesity in a population at high risk for type 2 diabetes. *J Pediatr* 136:365-369, 2000.
131. Fagot-Campagna A, Pettitt DJ, Engelgau MM, et al: Type 2 diabetes among North American children and adolescents: An epidemiologic review and a public health perspective. *J Pediatr* 136:664-672, 2000.
132. Wolever TMS: The glycemic index: Flogging a dead horse? *Diabetes Care* 20:452-456, 1997.
133. Coulston AM, Reaven GM: Much ado about (almost) nothing. *Diabetes Care* 20:241-243, 1997.
134. Brand Miller J, Colagiuri S, Foster-Powell K: The glycemic index is easy and works in practice. *Diabetes Care* 20:1628-1629, 1997.
135. Wolever TM, Bolognesi C: Prediction of glucose and insulin responses of normal subjects after consuming mixed meals varying in energy, protein, fat, carbohydrate and glycemic index. *J Nutr* 126:2807-2812, 1996.
136. Jenkins DJ, Wolever TM, Collier GR, et al: Metabolic effects of a low-glycemic-index diet. *Am J Clin Nutr* 46:968-975, 1987.
137. Jarvi AE, Karlstrom BE, Granfeldt YE, et al: Improved glycemic control and lipid profile and normalized fibrinolytic activity on a low-glycemic index diet in type 2 diabetic patients. *Diabetes Care* 22:10-18, 1999.
138. DeFronzo RA, Bonadonna RC, Ferrannini E: Pathogenesis of NIDDM. *Diabetes Care* 15:318-368, 1992.
139. Jenkins DJA, Wolever TMS, Kalmusky J, et al: Low glycemic index carbohydrate foods in the management of hyperlipidemia. *Am J Clin Nutr* 42:604-617, 1985.

140. Jenkins DJA, Wolever TMS, Kalmusky J, et al: Low-glycemic index diet in hyperlipidemia: Use of traditional starchy foods. *Am J Clin Nutr* 46:66-71, 1987.
141. Jenkins DJA, Wolever TMS, Buckley G, et al: Low-glycemic-index starchy foods in the diabetic diet. *Am J Clin Nutr* 48:248-254, 1988.
142. Collier GR, Giudici S, Kalmusky J, et al: Low glycaemic index starchy foods improve glucose control and lower serum cholesterol in diabetic children. *Diabet Nutr Metab* 1:11-19, 1988.
143. Brand JC, Colagiuri S, Crossman S, et al: Low-glycemic index foods improve long-term glycemic control in NIDDM. *Diabetes Care* 14:95-101, 1991.
144. Wolever TMS, Jenkins DJA, Vuksan V, et al: Beneficial effect of a low glycaemic index diet in type 2 diabetes. *Diabet Med* 9:451-458, 1992.
145. Wolever TMS, Jenkins DJA, Vuksan V, et al: Beneficial effect of low-glycemic index diet in overweight NIDDM subjects. *Diabetes Care* 15:562-564, 1992.
146. Fontvieille AM, Rizkalla SW, Penfornis A, et al: The use of low glycaemic index foods improves metabolic control of diabetic patients over five weeks. *Diabet Med* 9:444-450, 1992.
147. Frost G, Wilding J, Beecham J: Dietary advice based on the glycaemic index improves dietary profile and metabolic control in type 2 diabetic patients. *Diabet Med* 11:397-401, 1994.
148. Kiens B, Richter EA: Types of carbohydrate in an ordinary diet affect insulin action and muscle substrates in humans. *Am J Clin Nutr* 63:47-53, 1996.
149. Frost G, Leeds A, Trew G, et al: Insulin sensitivity in women at risk of coronary heart disease and the effect of a low glycemic diet. *Metabolism* 47:1245-1251, 1998.
150. Luscombe ND, Noakes M, Clifton PM: Diets high and low in glycemic index versus high monounsaturated fat diets: Effects on glucose and lipid metabolism in NIDDM. *Eur J Clin Nutr* 53:473-478, 1999.
151. Giacco R, Parillo M, Rivellese AA, et al: Long-term dietary treatment with increased amounts of fiber-rich low-glycemic index natural foods improves blood glucose control and reduces the number of hypoglycemic events in type 1 diabetic patients. *Diabetes Care* 23:1461-1466, 2000.
152. Frost G, Leeds AA, Dore CJ, et al: Glycemic index as a determinant of serum HDL-cholesterol concentration. *Lancet* 353:1045-1048, 1999.
153. Trout DL, Behall KM, Osilesi O: Prediction of glycemic index for starchy foods. *Am J Clin Nutr* 58:873-878, 1993.
154. Ludwig DS: Dietary glycemic index and obesity. *J Nutr* 130:280S-283S, 2000.

CHAPTER 7

Peripheral Neuropathy in the First 2 Years of Life: Diagnostic Evaluation Including Molecular Genetics

Atilano G. Lacson, MD, FRCPC
Clinical Associate Professor, Departments of Pathology and Pediatrics, University of South Florida, Tampa; Staff Pathologist, All Children's Hospital, Department of Pathology and Laboratory Medicine, St Petersburg, Fla

Maria Gieron-Korthals, MD
Professor, Departments of Pediatrics and Neurology, University of South Florida; Program Director, Pediatric Neurology, Tampa General Hospital, Tampa

O. Thomas Mueller, PhD
Associate Professor, Department of Pediatrics, University of South Florida, Tampa; Director, Molecular Genetics Clinical Laboratory, All Children's Hospital, St Petersburg, Fla

ABSTRACT

Inherited polyneuropathies present in the first 2 years of life are discussed with emphasis on clinical, pathologic, and molecular data. Early-onset polyneuropathies are relatively rare, sometimes life-threatening conditions that demand early recognition by clinical and pathologic examination. Histologic and ultrastructural overlaps among the various conditions are sometimes resolved by molecular genetic analysis. The growth in disease identification by genetic localization allows a more comprehensive understanding of the clinical and morphologic heterogeneity involving rearrangements of the same gene. Molecular mechanisms explaining the acquisition of such gene rearrangements are beginning to be unraveled.

Peripheral myelin disorders may be confused with primary axonal disorders, and electrophysiologic examination often helps to distinguish between these two. Furthermore, early-onset central nervous system disorders may present as peripheral polyneuropathies and confound the clinical picture. A tentative diagnosis can often be offered by pathologic examination and confirmed by biochemical enzyme analysis later. The differential clinical diagnostic considerations of early-onset polyneuropathies are offered, to help clinicians sort out these diseases in the most efficient manner.

Hereditary neuropathies are among the most common inherited diseases with an estimated frequency of 1 case per 2500 individuals.[1] However, despite this incidence, the wideranging symptoms and signs of hereditary neuropathies infrequently manifest during the newborn period or infancy.[2] Symptomatic peripheral polyneuropathies in newborn and young infants, although relatively rare, are serious conditions that can be immediately life-threatening or that can be chronically progressive, leading to long-term disability in later years. The identification of molecular derangements causing the major forms of hereditary peripheral neuropathies has progressed exponentially in recent years.

Among the hereditary neuropathies, alterations in 4 human genes are responsible for most clinical phenotypes.[3-13] Attempts at classification that encompass the clinical, genotypic, and morphological features of these conditions have generated some controversies,[14] whereas newly proposed classifications attempt to bridge these gaps.[9,15]

In this review we focus on peripheral polyneuropathies that present at birth or during the first 2 years of life, with an emphasis on selected early-onset neuropathies with clinical symptoms and signs that may share features with diseases affecting other parts of the nervous system; the clinical, pathologic, and molecular genetic differences currently known among these diseases; and recent molecular discoveries.

OVERVIEW OF CLINICAL, PATHOLOGIC, AND MOLECULAR FEATURES

Childhood peripheral neuropathies are of 2 major types: hereditary and acquired. Congenital hereditary neuropathy is the more common type, whereas acquired neuropathy is a sporadic type that shares many clinical features with inherited neuropathy. Among the hereditary neuropathies, Charcot-Marie-Tooth and its variants are the most common. The main characteristic that distinguishes hereditary from acquired neuropathies is the evidence of familial involvement in hereditary disorders. In this chapter we discuss hereditary peripheral neuropathies with onset during the neonatal and infantile period.

It is not uncommon for mild neuropathy of infantile onset to remain undiagnosed until later childhood or adulthood. Patients may have no clinical symptoms of neuropathy but have reduced conduction velocity, whereas other family members may have a fully developed clinical and electrophysiologic neuropathy. The main clinical characteristics of hereditary neuropathies with onset during the neonatal or infantile period are hypotonia, muscle weakness, and reduced or absent deep tendon reflexes. Hypotonia involves both the trunk and the extremities, and generally is not as severe as that in spinal muscular atrophy. Muscle weakness usually involves the legs more than the arms, and the distal muscles more than the proximal, but any pattern of weakness can be observed. Most of these infants have delayed gross motor development because of hypotonia and muscle weakness. Respiratory problems, sucking and swallowing difficulties, and orthopedic deformities, all of which are consequences of muscle weakness, are often present in these patients. Some of these neuropathies are progressive and some are not; in either case, intercurrent infections, particularly of the respiratory system, can exacerbate muscle weakness and, in some cases, can lead to death. Electrodiagnosis is the single most important diagnostic tool that a clinician can use to localize the problem to a specific segment of the lower motor neuron, to identify a type of neuropathy, and to assist with a further diagnostic study, whether this be a nerve biopsy or genetic testing.

A segmental sural nerve biopsy in conjunction with a muscle biopsy can help differentiate between an inherited or an acquired neuropathy in early life, particularly when closely correlated with the clinical findings.[16,17] In older children, a fascicular nerve biopsy may provide enough material for analysis. When a decision to perform a nerve or muscle biopsy is made, the clinical and electrophysiologic data must be made available to the examining pathologist. The nerve may show myelin alterations, axonal alterations, or both, with or without accompanying Schwann cell changes, fibroblast response, or associated blood-derived elements participating in an inflammatory or phagocytic reaction. Some inherited metabolic neuropathies often harbor specific cytoplasmic or axonal inclusions or alterations. Quantitative data often help in determining hypomyelination from hypermyelination by using the "g" ratio (axon diameter divided by total fiber diameter) among older children.[18] However, these ratios may not be obtainable when myelin is nearly absent among neonates and very young infants.[19] These nerve findings may help direct the workup further by eliminating diagnostic possibilities such as metabolic inherited neuropathy or toxic neuropathy.

On occasion, the nerve biopsy may show nondiagnostic features despite a clinical history consistent with a familial neuropathy. Molecular genetic confirmation may be the key to deciphering the clinical heterogeneity in these conditions. Advanced laboratory techniques allow molecular geneticists to detect critical gene rearrangements, including duplications, deletions, and point mutations, and thereby arrive at a diagnosis by using blood samples. An expanding list of mutations in several genes can help facilitate the molecular diagnosis among individual cases and families despite the variability in clinical expression,[20] thus avoiding the invasive procedures of nerve and muscle biopsies. Additionally, the application of molecular cytogenetic techniques (eg, the detection of PMP22 gene duplication using archival formalin-fixed tissues by fluorescence in situ hybridization techniques[21] and by polymerase chain reaction) will allow retrospective reclassification of these diseases.[22] With the completion of the human genome project, it is anticipated that more and more sophisticated tools for mutation identification will be designed for various categories of human diseases, including hereditary peripheral neuropathies.

EARLY-ONSET NEUROPATHIES

Table 1 lists neuropathies with an early onset between the newborn period and the end of the first decade of life. Only the more common conditions are discussed in the following sections.

CHARCOT-MARIE-TOOTH NEUROPATHY

Charcot-Marie-Tooth (CMT) neuropathy, also known as hereditary motor and sensory neuropathy (HMSN), shows 2 patterns of tissue involvement that allow the morphological separation of its variants. CMT1 (HMSN 1) involves progressive loss of myelin with secondary axonal loss and has 2 subtypes, A and B, whereas CMT2 (HMSN 2) involves primary axonal degeneration.[23]

CMT1A (HMSN 1A, Autosomal Dominant)

CMT1A is an autosomal dominant neuropathy that starts either before 1 year of age or during the first decade of life. When this disorder starts during infancy, the characteristic signs are hypotonia, leg weakness, and reduced deep tendon reflexes. Other early clinical features include a foot deformity, such as pes cavus or hammer

TABLE 1.
Neuropathies With an Early Onset

Disorder	Usual Onset	Early Symptoms	Tendon Reflexes	Average NCVs
CMT1A	1st decade	Distal weakness	Absent	15-20 m/s
CMT1B	1st decade	Distal weakness	Absent	15-20 m/s
CMT2C	1st decade	Vocal cord and distal weakness	Absent	>50 m/s
CMT R-Ax (Ouvrier)	1st decade	Distal weakness	Reduced	Axon loss
CMT2 (Cowchock)	1st decade	Distal weakness	Absent	Axon loss
CMT1-DSS (HMSN 3)	2 years	Severe weakness	Absent	<10 m/s
CHN	Birth	Severe weakness	Absent	<10 m/s
CMT4A	Childhood	Distal weakness	Reduced	Slow
CMT4B	2-4 years	Distal and proximal weakness	Absent	Slow
CMT4C	5-15 years	Delayed walking	Reduced	14-32 m/s
CMT4D (Lom)	1-10 years	Gait change	Absent	10-20 m/s
CMT4E	Birth	Infant hypotonia	Absent	9-20 m/s
CMT4F	1-3 years	Motor delay	Absent	Absent

Abbreviations: NCVs, Nerve conduction velocities; *CMT,* Charcot-Marie-Tooth; *DSS,* Dejerine-Sottas syndrome; *HMSN,* hereditary motor sensory neuropathy; *CHN,* congenital hypomyelinating neuropathy.

toes. The gait is often awkward and clumsy with a tendency to trip, and high steppage to compensate for foot drop may be observed. A symmetrical muscle weakness starts in the peroneal muscles, intrinsic muscles of the feet, and dorsiflexors of the ankles. Later, the hands become involved, and muscle weakness may progress proximally. Peroneal muscle atrophy can be present. Deep tendon reflexes are usually absent, and mild sensory symptoms may be present in the feet and hands. Some patients experience pain or other sensory disturbance, and others may have tremor in the hands. Peripheral nerves can be palpably enlarged and firm in about a quarter of the patients.[24] The clinical course of this neuropathy is very slowly progressive or relatively static, and a normal life expectancy is common. Patients often need orthoses or corrective procedures to improve the gait and foot deformities.

Electrodiagnostic studies show markedly decreased motor nerve conduction velocity (MNCV) to less than 20 m/s, and sensory nerve conduction velocity (SNCV) is also affected. The slow conduction may also be found in asymptomatic children; therefore, it is advisable to test the parents of any affected child for the presence of electrophysiologic abnormalities, which, when present, will help in genetic counseling.

A sural nerve biopsy in the early stages shows hypermyelination as a result of the overexpression of PMP22. In later stages, the nerve may show a decreased number of myelinated fibers (Fig 1, A). The repeated demyelination and remyelination results in the formation of typical "onion bulbs," which sometimes persist long after the axon has disappeared.[4] Ultrastructurally, the typical onion bulbs are formed by the concentric arrangement of Schwann cell cytoplasmic lamellae around demyelinated axons (Fig 1, B). Quantitative measurements confirm the axonal loss, particularly in older patients. Although primarily a myelin defect, a secondary loss of the largest myelinated fibers leads to axonal regenerative sprouting as evidenced by ultrastructural studies.[19]

In newborns and young infants, these typical changes may be absent. The onion bulbs are infrequent and poorly developed throughout the first few years of life, becoming more frequent and more complex with age.[18] A pseudoinflammatory change may be misinterpreted as evidence for chronic inflammatory demyelinating polyneuropathy[25] (Fig 1, C). The unmyelinated fibers are initially unaffected, but with time these show a relative increase in number, probably because of axonal regeneration.

Fluorescence in situ hybridization techniques with appropriate probes demonstrate the duplication of the PMP22 gene localized on chromosome 17p11-p12[21] (Table 2). The PMP22 gene encodes a small hydrophobic membrane glycoprotein highly expressed in and responsible for the development and maintenance of myelin in peripheral nerves. Approximately 70% of autosomal dominant forms of CMT1[26] are caused by a large tandem duplication of 1.5 megabase pairs of chromosome 17p11.2-12, thought to occur from unequal crossing over during germ cell meiosis.[6] The resulting overdosage of the PMP22 gene and possibly other genes in this region is hypothesized to cause the CMT phenotype by a mechanism involving hypermyelination. The rarity of PMP22 point mutations and elevated PMP22 mRNA levels in most CMT types support this hypothesis.

PMP22 missense mutations usually occur in more severe CMT1 cases associated with early demyelination and onion bulb formation. Other mutational mechanisms, including a hemizygous PMP22 mutation together with the 1.5-Mb deletion in an autosomal recessive form of CMT1, have also been described.[27] Apparently, point mutations in PMP22 affect intracellular trafficking, resulting in

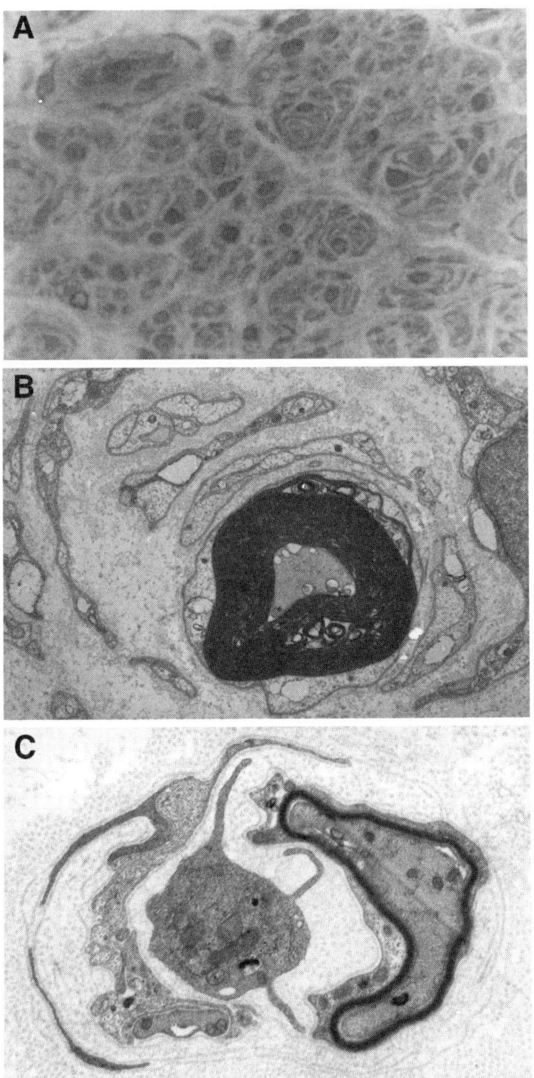

FIGURE 1.

A, Photomicrograph of sural nerve biopsy shows the paucity of myelinated axons in fairly advanced case of CMT1A. Note the plethora of onion bulbs (toluidine blue, epon-embedded tissue; original magnification, ×400). **B,** Electron micrograph of sural nerve shows a typical onion bulb with lamellae of Schwann cell cytoplasm arranged concentrically around a hypermyelinated axon (uranyl acetate-lead citrate; original magnification, ×4000). **C,** Electron micrograph of CMT1A sural nerve with macrophage adjacent to a partially demyelinated axon, with onion bulb (uranyl acetate-lead citrate; original magnification, ×2500).

TABLE 2.
Genes Involved in Hereditary Neuropathies

Type	Inheritance	Frequency	Subtype	Genetic Mutation	Chromosome Map Locus	Gene Mutation/Abnormality
CMT1	Autosomal dominant	35%-40%	CMT1A	PMP22	17p11-p12	1.5-Mb duplication or missense mutations
		2.5%-5%	CMT1B	MPZ	1q22-q23	Heterozygous mutations
	Autosomal dominant or recessive	?	CMT1C	?	?	
			Other	EGR2	10q21-q22	Missense mutations
CMT2	Autosomal dominant	20%-40%	CMT2A	?	1p36-35	
			CMT2B	?	3q13-q22	
			CMT2C	?	?	
			CMT2D	?	7p14	
			CMT2?	MPZ	1q22-q23	Missense mutations
CMT4	Autosomal recessive	Rare	CMT4A		8q13-q21	
			CMT4B	MTMR2	11q23	
			CMT4C	?	5q23-q33	
			CMT4D	?	8q24	
			CMT4E	EGR2	10q21-q22	

CMTX	X-linked dominant X-linked recessive	10%-20%	Connexin 32	Xq13.1	Missense and nonsense mutations, insertions, deletions
DSS	Sporadic, dominant		PMP22	17p11	Heterozygous and homozygous missense mutations
	Sporadic		EGR2	10q21-q22	Missense mutations
	Sporadic		MPZ	1q22-q23	Heterozygous and homozygous missense mutations
CHN	Dominant or recessive		EGR2	10q21-q22	Homozygous mutations
			MPZ	1q22-q23	Missense and nonsense mutations
HNPP			PMP22	17p11	1.5-Mb deletion or nonsense mutations

Abbreviations: CMT, Charcot-Marie-Tooth; *PMP22,* peripheral myelin protein 22 gene; *MPZ,* myelin protein zero gene; *EGR2,* early growth response 2 gene; *MTMR2,* myotubularin-related protein 2 gene; *DSS,* Dejerine-Sottas syndrome; *CHN,* congenital hypomyelinating neuropathy; *HNPP,* hereditary neuropathy with liability to pressure palsies; *Mb,* megabase.

accumulation of both the mutant protein and its normal counterpart in the endoplasmic reticulum and intermediate compartment, resulting in severe shortages at the membrane available for myelination.[28]

Most duplications and deletions arise during meiotic recombination after misalignment and unequal crossing over between the proximal and distal duplicated CMT1A-REP gene elements.[29] The REP elements apparently contain a recombination hotspot whose sequence suggests a transposon-like element. This element promotes recombination at levels 50 times greater than in surrounding sequences within the REP element.[30]

The phenotype of CMT patients with PMP22 point mutations is more severe than those of the more common 17q duplications. Most mutations were missense mutations located in the transmembrane domain of the gene.[12] Morphometric assessments including measurements of the "g" ratio (vide supra) are useful in distinguishing the dominantly inherited duplication-positive CMT1A from other forms of CMT. In CMT1A, a "g" ratio less than 0.20 confirms a hypermyelinated state associated with PMP22 overexpression, whereas a higher "g" ratio (eg, 0.71) suggests hypomyelination seen in autosomal recessive missense mutations of PMP22 or P0 (MPZ) mutations.[18,31]

It is generally accepted that the disabilities noted in demyelinating polyneuropathies correlate directly with axonal loss secondary to the myelin disorder. Thus, the molecular mechanisms underlying Schwann cell and axon interactions become very important[32-34] and need to be studied further to facilitate the development of rational therapeutic approaches.

CMT1B (HMSN 1B)

CMT1B neuropathy presents with signs and symptoms similar, if not identical, to those of CMT1A; unlike CMT1A, the genetic abnormality involves either missense or heterozygous frameshift mutations of the extracellular domain of myelin protein zero (Table 2). The myelin protein zero (MPZ or P0) encodes a protein that is the major component of peripheral nerve myelin. Frameshift mutations of this protein in the extracellular and transmembrane domains may lead to severe clinical symptoms of Dejerine-Sottas syndrome (DSS), whereas nonsense mutations involving the intracellular domain may lead to an infantile presentation of congenital hypomyelinating neuropathy (CHN).[3] Thus, these 2 disorders seem to be variants of CMT1B, although PMP22 point mutations have also been demonstrated in children with the DSS phenotype.[10]

Studies suggest that the proteins P0 and PMP22 form a complex in the myelin membrane, and thus mutations in either gene can give rise to peripheral neuropathies.[35]

CMT1 and Dejerine-Sottas Syndrome (DSS, HMSN 3, Hypertrophic Neuropathy of Infancy)

CMT1 and DSS likely represent a spectrum of entities that vary both clinically and pathologically. On one end of the spectrum there is DSS, with a characteristic demyelination-remyelination sequence leading to the formation of onion bulbs, while on the other end there is a disorder with a total absence of the peripheral nervous system myelin, represented by congenital amyelinating neuropathy (CAN). Disorders of hypomyelination fall in between the two extreme ends. The concept of hypomyelination implies a congenital onset of a disease process that is usually nonprogressive, unless some other pathologic process such as axonal degeneration intervenes. Hence, the basic mechanism in the above group of congenital peripheral neuropathy is a defect in myelination, which in turn may be the result of a different pathologic process.[36,37] Hypomyelination can result from a defective axonal influence on the Schwann cell, from abnormalities of the Schwann cell itself, or from a deficiency of myelin precursors.[36] There has been a long debate in the literature concerning classification and pathophysiology of DSS and congenital hypomyelinating neuropathy (CHN). Some have argued that these represent 2 distinct entities with unique clinical and pathologic features, CHN being a disorder of myelin formation whereas DSS is a demyelinating disorder. Others, including the authors of this article, have suggested that CHN falls within the DSS spectrum. Recent developments in the molecular genetics further support a notion that those two might be on a continuum of myelinopathies that differ in severity but have a common underlying pathologic defect in myelination.[36-40] Vance[15] proposed the most up-to-date classification of CMT, in which a disorder is described by its primary clinical manifestations, its gene, locus, or actual mutation.

DSS. DSS is a recessively inherited neuropathy that has its onset usually in infancy. Children manifest delayed early motor milestones, and independent walking might not be achieved until 3 or 4 years of age. After an initial improvement and often after a peak performance between 8 and 15 years of age, there is a gradual decline in motor function; some patients lose the ability to walk in adult life. When the onset of DSS is during infancy, hypotonia and muscle weakness are characteristic features, with weakness affecting the hands and feet and eventually ascending to affect the more proximal muscles. Muscle atrophy is not a striking feature but the nerves are enlarged, and some distal sensory loss may be present, as well as ataxia of the trunk and extremities. Short stature and scoliosis may be associated with this type of neuropathy.

Motor and sensory NCV is slow. It is important to check the NCV in other members of the family because a subclinical disease with slow MNCV coexists, and if present indicates a dominant type of inheritance.

The distal portions of the nerves are often enlarged. Sural nerve biopsy specimens show a high "g" ratio, often greater than 0.85.[41] The axons show a shift to the smaller sizes, with pronounced myelin loss. Teased fibers demonstrate frequent segmental and consecutive internodal demyelination associated with typical onion bulb formation composed of lamellae of Schwann cell cytoplasmic processes, basal lamina, or both, as well as circumferentially arranged Schwann cell nuclei (Fig 2).[19]

DSS may be caused by either PMP22 or P0 mutations through a variety of mechanisms,[11] including homozygous PMP22 duplications, mutations, and homozygous P0 null alleles, accounting for the relative severity of this disorder (Table 2). Takashima et al[42] describe 2 siblings with DSS who have heterozygous P0 mutations. The mutations in the parents were not found, suggesting gonadal mosaicism. Most reports of PMP22 mutations in DSS describe mis-

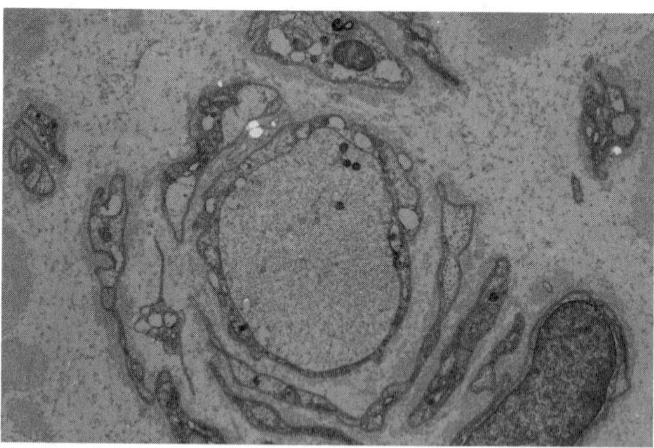

FIGURE 2.
A typical onion bulb around a completely demyelinated axon in a case of Dejerine-Sottas disease (electron micrograph; original magnification, ×8000).

sense point mutations, suggesting a dominant mode of inheritance; however, at least one report described autosomal recessive inheritance in a family with 3 affected siblings where both parents were unaffected and carried a novel PMP22 mutation, arg157trp.[43] Furthermore, a 17q duplication similar to that described for most CMT cases has also been described in patients who seem to fit the clinical description of DSS.[44]

CHN. CHN is a rare type of congenital neuropathy with an autosomal recessive inheritance. It is characterized by a nonprogressive course, weakness, areflexia, hypotonia, slow NCVs, often an increased level of cerebrospinal fluid protein, and hypomyelination of the peripheral nerve.[38] Morphologically, nerve changes can be of different severity; thus, this congenital neuropathy can be divided into CAN, and a larger group of CHN. Within the amyelinating group, there is substantial heterogeneity as well; cases with a total absence of peripheral myelin, and others in which some myelinated fibers were seen on nerve biopsy specimens, have been reported. Cases of CAN that presented with lethal arthrogryposis multiplex congenita (AMC) and cases without such an association have been reported.[36,40,45-49] The absence of AMC is consistent with a postnatal onset of symptoms, probable dominant inheritance, and longer survival. In distinction, the presence of AMC with CAN suggests a disruption in the early stages of Schwann cell development, leading to severe abnormalities and a short or no survival.[36,46] To illustrate, we encountered a stillborn baby girl of 26 weeks' gestational age with arthrogryposis whose peripheral nerves and distal spinal roots showed a virtual absence of myelin (Fig 3, A), compared with the normal peripheral nerves of another baby girl born at 32 weeks' gestation with arthrogryposis caused by nemaline rod myopathy (Fig 3, B).

CHN can further be classified, based on the age of onset, into neonatal and infantile forms.[37,46] In infantile-onset CHN, symptoms usually occur within the first year of life, with delayed motor development preceding the onset of hypotonia and muscle weakness. Other clinical manifestations include absent or markedly reduced deep tendon reflexes, and respiratory difficulty secondary to involvement of the diaphragm. The cranial nerves are usually spared, although patients have difficulty sucking and swallowing and gain weight poorly. These patients have a better prognosis, often walking with support by 4 years of age, and continue making developmental progress beyond early childhood despite the presence of significant ataxia in some. Ataxia, which significantly contributes to disability, is probably caused by the reduced proprio-

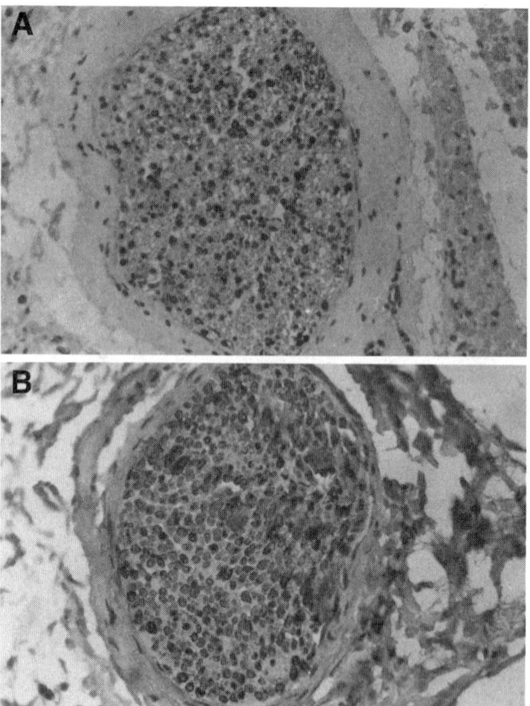

FIGURE 3.
A, Intramuscular nerve of a 26-week gestation stillbirth with congenital amyelinating neuropathy. Notice the paucity to total absence of myelin (myelin basic protein immunoperoxidase stain; original magnification, ×250). **B,** Intramuscular nerve of a 32-week gestation neonate with arthrogryposis caused by nemaline rod myopathy. Notice the presence of normal myelin profiles (myelin basic protein immunoperoxidase stain; original magnification, ×250).

ception that results from peripheral neuropathy. Children with a neonatal onset of CHN have profound weakness and hypotonia. Their prognosis is much worse, although the disease is not always fatal, and clinical improvement is possible if respiratory and infectious complications can be managed successfully.[38] The neonatal form of CHN may also be associated with arthrogryposis.[45,46] As noted above, occasional patients show long-term improvement, such as the neonatal case reported by Levy et al[47] in which the patient showed nearly complete recovery at the age of 26 months, and the neonatal case reported by Ghamdi et al[48] in which the patient's last examination at 19 months of age was completely normal, including normal motor milestones.

In both neonatal- and infantile-onset CHN, the NCV is either not recordable or extremely slow, often less than 5 m/s, and does not change even though motor function may improve.

The nerves as a rule are not grossly enlarged. A high or often unrecordable "g" ratio indicates severe myelin paucity.[19] Often, these axons show atypical onion bulbs composed of concentric lamellae of Schwann cell basal lamina.[49] Each nerve fascicle shows markedly diminished numbers and thinning of myelin sheaths associated with endoneural fibrosis, "naked" axons, proliferated Schwann cells, absence of inflammatory cells (Fig 4, A), and atypical onion bulbs (Fig 4, B). Ultrastructural analysis suggests that the condition results from impaired myelin develop-

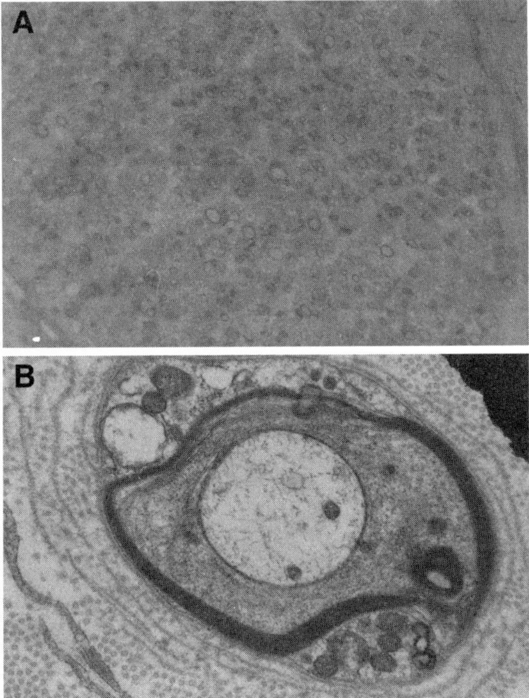

FIGURE 4.
A, Oil-immersion photograph of epon-embedded nerve from a 4-month-old boy with congenital hypomyelinating neuropathy. Notice the paucity of myelinated axons, many of which have thin myelin sheaths (toluidine blue; original magnification, ×1000). **B,** Atypical (basal lamina) onion bulb surrounding a partially demyelinated axon in the same case of congenital hypomyelinating neuropathy (electron micrograph; original magnification, ×8000).

ment.[19,49] The "reversible" cases are thought to be caused by a chronic inflammatory demyelinating neuropathy in utero, an abnormal expression of a developmental gene, or a reversible enzyme deficiency (eg, cytochrome oxidase).[48]

The genetic basis for this condition is complex. Some cases were shown to be caused by mutations of the MPZ gene (see above). The early growth response 2 gene (EGR2 or Krox-20) encodes a transcription factor that is one of the key regulation elements controlling the differentiation of Schwann cells from a promyelinating to myelinating stage (Table 2).[28] Mutations in this gene were found in a family with autosomal dominant CMT1.[50] Bellone et al[51] also described a heterozygous missense mutation in EGR2 (D305V) in a severe case of CMT1. A family with multiple siblings affected by CHN was found to have heterozygous mutations in the EGR2 gene. The EGR2 gene has a DNA-binding zinc finger domain, and mutations in this gene region that affect its DNA binding were found to directly correlate with disease severity.[11]

OTHER FORMS OF CMT

CMT2 (HMSN 2)

CMT2 neuropathy is inherited in an autosomal dominant pattern and shares common characteristics with CMT1 (HMSN 1), except that the symptoms usually start during early childhood and occasionally in the first 2 decades of life or even in middle age. The early childhood onset can occur before 2 years of age. The initial presentation might be that of motor disability with a toe gait, and some muscle wasting may be present before development of the more typical features. These features include striking muscle atrophy with the characteristic "stork legs," and pes cavus may also be present. The hands are usually less affected than the feet, and the peripheral nerves are not enlarged.[23,24] The tendon reflexes are depressed in the legs and usually normal in the arms. Some patients experience cramps in the leg or foot muscles.

The NCV is normal in the arms and only mildly decreased in the peroneal nerves while SNCV is normal. Electromyography (EMG) examination may show large motor unit potentials and fasciculations suggestive of anterior horn cell involvement.

Sural nerve biopsy specimens often show a nonspecific picture of overall reduction in large myelinated axons. Quantitative analysis of the teased nerve fibers is most helpful in these cases. An occasional onion bulb may be detected,[23] but this finding is not characteristic. Familial analysis in most of these clinical forms shows distinct chromosomal linkage (Table 2). One form

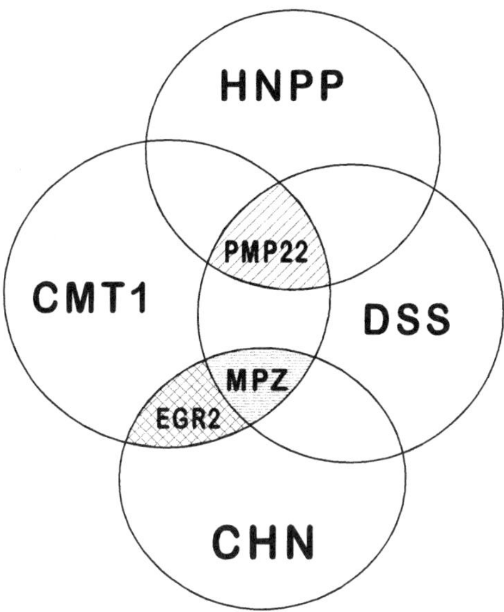

FIGURE 5.
Spectrum of myelinopathies associated with mutations of peripheral myelin protein 22 gene *(PMP22)*, myelin protein zero gene *(MPZ)*, and early growth response 2 gene *(EGR2)*. A gene symbol (eg, PMP22) in the region where the *circles* overlap indicates that each of these neuropathies are associated with mutations involving that particular gene. *Abbreviations: HNPP,* Hereditary neuropathy with liability to pressure palsies; *CMT,* Charcot-Marie-Tooth; *DSS,* Dejerine-Sottas syndrome; *CHN,* congenital hypomyelinating neuropathy. (Reprinted with permission from the *Annual Review of Medicine*, volume 50, courtesy of Warner LE, Garcia CA, Lupski JR: Hereditary peripheral neuropathies: Clinical forms, genetics, and molecular mechanisms. *Annu Rev Med* 50:263-275. © 1999 by Annual Reviews [www.AnnualReviews.org].)

appears to be associated with a missense mutation of the MPZ (P0) gene.[52,53]

To help explain the tremendous genetic heterogeneity and correlate it with the aforementioned clinical phenotypes, Figure 5 shows the overlap demonstrated between the clinical phenotypes and the genotypes that express these.[11]

Two new forms of familial autosomal recessive axonal sensorimotor neuropathy were recently described. The first form presents with neonatal hypotonia, weakness, and respiratory failure and a lethal outcome before the end of the first year. Pathologically, there is depletion of large and medium-sized myelinated axons with ultrastructural evidence of axonal atrophy.[54] Another familial form is associated with sideroblastic anemia, optic atrophy, and progressive sensorineural hearing loss.[55]

CMT-X (HMSN, X-linked Recessive)

CMT-X is caused by mutations in the CX32 gene (connexin) and phenotypically resembles CMT2,[56] with absent male-to-male transmission. Female carriers may also manifest the disease but in a less severe form. This disorder represents the second most common form of CMT, with an incidence of 1 in 3000.[57] The age of onset varies. Symptoms of CMT-X may manifest early, as is seen in a congenital, occasionally severe form with a DSS phenotype,[58] or may be delayed until the third decade.[59] The symptoms involve the longest nerves first (length-dependent distribution), but all patients experience weakness from mild to severe, leading to muscle atrophy and loss of deep tendon reflexes.[23] Distal sensory loss is common. Female heterozygotes generally have symptoms that are of intermediate severity as compared with those of affected males, but severely affected females have been described.[58]

Electrodiagnostic findings have suggested a primary demyelinating process[60] or a primary axonal degeneration similar to that in CMT2.[61] Careful analysis of the electrophysiologic abnormalities reveals a nonuniform slowing of the conduction velocities, suggesting a primary demyelinating process that precedes the development of axonal loss. This demyelinating process can only be detected through measurements of different segments of each individual nerve as well as comparisons of different nerves to each other.[62] Similarly, nerve biopsy specimens may show seemingly predominant axonal degeneration with increased axon clusters,[63] particularly in the distal portions of the nerve. However, reduced myelination with onion bulb formation has also been observed.[64,65]

More than 160 mutations of the CX32 gene have been described.[12,66] The connexins are a group of related proteins that exist in gap junctions and form intracellular channels. Connexin 32 (CX32) is one such protein that is present in paranodal and Schwann cells of the peripheral nervous system, but not in the compact myelin of the CNS. This gene was mapped to human Xq13 by somatic cell hybridization and in situ hybridization (Table 2).[67] The finding that gene mutations encoding CX32 cause the X-linked form of CMT disease was first described by Bergoffen et al[68] and further supported by the data of Bone et al.[69] The mutations in CX32 consist largely of missense mutations, which have a milder phenotype, as well as nonsense mutations, deletions, and insertions that are relatively more severe.[12,57]

CMT4B (HMSN With Focally Folded Myelin Sheaths)

CMT4B, a variant of CMT4, is an autosomal recessive demyelinating polyneuropathy characterized by infantile onset and survival from 27 to 39 years.[70] The main clinical features of CMT4B are delayed walking, progressive symmetric distal and proximal muscle weakness including facial weakness, and foot deformities in the form of pes equinovarus. Patients have distal sensory impairment in the upper and lower limbs with absent tendon reflexes. Intellectually they are normal. Examination of the cerebrospinal fluid reveals a slightly elevated protein concentration. EMG shows absent sensory nerve action potentials, and compound muscle action potentials that are either reduced in amplitude or absent. Motor nerve conduction ranges from 14 to 17 m/s.

Sural nerve biopsy specimens often show a depletion of myelinated fibers with focal segmental demyelination with or without onion bulb formation. Residual myelin often shows redundant loops and folds wrapped around the axon irregularly.

The finding of mutations involving the myotubularin-related protein-2 (MTMR2)[71] confirmed previous studies linking the disease to the chromosome 11q23 region (Table 2).[72,73] The dominant form of the disease has been shown to have point mutations in the P0 gene.[74]

EARLY-ONSET CNS DISORDERS WITH PERIPHERAL NEUROPATHY

When dealing with a demyelinating neuropathy in infancy, one must consider metabolic disorders along with the hereditary motor and sensory neuropathies described above. Among these are 2 progressive degenerative CNS disorders, metachromatic leukodystrophy (MLD) and Krabbe disease, that have involvement of the peripheral nerves, with marked slowing of the conduction velocity as the disorders progress.

MLD

The classic infantile form of MLD is an autosomal recessive disorder with onset of symptoms during the second year of life. The presenting symptoms are loss of ability to stand and walk, hypotonia, and decreased deep tendon reflexes. As the disease progresses, there is deterioration in intellectual function, progressive optic atrophy with blindness, and finally decerebrate rigidity. The condition follows a steady downhill course and usually leads to death by about 5 years of age. The diagnosis can be established with the aid of nerve conduction studies, which already in the early stages shows a marked slowing of the MNCV. Brain neuroimaging shows abnormal signal changes in the white matter.

There is a marked reduction or total absence of the enzyme aryl sulfatase A (ARSA) in the leukocytes. The gene for ARSA is located on chromosome 22q13.31. Several different mutations have been identified in the DNA that relate to different clinical phenotypes.[75] Although most alterations in the gene are small base substitutions or deletions, 2 mutations each account for approximately 25% of all ARSA alterations: P426L and 459+1G→A.[76] Other mutations are associated with phenotypes of different severity. Furthermore, a high level of phenotypic diversity is present even among individuals with the same genotype.[77]

The peripheral nerves in biopsy specimens of the skin, conjunctiva, muscle, and sural nerve show widespread myelin loss with Schwann cell atrophy, demyelination, and scattered granular inclusions in the Schwann cell cytoplasm (Fig 6, A).[78-80] These periodic acid–Schiff (PAS) positive, diastase digestion–resistant inclusions stain brown with any of the Romanowsky stains (eg, crystal violet) and may be seen in nonneural tissues such as circulating lymphocytes and sweat gland epithelial cells.[80] Ultrastructural examination reveals complex, membrane-bound, lipid inclusions representing intralysosomal accumulation of unmetabolized cerebroside sulfatides[78]; often, these take the form of lamellar bodies termed "tuffstone" or "prismatic" bodies (Fig 6, B). Prenatal diagnosis is possible by measurements of ARSA in the amniotic fluid with subsequent tissue confirmation.[81]

KRABBE DISEASE AND OTHER CNS DISORDERS

Krabbe disease, also known as globoid cell leukodystrophy, usually starts in the second half of the first year of life with deterioration of motor and intellectual function, followed by a more rapid progression than that seen with MLD, often leading to death within months. Later-onset variants have also been described. The diagnosis can be confirmed by the demonstration of a markedly slow NCV and deficiency of galactocerebrosidase enzyme in the leukocytes. The gene for Krabbe disease has been located on chromosome 14.[82] Rafi et al[83] described a mutation found relatively often in patients with Krabbe disease, a C502T polymorphism that results in a 20-kb deletion from the middle of exon 10 to exon 17. De Gasperi et al[84] reported that the galactocerebrosidase gene in approximately half of families with late-onset Krabbe disease was compound heterozygous for the 20-kb gene deletion. Peripheral nerves in biopsy specimens of skin, conjunctivae, muscle, and nerve show the characteristic thin, needle-shaped, clear, membrane-bound inclusions in the Schwann cell cytoplasm (Fig 7).[85-89]

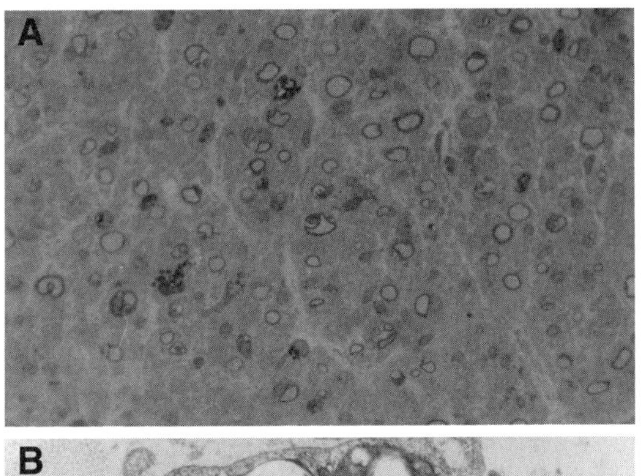

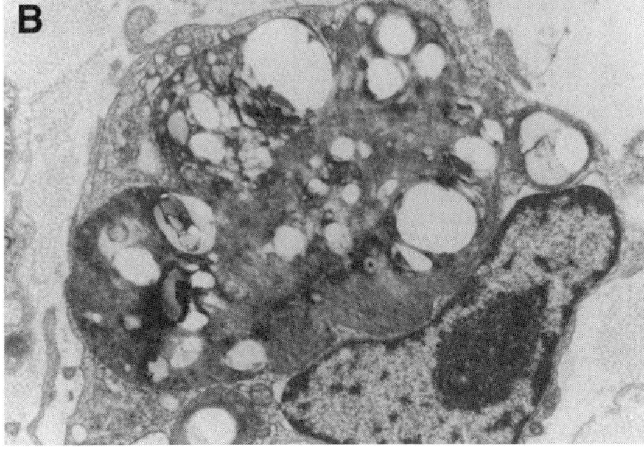

FIGURE 6.
A, Epon-embedded photograph of sural nerve from a patient with metachromatic leukodystrophy (MLD). Note the diminished number of myelinated axons and thin myelin sheaths. Granular inclusions in the Schwann cell cytoplasm indicate a storage disorder (toluidine blue; original magnification, ×1000). **B**, An endoneurial macrophage containing "prismatic" bodies typical of excess sulfatides in MLD (electron micrograph; original magnification, ×10,000).

Moreover, macrophages within the nerve tissue may show similar inclusions. Involvement of the lower motor neuron and specifically peripheral nerves can occur in many other rare degenerative CNS disorders. Peripheral neuropathy with a marked slowing of NCV, suggestive of demyelination, can be found in Cockayne and Leigh syndromes,[90,91] whereas hypotonia can be present in the gangliosidoses and familial dysautonomia.[24]

CLINICAL DIFFERENTIAL DIAGNOSIS

Hypotonia or floppiness is one of the common problems encountered by pediatricians and neurologists who care for children.

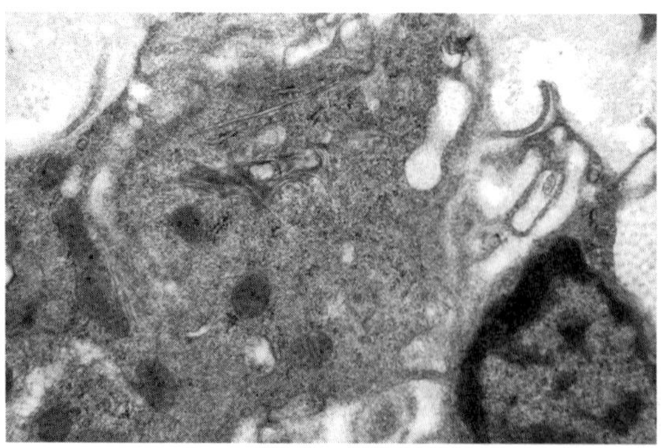

FIGURE 7.
An endoneurial macrophage showing needle-like inclusions seen typically in cases of Krabbe leukodystrophy (electron micrograph; original magnification, ×12,000).

Although hypotonia is a common feature of congenital peripheral neuropathy (CPN), it is also a nonspecific sign that can be present in CNS, peripheral nervous system (PNS), and mixed CNS and PNS disorders. Therefore, a clinician should develop the differential diagnosis for every case in which hypotonia is present. We will use the anatomical approach and consider every level of the CNS and every component of the lower motor neuron where the lesion can cause hypotonia (Fig 8). With this approach the clinician can narrow the differential diagnosis to 1 or 2 entities and plan further workup and management that is most efficient and cost-effective.

Lesions of the brain that are located in the cerebrum, basal ganglia, or cerebellum can cause hypotonia in a child more often than do lesions of the spinal cord or lower motor neuron. The prototype of central hypotonia is atonic cerebral palsy or atonic diplegia, which may or may not be associated with mental retardation. The important differential point is that deep tendon reflexes are brisk and pathologic reflexes are often present in central hypotonia, whereas reflexes are either reduced or absent in CPN. Lesions of the basal ganglia can be responsible for athetoid cerebral palsy. The abnormal movements such as dystonia or choreoathetosis that are associated with athetoid cerebral palsy are absent in CPN. Lesions of the cerebellum can cause ataxic cerebral palsy with ataxia and decreased, pendular-type deep tendon reflexes; these signs are absent in CPN. Some CNS degenerative white matter disorders such as metachromatic and Krabbe leukodystrophies progress to involve the PNS, causing neuropathy. Although clinically these disorders share some common features with CPN, they also differ from CPN by the presence of abnormalities on magnetic resonance imaging of the brain, specific enzyme deficiencies, and a relentlessly progressive course. Injuries to the spinal cord during either difficult labor or breech delivery can result in hypotonia and

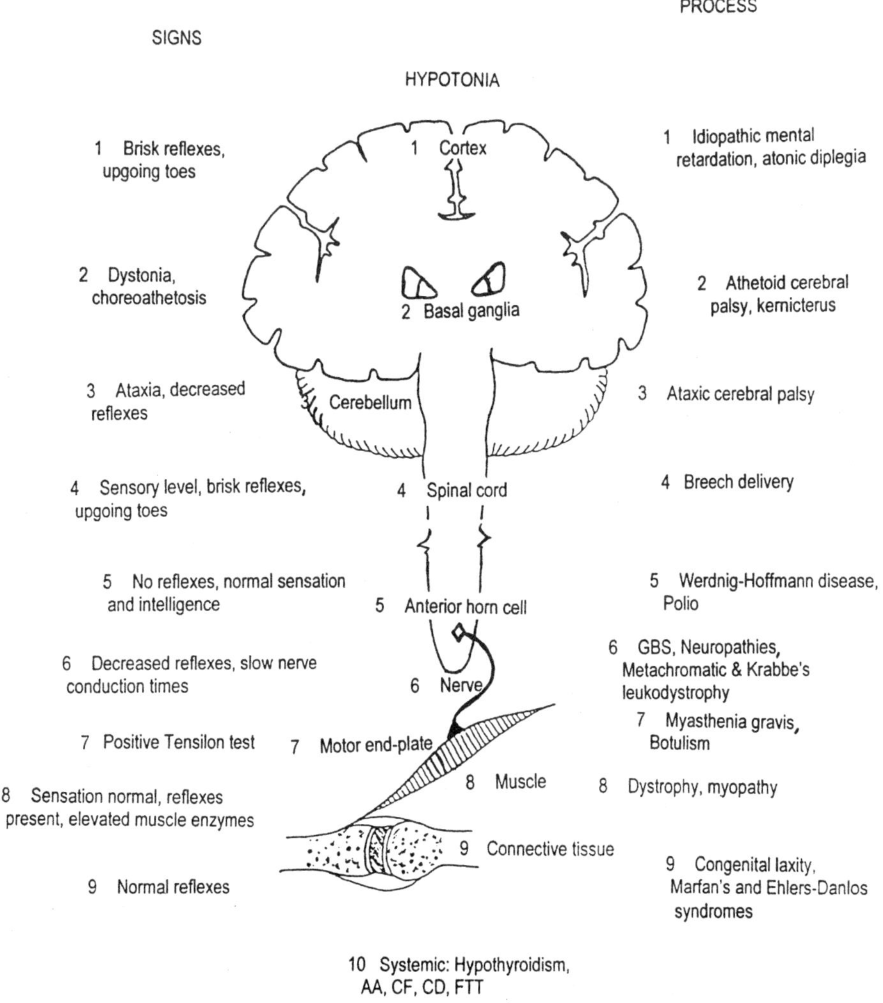

FIGURE 8.
Hypotonia and the level of nervous system dysfunction. *Abbreviations: GBS,* Guillain-Barré syndrome*; AA,* amino acid disorders; *CF,* cystic fibrosis; *CD,* celiac disease; *FTT,* failure to thrive.

respiratory distress because the lesion is usually high in the cervical region. Respiratory distress does not usually progress over time. A discrete sensory level impairment, abnormal deep tendon reflexes, and pathologic reflexes are often present in patients with birth-related spinal cord injury. Examples of pathologic processes that affect the anterior horn cell of the spinal cord, where the lower motor neuron starts, are spinal muscular atrophy (SMA) type I or Werdnig-Hoffmann disease, and poliomyelitis. Werdnig-Hoffmann disease is the single most important entity that should be included in the differential diagnosis because it can mimic some of the CPNs. In infants with Werdnig-Hoffman disease, however, weakness is more proximal than distal, and the chest is bell-shaped because of weakness of the intercostal muscles and preserved diaphragmatic breathing. Tongue fasciculations are often present, and both weakness and respiratory difficulties are progressive. Nerve conduction studies show a normal to mildly decreased MNCV in severe cases, and EMG shows a decreased interference pattern with polyphasic potentials and fibrillations. DNA analysis is commercially available and will show deletions of the survival motor neuron telomeric gene (SMN-T), which confirms the diagnosis in 95% of type I, about 90% of type II, and about 80% of type III variants of SMA disease. When the results of genetic testing and electrophysiologic testing are abnormal, there is no need to do any further testing, such as a muscle biopsy, which often yields inconclusive results in the neonatal period.

Poliomyelitis is an acquired disease that can occur at any age. The first symptoms are fever, malaise, and meningismus, giving rise to hypotonia, areflexia, and muscle weakness, which is characteristically asymmetrical. Cerebrospinal fluid examination shows pleocytosis and an elevated level of protein. At the spinal root and nerve level, examples of pathologic processes that cause hypotonia, weakness, respiratory distress, and reduced or absent deep tendon reflexes include earlier discussed hereditary motor and sensory neuropathies, and acquired diseases such as Guillain-Barré syndrome (GBS). GBS must be differentiated from CPN, which at times can be a difficult clinical task. GBS is a rare disorder during infancy, and there are only individual case reports of patients with neonatal onset.[92] The clinical course of GBS is that of progressive weakness, followed by a plateau of variable duration, and then either complete or partial recovery. Autonomic symptoms are often present and contribute to the morbidity and mortality of GBS. Nerve conduction studies are very helpful and show decreased amplitudes of motor evoked potentials and decreased MNCV.

Examples of disease processes at the neuromuscular junction are myasthenia gravis and botulism. Transient infantile and congenital myasthenia must be differentiated from CPN. A positive history of maternal myasthenia during pregnancy or a family history of myasthenia, a fluctuating course, fatigability during feeding, the presence of eyelid ptosis, and a positive Tensilon test are all consistent with a diagnosis of myasthenia. Repetitive nerve stimulation shows a characteristic decremental response in myasthenia gravis. Botulism can occur during infancy and can be excluded by finding no history of feeding honey, an absence of autonomic signs such as fixed dilated pupils, and an absence of ptosis. Muscle disease or myopathy can result in hypotonia and muscle weakness. Two major types of myopathies occur during infancy: congenital myopathy and muscular dystrophy. Examples of dystrophy are congenital muscular dystrophy and myotonic dystrophy, and examples of congenital myopathy are centronuclear, mitochondrial, and fiber-type disproportion myopathy. All of these disorders can lead to profound hypotonia and weakness. Three muscle disorders can manifest at birth with hypotonia and respiratory distress: myotonic dystrophy, centronuclear myopathy, and fiber-type disproportion myopathy. Metabolic myopathies such as hyperkalemic periodic paralysis should be considered in the differential diagnosis because the attacks of weakness may begin during infancy. A positive family history for muscular dystrophy or other myopathies, the presence of ocular involvement or skeletal anomalies as seen in congenital myopathies, normal sensation, normal deep tendon reflexes, elevated creatine kinase and lactic acid levels, and a characteristic myopathic EMG help to differentiate muscle disorders from neuropathies.

Extraneural disorders such as connective tissue disorders or systemic disorders can contribute to the floppy infant syndrome as well. Examples of connective tissue disorders are congenital joint laxity, Marfan syndrome, and Ehlers-Danlos syndrome. Usually, a positive family history of a similar disorder is present, muscle weakness and respiratory distress are not present, and ligament laxity is prominent. Ligament laxity causes decreased resistance to passive range of movement and often is interpreted as hypotonia. Among systemic disorders and syndromes, amino acid and organic acid disorders, cystic fibrosis, celiac disease, failure to thrive, hypothyroidism, Down syndrome, and Prader-Willi syndrome can sometimes mimic CPN. Usually these disorders are distinguished from neuropathy by the presence of a clear-cut period of normalcy preceding the onset of symptoms, the presence of metabolic or hormonal abnormalities, the presence of dysmorphic syndromic features, the absence of progressive respiratory symptoms, and normal deep tendon reflexes.

REFERENCES

1. Skre H: Genetic and clinical aspects of Charcot-Marie Tooth's disease. *Clin Genet* 6:98-118, 1974.
2. Ouvrier RA, McLeod JG, Pollard JD, eds: Historical perspective, in *Peripheral Neuropathy in Childhood. International Review of Child Neurology Series.* London: MacKeith Press, 1999, pp 10-11.
3. Warner LE, Mancias P, Butler IJ, et al: Molecular mechanisms for Charcot-Marie-Tooth disease and related demyelinating peripheral neuropathies. *Cold Spring Harbor Symp Quant Biol* 61:659-671, 1996.
4. Ouvrier R: Correlation between the histopathologic, genotypic, and phenotypic features of hereditary peripheral neuropathies in childhood. *J Child Neurol* 11:133-146, 1966.
5. Roa BB, Warner LE, Garcia CA, et al: Myelin protein zero (MPZ) gene mutations in nonduplication type 1 Charcot-Marie-Tooth disease. *Hum Mutat* 7:36-45, 1996.
6. Lupski JR: Charcot-Marie-Tooth disease: A gene-dosage effect. *Hosp Pract* 32:83-95, 1997.
7. Mendell JR: Charcot-Marie-Tooth neuropathies and related disorders. *Semin Neurol* 18:41-47, 1998.
8. Martini R: P0-deficient knockout mice as tools to understand pathomechanisms in Charcot-Marie-Tooth 1B and P0-related Dejerine-Sottas syndrome. *Ann N Y Acad Sci* 883:273-280, 1999.
9. Anonymous: 3rd Workshop of the European CMT Consortium: 54th ENMC International Workshop on genotype/phenotype correlations in Charcot-Marie-Tooth type 1 and hereditary neuropathy with liability to pressure palsies, Naarden, The Netherlands, Nov 28-30, 1997. *Neuromuscul Disord* 8:591-603, 1998.
10. Keller MP, Chance PF: Inherited neuropathies: From gene to disease. *Brain Pathol* 9:327-341, 1999.
11. Warner LE, Garcia CA, Lupski JR: Hereditary peripheral neuropathies: Clinical forms, genetics, and molecular mechanisms. *Annu Rev Med* 50:263-275, 1999.
12. Nelis E, Timmerman V, De Jonghe P, et al: Molecular genetics and biology of inherited peripheral neuropathies: A fast-moving field. *Neurogenetics* 2:137-148, 1999.
13. Pareyson D: Charcot-Marie-Tooth disease and related neuropathies: Molecular basis for distinction and diagnosis. *Muscle Nerve* 22:1498-1509, 1999.
14. Pleasure D: Hereditary motor and sensory neuropathy: The plot thickens (editorial). *Arch Neurol* 56:1195, 1999.
15. Vance JM: The many faces of Charcot-Marie-Tooth. *Arch Neurol* 57:638-640, 2000.

16. Appenzeller O, Snyder R, Kornfeld M: Sural nerve biopsies in pediatric neurological disorders. *Dev Med Child Neurol* 12:42-48, 1970.
17. Schroeder JM: Recommendations for the examination of peripheral nerve biopsies. *Virchows Arch* 432:199-205, 1998.
18. Gabreels-Festen AA, Joosten EM, Gabreels FJ, et al: Early morphological features in dominantly inherited demyelinating motor and sensory neuropathy (HMSN type I). *J Neurol Sci* 107:145-154, 1992.
19. Guzzetta F, Rodriguez J, Deodato M, et al: Demyelinating hereditary neuropathies in children: A morphometric and ultrastructural study. *Histol Histopathol* 10:91-104, 1995.
20. Garcia CA: A clinical review of Charcot-Marie-Tooth. *Ann N Y Acad Sci* 883:69-75, 1999.
21. Liehr T, Grehl H, Rautenstrauss B: Molecular diagnosis of PMP22-associated neuropathies using fluorescence in situ hybridization (FISH) on archival peripheral nerve tissue preparations. *Acta Neuropathol* 94:266-271, 1997.
22. Thiex R, Schroder JM: PMP-22 gene duplications and deletions identified in archival, paraffin-embedded sural nerve biopsy specimens: Correlation to structural changes. *Acta Neuropathol (Berl)* 96:13-21, 1998.
23. Dyck PJ, Chance PF, Lebo RV, et al: *Peripheral Neuropathy*, ed 3. Philadelphia, WB Saunders, 1993, pp 1094-1136.
24. Dubowitz V: Disorders of the lower motor neurone. Hereditary motor neuropathies, in Dubowitz V (ed): *Muscular Disorders of Childhood*, ed 2. London, WB Saunders, 1995, pp 370-397.
25. Vital A, Vital C, Julien J, et al: Occurrence of active demyelinating lesions in children with hereditary motor and sensory neuropathy (HMSN) type I. *Acta Neuropathol* 84:433-436, 1992.
26. Nelis E, Van Broeckhoven CV, De Jonghe P, et al: Estimation of the mutation frequencies in Charcot-Marie-Tooth disease type II and hereditary neuropathy with liability to pressure palsies: A European collaborative study. *Eur J Hum Genet* 4:25-33, 1996.
27. Numakura C, Lin C, Oka N, et al: Hemizygous mutation of the peripheral myelin protein 22 gene associated with Charcot-Marie-Tooth disease type 1. *Ann Neurol* 47:101-103, 2000.
28. Kamholz J, Awatramani R, Menichella D, et al: Regulation of myelin-specific gene expression. Relevance to CMT1. *Ann N Y Acad Sci* 883:91-108, 1999.
29. Stronach EA, Clark C, Bell C, et al: Novel PCR-based diagnostic tools for Charcot-Marie-Tooth type 1A and hereditary neuropathy with liability to pressure palsies. *J Peripher Nerv Syst* 4:117-122, 1999.
30. Reiter LT, Hastings PJ, Nelis E, et al: Human meiotic recombination products revealed by sequencing a hotspot for homologous strand exchange in multiple HNPP deletion patients. *Am J Hum Genet* 62:1023-1033, 1998.
31. Gabreels-Festen A, Van de Wetering R: Human nerve pathology caused by different mutational mechanisms of the PMP22 gene. *Ann NY Acad Sci* 883:336-343, 1999.

32. Bjartmar C, Yin X, Trapp BD: Axonal pathology in myelin disorders. *J Neurocytol* 28:383-395, 1999.
33. Griffin JW, Sheikh K: Schwann cell-axon interactions in Charcot-Marie-Tooth disease. *Ann N Y Acad Sci* 883:77-91, 1999.
34. Hanemann CO, Gabreels-Festen AAWM, Stoll G, et al: Schwann cell differentiation in Charcot-Marie-Tooth disease type IA (CMT1A): Normal number of myelinating Schwann cells in young CMT1A patients and neural cell adhesion molecule expression in onion bulbs. *Acta Neuropathol* 94:310-315, 1997.
35. D'Urso D, Ehrhardt P, Muller HW: Peripheral myelin protein 22 and protein zero: A novel association in peripheral nervous system myelin. *J Neurosci* 19:3396-3403, 1999.
36. Charnas L, Trapp B, Griffin J: Congenital absence of peripheral myelin: Abnormal Schwann cell development causes lethal arthrogryposis multiplex congenita. *Neurology* 38:966-974, 1988.
37. Karch SB, Urich H: Infantile polyneuropathy with defective myelination: An autopsy study. *Dev Med Child Neurol* 17:504-511, 1975.
38. Phillips JP, Warner LE, Lupski JR, et al: Congenital hypomyelinating neuropathy: Two patients with long-term follow-up. *Pediatr Neurol* 20:226-232, 1993.
39. Kasman M, Bermstein L, Schulman S: Chronic polyradiculoneuropathy of infancy: A report of three cases with familiar incidence. *Neurology* 26:565-573, 1976.
40. Hakamada S, Kumagai T, Hera K, et al: Congenital hypomyelinating neuropathy in a newborn. *Neuropediatrics* 14:182-183, 1983.
41. Gabreels-Festen AAWM, Bolhuis PA, Hoogendijk JE, et al: Charcot-Marie-Tooth disease type 1A: Morphological phenotype of the 17p duplication versus PMP22 point mutations. *Acta Neuropathol* 90:645-649, 1995.
42. Takashima H, Nakagawa M, Kanzaki A, et al: Germline mosaicism of MPZ gene in Dejerine-Sottas syndrome (HMSN III) associated with hereditary stomatocytosis. *Neuromuscul Disord* 9:232-238, 1999.
43. Parman Y, Plante-Bordeneuve V, Guiochon-Mantel A, et al: Recessive inheritance of a new point mutation of the PMP22 gene in Dejerine-Sottas disease. *Ann Neurol* 45:518-522, 1999.
44. Silander K, Meretoja P, Juvonen V, et al: Spectrum of mutations in Finnish patients with Charcot-Marie-Tooth disease and related neuropathies. *Hum Mutat* 12:59-68, 1998.
45. Boylan KS, Ferriero DM, Greco CM, et al: Congenital hypomyelination neuropathy with arthrogryposis multiplex congenita. *Ann Neurol* 31:337-340, 1992.
46. Seitz RJ, Wechsler W, Mosny DS, et al: Hypomyelination neuropathy in a female newborn presenting as arthrogryposis multiplex congenita. *Neuropediatrics* 17:132-136, 1986.
47. Levy BK, Fenton GA, Loaiza S, et al: Unexpected recovery in a newborn with severe hypomyelinating neuropathy. *Pediatr Neurol* 16:245-248, 1997.

48. Ghamdi M, Armstrong DL, Miller G: Congenital hypomyelinating neuropathy: A reversible case. *Pediatr Neurol* 16:71-73, 1997.
49. Lyon G: Ultrastructural study of a nerve biopsy from a case of early infantile chronic neuropathy. *Acta Neuropathol* 13:131-142, 1969.
50. Warner LE, Mancias P, Butler IJ, et al: Mutations in the early growth response 2 (EGR2) gene are associated with hereditary myelinopathies. *Nat Genet* 18:382-384, 1998.
51. Bellone E, Di Maria E, Soriani S, et al: A novel mutation (D305V) in the early growth response 2 gene is associated with severe Charcot-Marie-Tooth type 1 disease. *Hum Mutat* 14:353-354, 1999.
52. Marrosu MG, Vaccargiu S, Marrosu G, et al: Charcot-Marie-Tooth disease type 2 associated with mutation of the myelin protein zero gene. *Neurology* 50:1397-1401, 1998.
53. Senderek J, Hermanns B, Lehmann U, et al: Charcot-Marie-Tooth neuropathy type 2 and P0 point mutations: Two novel amino acid substitutions (Asp61Gly; Tyr119Cys) and a possible "hotspot" on Thr124Met. *Brain Pathol* 10:235-248, 2000.
54. Vedanarayanan V, Smith S, Subramony S, et al: Lethal neonatal autosomal recessive axonal sensorimotor polyneuropathy. *Muscle Nerve* 21:1473-1477, 1998.
55. Eckhardt SM, Hicks EM, Herron B, et al: New form of autosomal-recessive axonal hereditary sensory motor neuropathy. *Pediatr Neurol* 19:234-235, 1998.
56. Birouk N, Le Guern E, Maisonobe T, et al: X-linked Charcot-Marie-Tooth disease with connexin 32 mutations. *Neurology* 50:1074-1082, 1998.
57. Martyn CN, Martyn HR: Epidemiology of peripheral neuropathy. *J Neurol Neurosurg Psychiatry* 62:310-318, 1997.
58. Lin GS, Glass JD, Shumas S, et al: A unique mutation in connexin 32 associated with severe, early onset CMTX in a heterozygous female. *Ann NY Acad Sci* 14:481-484, 1999.
59. Ionasescu VV, Searby C, Ionasescu R, et al: Mutations of the noncoding region of the connexin 32 gene in X-linked dominant Charcot-Marie-Tooth neuropathy. *Neurology* 47:541-544, 1996.
60. Lewis RA, Shy ME: Electrodiagnostic findings in CMTX: A disorder of the Schwann cell and peripheral myelin. *Ann N Y Acad Sci* 883:504-507, 1999.
61. Hahn AF, Brown WF, Koopman WJ, et al: X-linked dominant hereditary motor and sensory neuropathy. *Brain* 113:1511-1525, 1990.
62. Lewis RA: The challenge of CMTX and connexin 32 mutations. *Muscle Nerve* 23:147-149, 2000.
63. Sander S, Nicholson GA, Ouvrier RA, et al: Charcot-Marie-Tooth disease: Histopathological features of the peripheral myelin protein (PMP22) duplication (CMT1A) and connexin 32 mutations (CMTX1). *Muscle Nerve* 21:217-225, 1998.
64. Fischbeck KH, ar-Rushdi N, Pericak-Vance M, et al: X-linked neuropathy: Gene localization with DNA probes. *Ann Neurol* 20:527-532, 1986.

65. Rozear MP, Pericak-Vance MA, Fischbeck KH, et al: Hereditary motor and sensory neuropathy, X-linked: A half century follow-up. *Neurology* 37:1460-1465, 1987.
66. Abrams CK, Oh S, Ri Y, et al: Mutations in connexin 32: The molecular and biophysical bases for the X-linked form of Charcot-Marie-Tooth disease. *Brain Res Brain Res Rev* 32:203-214, 2000.
67. Raimondi E, Gaudi S, Moralli D, et al: Assignment of the human connexin 32 gene (GJB1) to band Xq13. *Cytogenet Cell Genet* 60:210-211, 1992.
68. Bergoffen J, Scherer SS, Wang S, et al: Connexin mutations in X-linked Charcot-Marie-Tooth disease. *Science* 262:2039-2042, 1993.
69. Bone LJ, Dahl N, Lensch MW, et al: New connexin 32 mutations associated with X-linked Charcot-Marie-Tooth disease. *Neurology* 45:1863-1866, 1995.
70. Gambardella A, Bono F, Muglia M, et al: Autosomal recessive hereditary motor and sensory neuropathy with focally folded myelin sheaths (CMT4B). *Ann N Y Acad Sci* 883:47-55, 1999.
71. Bolino A, Muglia M, Conforti FL, et al: Charcot-Marie-Tooth type 4B is caused by mutations in the gene encoding myotubularin-related protein-2. *Nat Genet* 25:17-19, 2000.
72. Gambardella A, Bolino A, Muglia M, et al: Genetic heterogeneity in autosomal recessive hereditary motor and sensory neuropathy with focally folded myelin sheaths (CMT4B). *Neurology* 50:799-801, 1998.
73. Bolino A, Brancolini F, Bono F, et al: Localization of a gene responsible for autosomal recessive demyelinating neuropathy with focally folded myelin sheaths to chromosome 11q23 by homozygosity mapping and haplotype sharing. *Hum Genet* 5:1051-1054, 1996.
74. Nakagawa M, Suehara M, Saito A, et al: A novel MPZ gene mutation in dominantly inherited neuropathy with focally folded myelin sheaths. *Neurology* 52:1271-1274, 1999.
75. Kolodny EH: Metachromatic leukodystrophy and multiple sulfatase deficiency: Sulfatide lipidosis, in Rosenberg RN, Prusiner SB, DiMauro S, et al (eds): *The Molecular and Genetic Basis of Neurological Disease*. Boston, Butterworth-Heinemann, 1993, pp 497-503.
76. Gort L, Coll MJ, Ghabas A: Identification of 12 novel mutations and two new polymorphisms in the arylsulfatase A gene: Haplotype and genotype-phenotype correlation studies in Spanish metachromatic leukodystrophy patients. *Hum Mutat* 14:240-248, 1999.
77. Polten A, Fluharty AL, Fluharty CB, et al: Molecular basis of different forms of metachromatic leukodystrophy. *N Engl J Med* 324:18-22, 1991.
78. Duckett S, Cracco J, Graziani L, et al: Inclusions in the sural nerve in metachromatic leukodystrophy. *Acta Neurol Latinoam* 21:184-193, 1975.
79. Martinez AC, Ferrer MT, Fueyo E, et al: Peripheral neuropathy detected on electrophysiological study as first manifestation of metachromatic leucodystrophy in infancy. *J Neurol Neurosurg Psychiatry* 38:169-174, 1975.

80. Ikeda K, Goebel HH, Burck U, et al: Ultrastructural pathology of human lymphocytes in lysosomal disorders: A contribution to their morphological diagnosis. *Eur J Pediatr* 138:179-185, 1982.
81. Wiesmann UN, Meier C, Spycher MA, et al: Prenatal metachromatic leukodystrophy. *Helv Paediatr Acta* 30:31-42, 1975.
82. Zlotogora J, Chakraborty S, Knowlton RG, et al: Krabbe disease locus mapped to chromosome 14 by genetic linkage. *Am J Hum Genetics* 47:37-44, 1990.
83. Rafi MA, Luzi P, Chen YQ, et al: A large deletion together with a point mutation in the GALC gene is a common mutant allele in patients with infantile Krabbe disease. *Hum Mol Genet* 4:1285-1289, 1995.
84. De Gasperi R, Sosa MAG, Sartorato EL, et al: Molecular heterogeneity of late-onset forms of globoid-cell leukodystrophy. *Am J Hum Genet* 59:1233-1242, 1996.
85. Schlaepfer WW, Prensky AL: The peripheral neuropathy of globoid cell leukodystrophy. *Trans Am Neurol Assoc* 94:344-346, 1969.
86. Joosten EM, Krijgsman JB, Gabreels-Festen AA, et al: Infantile globoid cell leucodystrophy (Krabbe's disease). Some remarks on clinical, biochemical and sural nerve biopsy findings. *Neuropadiatrie* 5:191-209, 1974.
87. Matsumoto R, Oka N, Nagahama Y, et al: Peripheral neuropathy in late-onset Krabbe's disease: histochemical and ultrastructural findings. *Acta Neuropathol* 92:635-639, 1996.
88. Ida H, Rennert OM, Watabe K, et al: Pathological and biochemical studies of fetal Krabbe disease. *Brain Dev* 16:480-484, 1994.
89. Goebel HH, Kimura S, Harzer K, et al: Ultrastructural pathology of eccrine sweat gland epithelial cells in globoid cell leukodystrophy. *J Child Neurol* 8:171-174, 1993.
90. Moosa A: Peripheral neuropathy in Leigh's encephalomyelopathy. *Dev Med Child Neurol* 17:621-624, 1975.
91. Moosa A, Dubowitz V: Peripheral neuropathy in Cockayne's syndrome. *Arch Dis Child* 45:674-677, 1970.
92. Al-Qudah AA, Shahar E, Logan WJ, et al: Neonatal Guillain-Barré syndrome. *Pediatr Neurol* 4:255-256, 1988.

CHAPTER 8

Fetal Growth Programs Future Health: Causes and Consequences of Intrauterine Growth Retardation

Frank B. Diamond, Jr, MD
Professor of Pediatrics, University of South Florida College of Medicine, Tampa

Intrauterine growth retardation (IUGR) has been variously defined as a birth weight of less than 2500 g at term, or a weight or length that is less than the 10th percentile or below 2 SD for gestational age. These criteria have been primarily determined by the increased morbidity and mortality of infants whose size at birth is below these limits.[1] Infants who are small at birth relative to placental size or short in relation to head size have also experienced altered patterns of intrauterine growth.[2] Studies seeking to define IUGR are confounded by population differences in ethnicity, parity, socioeconomic status, geographic location, and altitude. Advances in perinatal care that alter outcomes and a secular trend of increasing heights over generations also affect growth reference values and cutoff points. Because 3% of healthy constitutionally small infants will fall below the statistical growth norms at birth, it is important to distinguish the pathologically fetal growth-restricted (FGR) infant from the healthy genetically small infant (small for gestational age, SGA). An estimated 28% to 70% of IUGR infants are simply constitutionally small, whereas only about 30% are truly pathologically growth restricted.[3] FGR represents a continuum of intrauterine stunting. The odds ratio of fetal loss relative to baseline birth weight increases from 1.9 for infants whose birth weights are below the 10th to 15th percentiles, to 2.8 for those whose birth weights are below the 5th to 10th percentiles, and to 5.6 for newborns with birth weights below the 5th percentile.[4] Ponderal index (wt-kg^3/ht) combines the determination of both height and weight. Low birth weight (LBW) infants exposed to an early gestational insult are often proportionately growth retarded with a normal ponderal index, whereas those affected later in pregnancy have asymmetric growth retardation, low ponderal index, and adaptive sparing of brain (head) size.[5]

NORMAL PATTERNS OF FETAL GROWTHS

Gestational age is defined obstetrically as the time elapsed from the first day of the last menstrual period, and term delivery occurs, on average, 280 days or 40 weeks from this date. The embryonic period begins 2 weeks after fertilization and extends 8 weeks to the start of the fetal period; at this time the fetus-embryo measures about 4 cm in length.[6] By the end of the first trimester, fetal crown-rump length has increased to 6 to 7 cm. At midpregnancy, the fetus weighs slightly more than 300 g. Fetal weight then increases linearly until the 37th week at a rate of approximately 15 g/kg per day, increasing 12-fold between 14 and 28 weeks (Fig 1).[7,8] Fetal fat mass quadruples in the third trimester when fetal and placental weight gain may account for as much as 50% of maternal weight gain.[8] Fetal crown-rump length attains 28 cm by 32 weeks, 32 cm by 36 weeks, and 36 cm at term, at which time fetal weight approximates 3400 g.[6] At birth, male weight exceeds female weight by approximately 100 g. These auxologic changes are documented in various populations by intrauterine growth curves that represent cross-sectional measurements of individual infants at birth, rather than sequential determinations over time.

ASSESSMENT OF PRENATAL GROWTH

Recognition of IUGR requires comparisons of fetal growth with standards of normally growing fetuses by gestational age, and requires accurate dating of pregnancy. Tape measurement of symphysis fundal height is the standard clinical method to screen prenatal growth. When this determination is less than expected for gestational age, an ultrasound is performed. Ultrasonographic measurement of crown-rump length is the most sensitive method for dating pregnancy in the first trimester before fetal stretching and bending begins.[9] Measurement of biparietal diameter is reliable in the second trimester, but less so in the third when hereditary factors influence head growth.[9] Breech position, multiple gestation, or oligohydramnios limit the usefulness of biparietal diameter. Abdominal circumfer-

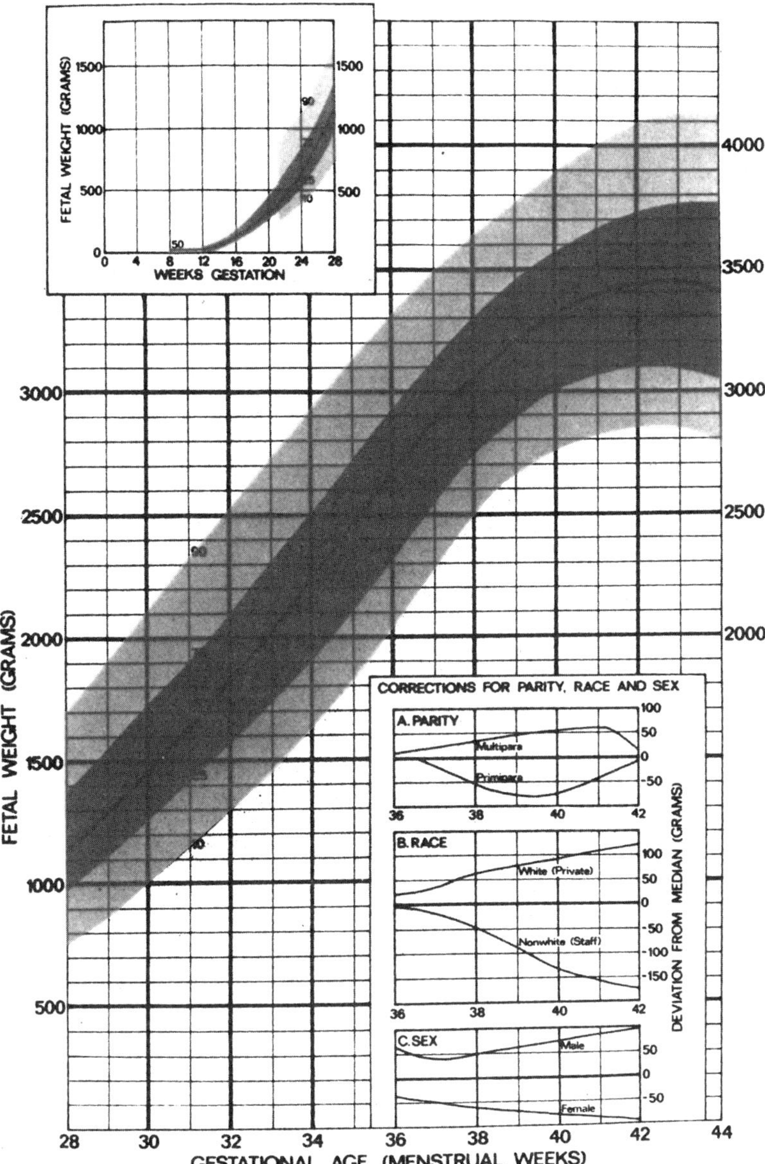

FIGURE 1.
Tenth to 90th percentiles of fetal weight gain at sea level from 28 to 44 weeks' gestation for 31,202 infants and abortuses. **Insert** shows effects of parity, race, and sex on fetal growth. (Courtesy of Brenner WE, Edelman DA, Hendricks CH: A standard for fetal growth for the United States of America. *Am J Obstet Gynecol* 126:555-564, 1976.)

ence at the level of bifurcation of the portal vein estimates subcutaneous abdominal fat and liver size, important indices of fetal nutritional health, and is considered the best ultrasonographic method to screen for IUGR.[9] However, care must be taken when comparing changes in abdominal circumference over time, because measurement errors may create false-positive diagnoses of fetal growth restriction with advancing gestational age.[10] Subcutaneous fat seen sonographically on transverse abdominal section as a well-demarcated echogenic border (the in utero equivalent of skinfold thickness) and measurement of the transcerebellar diameter have also been used to predict low birth weight.[11] Femur length, less influenced by nutritional deficits than abdominal circumference, is reduced in IUGR; it is altered in skeletal dysplasias and chromosomal abnormalities.[9]

Placental blood flow as assessed by Doppler studies of vascular velocity in fetal vessels correlates with fetal hypoxia and acidosis. Pulsatility of the umbilical artery (increased systolic-to-diastolic ratio), reflecting increased placental vascular resistance, has been used to predict chronic fetal hypoxia and growth retardation.[12]

PLACENTA AND AMNIOTIC FLUID IN IUGR

The placenta provides oxygen and nutrients to the developing fetus, with most placental growth occurring in the first half of gestation.[13] Second-trimester placental volume correlates with fetal weight at term, whereas fetal capillary surface area reflects maternal prepregnancy weight.[13] When the development of the placenta and its spiral arteries is restricted, fetal growth is limited. Infants of LBW mothers have lower placental weights, suggesting maternal "constraint" of fetal growth. Thus, a smaller placenta may result from uterine or ovarian underdevelopment that occurred during the mother's own intrauterine life.[14,15] Consistent with these findings is the experimental observation that transfer of the embryo of a smaller breed into the uterus of a larger one results in increased size at birth.[16]

Oxygen compromise stimulates placental growth and increases capillary volumes during implantation in mothers gestating at higher altitudes; maternal anemia (reduced oxygen-carrying capacity) correlates positively with placental size.[14]

Maternal undernutrition in early pregnancy also promotes placental growth, whereas high first-trimester carbohydrate intake or low third-trimester animal protein intake reduces placental size and birth weight.[17] Reduced dietary intake of animal protein relative to carbohydrates also predisposes to higher adult blood pressure (vide infra).[17] The placenta produces lactate and ammonia for both fetal and maternal circulations, and transports amino acids from mother to fetus. Reduced fetal leucine levels caused by increased protein catabolism or reduced placental transport are seen in IUGR pregnancies.[18]

As pregnancy advances, increased maternal blood flow to placental intravillous spaces is accompanied by endovascular invasion of trophoblast cells and deposition of fibrin. Placental thrombosis and atherosclerosis of spiral arteries are seen in pregnancies complicated by IUGR, with or without preeclampsia.[19] Recent investigation has focused on evaluation of peptide regulators of fetoplacental coagulation that may influence in utero hemostasis. For example, higher levels of plasminogen activator inhibitor type-1 and type-2 are found in uterine venous blood and cytotrophoblast isolates from IUGR compared with normal pregnancies.[20] Increased local synthesis of plasminogen activator inhibitor may restrict endovascular trophoblast invasion and increase fibrin deposition, reducing uteroplacental blood flow. Other proteins involved in coagulation that have been investigated in IUGR pregnancies are listed in Box 1. Angiogenesis is also affected by oxygen-sensitive vascular growth factors during pregnancy. Hypoxia upregulates vascular endothelial growth factor while downregulating endothelial inhibitory placental growth factor released from the trophoblast

BOX 1.
Vasoactive Compounds in Placental Circulation

Vasodilators and Inhibitors of Platelet Aggregation
- Parathyroid hormone-related peptide (PTHrP)
- Prostacyclin
- Annexin V
- Antithrombin (AT)
- Fibrinogen C4-binding protein (C4b-BP)
- Platelet-activating factor acetylhydrolase

Vasoconstrictors and Stimulators of Platelet Aggregation
- Endothelin
- Thromboxane A2
- Phosphatidylserine
- Thrombin-antithrombin complex (TAT)
- Tissue factor inhibitor free antigen (TFP1-Fag)
- Protein S free antigen

bilayer and villous mesenchyme.[21] Relatively high intervillous oxygen levels in IUGR, "placental hyperoxia," may alter angiogensis through reciprocal changes in vascular endothelial growth factor and placental inhibitory growth factor expression.[21] Levels of epidermal growth factor are also reduced in urine of FGR infants.[22]

ENDOCRINOLOGY OF FETAL GROWTH

GROWTH HORMONE

In the fetus, pituitary-derived growth hormone (GH) levels increase from 50 ng/mL at 3 months' gestation to 150 ng/mL by midpregnancy, then gradually decrease toward term (20 ng/mL in umbilical blood) as central inhibitory controls mature.[23] GH receptors, widely dispersed but present in low abundance in early pregnancy, increase in late gestation and after parturition. Concentrations of GH binding protein (GHBP), the extracellular domain of the GH receptor, are reduced in fetal blood.[24] This finding helps to explain the transition from relatively GH-independent fetal growth to GH-dependent postnatal growth. Clinically, children with isolated GH deficiency or anencephaly show relatively minor growth deficits of about -0.8 ± 1.4 SD below the mean in length, whereas infants with GH insensitivity caused by GH receptor defects measure approximately -1.6 ± 2.0 SD below the mean.[25] Similarly, transgenic mice expressing high levels of pituitary GH or GH-releasing hormone (GHRH) are not large at birth, but overgrow by 14 to 21 days of age.[26]

In the maternal circulation, pituitary-derived GH (hGH-N) predominates in early gestation, but is suppressed in the second half of pregnancy by secretion of a placental GH variant (hGH-V, PGH), which also binds to fetal and maternal GH receptors. The amino acid sequence of the mature PGH protein differs from that of hGH-N by 13 amino acids and appears in mothers' blood at 10 to 12 weeks.[27] Concentrations increase by the third trimester to 15 to 25 ng/mL. Unlike hGH-N, PGH is released in a tonic, not pulsatile fashion, and is regulated independently of GHRH.[27] PGH induces maternal insulin-like growth factor-1 (IGF-1), which stimulates maternal uterine and breast growth and correlates with fetal femur length and birth weight.[27,28] The actions of PGH on maternal metabolism are also modulated by GHBP, whose levels in pregnant serum approximate or exceed those of the nonpregnant state depending on gestational age.[29] GHBP levels decline as pregnancy progresses, correlate positively with mothers' weight and body mass index (BMI), and relate inversely to maternal glucose values.[27]

GHBP is increased, whereas PGH and IGF-1 are reduced in IUGR pregnant serum. Altogether, maternal GH-related factors account for up to 40% of the variance in fetal birth weight.[30]

HUMAN PLACENTAL LACTOGEN

Human placental lactogen (hPL), synthesized in the syncytiotrophoblast, is transcribed from highly homologous hPL-A and hPL-B genes, encoding proteins with 85% identity to hGH-N and 17% to human prolactin.[31] hPL is secreted differentially into both maternal and fetal circulations: maternal concentrations correlate with placental mass, are first detected at mid-first trimester, and increase to 5 to 7 μg/mL by mid-third trimester; fetal levels increase from a mean of 5 ng/mL at 20 weeks to 20 to 30 ng/mL at parturition.[31] The possible hPL regulation of IGF synthesis in fetal liver is suggested by a high correlation of hPL and IGF levels in sera obtained by direct in utero umbilical cord puncture.[32] hPL receptors are widely expressed in early gestation, suggesting that hPL is active in tissue differentiation.[31] Placental lactogen exerts direct anabolic effects on fetal metabolism; in vitro hPL stimulates amino acid uptake and DNA synthesis in myoblasts, fibroblasts, and hepatocytes, induces islet cell formation and insulin production, stimulates dehydroepiandrosterone sulfate secretion from fetal adrenal, and promotes production of surfactant from lung cells.[31]

IGFs

The glucose-insulin-IGF axis is the primary regulator of fetal growth.[33] IGF-1 mRNA is present in the placenta and in all fetal tissues beginning in early embryogenesis, although it appears to exert its effect as a growth stimulator in later fetal life.[33] IGF-1 levels increase 400% between 25 to 31 weeks and term, while IGF-2 values remain relatively constant.[34] IGF-1 levels correlate with birth size, and circulating levels are reduced in fetal blood of IUGR infants.[33] In studies of fetal rats rendered IUGR by uterine artery ligation, tissue IGF-1 responsible for paracrine growth stimulation is also reduced.[35] Postnatally, the null state for IGF-1 in the mouse is lethal. Affected animals are growth retarded, infertile, and have multiple organ failure. Neurologic sequelae suggest a role of IGF-1 in axonal growth and myelinization.[36] The Cre/lox P conditional knockout mouse has selective absence of liver-generated IGF-1, resulting in a 75% reduction in circulating IGF-1 values. Despite this deficit, the animals grow normally, demonstrating the primacy of tissue/paracrine IGF-1 in this species.[37]

Nutrient flux, glucose availability, and circulating insulin are the principal regulators of fetal IGFs, with GH and thyroid hormone subserving lesser roles until after parturition. For example, fetal pancreatectomy reduces IGF-1 levels with resultant IUGR, whereas fetal infusion of glucose or insulin augments fetal IGF levels.[38] IGF-2 predominates as a growth mediator during early gestation at the time of organogenesis and embryo growth, with a shift in later pregnancy to the more nutrient-sensitive IGF-1 influence on fetal growth. Fetal IGFs act to direct nutrient flow from placenta to fetus. In fetal sheep, for example, IGF-1 inhibits placental lactate production and metabolism of fetal amino acids, increasing fetal substrate supply.[25]

Mice with gene knockouts of either IGF-1 or IGF-2 are 40% smaller at birth than normal, whereas elimination of both growth factors stunts rodents to 30% of normal newborn size, suggesting independent fetal growth-promoting effects of both IGF-1 and IGF-2 (Fig 2).[39] Insulin knockout mice show growth retardation of only

Mutation	Size		
•I	80%		
•IGF-1	60%	30% (IGF-1 + IGF-2)	
•IGF-2	60%		
•IR	90%	30% (IR + IGF-1R)	30% (IR + IGF-1R + IGF-2R/M6P)
•IGF-1R	45%		
•IGF-2R/M6P	140%	100% (IGF-1R + IGF-2R/M6P)	

FIGURE 2.
The additive effect of mutating both IGF-1 and IGF-2 genes in "knock-out" mouse models suggests that each growth factor acts independently on fetal growth. *Abbreviations: I,* Insulin; *IGF-1* and *IGF-2,* insulin-like growth factors 1 and 2; *IR,* insulin receptor; *IGF-1R,* IGF-1 receptor; *IGF-2R/M6P,* IGF-2 receptor. (Courtesy of Accili D, Nakae J, Kim JJ, et al: Targeted gene mutations define the roles of insulin and IGF-1 receptors in mouse embryonic development. *J Pediatr Endocrinol Metab* 12:475-485, 1999. Reproduced by permission of Freund Publishing House Ltd.)

10% to 20%, suggesting a "permissive" rather than direct effect of insulin on intrauterine growth. Receptor knockout studies illustrate that IGF-1 acts exclusively through the IGF-1 receptor, whereas IGF-2 growth effects are mediated through the insulin and IGF-1 receptors.[39] A distinct IGF-2 receptor sequesters ligand and clears it from the circulation. Knockout of both the insulin receptor and IGF-1 receptor results in a 70% reduction in neonatal size, whereas deletion of the IGF-2 receptor gene responsible for clearing IGF-2 from the circulation results in increased circulating levels of IGF-2 and a newborn mouse 40% larger than normal.[39]

Although maternal IGF-1 does not cross the placenta, it influences cross-placental nutrient transfer.[40] IGF-1 administration to pregnant rats increases maternal mRNA of GLUT-1 and GLUT-3, glucose transporters from mother to placenta and placenta to fetus, respectively.[41] In sheep, maternal infusion of IGF-1 increases fetal glucose levels and placental lactate flow to the fetus.[42] Maternal IGF-1 levels are low in human gestations complicated by IUGR with growth restriction and placental dysfunction (abnormal umbilical artery pulsatility index), but normal in mothers of SGA infants with normal pulsatility index.[43] Reduction of maternal IGF-1 in growth-restricted pregnancies may adaptively prevent acidosis induced by glucose delivery to a hypoxic fetus or primarily reflect placental injury.[43]

The role of the IGF-1 system in prenatal (and postnatal) growth is illustrated clinically by a case report of a teenage boy with severe IUGR that persisted postnatally (–6.9 SD), who was found to be homozygous for a partial deletion of the IGF-1 gene. The patient's birth weight and birth length were –3.9 and –5.4 SD below the mean, respectively, and his head circumference was –4.9 SD. Placental weight was –1.3 SD. The patient was deaf, microcephalic, and mentally retarded, suggesting the importance of IGF-1 in human neurodevelopment.[44]

IGF BINDING PROTEINS

The presence of IGF binding protein (IGFBP) mRNA in multiple fetal tissues suggests the importance of these proteins in growth regulation and development.[45] IGFBP-3 levels are reportedly lower in IUGR than is appropriate for gestational age (AGA) infants, whereas fetal levels of both IGFBP-1 and IGFBP-2 levels are increased.[33] IGFBP-1 sequesters delivery of IGFs to fetal tissues inhibiting somatic growth; its increased levels likely reflect the hypoinsulinemia and substrate limitation characteristic of IUGR. IGFBP-1 levels correlate negatively with birth weight.[27]

Maternal IGFBP-1, synthesized in the decidualized endometrium under the control of progesterone, increases by the end of the first trimester and continues to increase to term.[46] Its levels adjusted for BMI are increased in pregnancies affected by fetal growth restriction but not those caused by constitutional/genetic small-for-dates gestation.[42] Maternal IGFBP-3 is proteolyzed by a pregnancy-specific protease that appears during the first trimester. IGFBP-3 levels in pregnant serum assessed by Western ligand blot decrease by 6 weeks' gestation and do not normalize until the end of the first week postpartum.[47] Proteolytically altered IGFBP-3 has reduced affinity for IGF-1, increasing the bioavailability of the growth factor, although IGFBP-3 levels do not correlate with birth weight.[39] When evaluated prospectively by Western ligand blot in IUGR pregnancies that were either FGR or SGA, IGFBP-3 levels increased in mothers of FGR compared with SGA and control infants, and the proteolysis of IGFBP-3 was not altered.[39] IGFBP-2 levels gradually decrease as pregnancy proceeds, and levels are increased in pregnancies in which fetal growth restriction occurs.

LEPTIN

Leptin, a 16-kd protein hormone synthesized in adipose tissue, acts on hypothalamic centers to regulate satiety and energy metabolism.[48] The product of the *ob* gene, leptin mRNA is also expressed in placenta, suggesting an effect on placental function and perhaps on intrauterine growth.[49] SGA infants have lower neonatal serum leptin levels than do AGA newborns, likely reflecting their reduced fat mass.[50] Leptin measured in umbilical vein blood correlates with birth weight and length, placental weight, and cord concentrations of insulin.[51] Cord leptin levels also vary inversely with weight gain from birth to 4 months of age independent of birth weight. In one study, infants who demonstrated an increasing rate of weight gain by 4 months of age had lower cord leptin levels than those with little change in weight SD score or those whose rate of weight gain slowed.[52]

ETIOLOGY OF IUGR

Box 2 lists fetal and maternal/placental causes of IUGR. Fetal disorders include chromosomal abnormalities and embryopathies such as renal agenesis or neural tube defects. Deletions or duplications of chromosomal material disrupt cell division, causing intrauterine stunting; for example, average birth weight is reduced 300 g by the presence of each additional (multiple) X chromosome.[53] Uniparental disomy of several chromosomes has also been recognized as a cause of IUGR. This may result from genomic imprinting, or from the unmasking of an autosomal recessive disorder caused when a protective normal gene from one parent is lost, leaving a pair of mutated chromosomes of the other parent. In the mouse, several imprinted genes involving IGF-2 influence fetal growth, including igf2, igf2r, Grb10, and H19.[54]

In humans, IUGR is associated with maternal uniparental disomy for chromosome 6, unmasked by congenital adrenal hyperplasia resulting from homozygosity for the I172N exon 4 mutation.[55] UPDmat14 is associated with low birth weight, early onset of puberty, short stature, and small hands.[56] UPDmat22 also results in IUGR. Nonmosaic trisomy of the placenta and maternal uniparental heterodisomy for chromosome 22 in peripheral blood suggests a conceptus with maternal trisomy caused by meiotic nondisjunction and trisomy rescue by loss of the paternal homologue.[57] Classic Russell-Silver syndrome is recognized clinically by the history of severe IUGR, and physical findings including asymmetric limbs, trunk, or body, triangular faces with high forehead tapering to a small pointed jaw, clinodactyly, postnatal growth retardation, and genital anomalies, hernia, or undescended testes. Uniparental disomy has been identified in about 7% of cases of Russell-Silver syndrome.[58]

Polymorphisms at the variable number of tandem repeat (VNTR) locus of the insulin gene (INS) promoter region have been associated with size at birth.[59] The INS VNTR III allele has been associated with reduced transcription of INS in fetal pancreas and with the placental gene encoding IGF-2.[60] In 758 children who underwent genotyping, INS VNTR was significantly associated with head circumference at birth across all 2 genotypes of allelic sizes class I and III.[59] Trends for association of birth weight and length with INS VNTR were most evident in children who did not cross growth channels downward nor upward in the first 2 years of life. In this group, the postnatal growth pattern likely reflects fetal genetic influence more than intrauterine environment or maternal constraint. INS VNTR may also influence rates of weight gain between birth and 2 years of age independent of effects on birth weight.[59]

Extrinsic factors that compromise fetal growth include any process that disrupts uteroplacental blood supply or alters normal placental function, such as maternal hypertension, or placental abruption, infarction, or malformation. Placental damage is suggested by the finding of increased fetal erythroblasts relative to nucleated red blood cells in maternal blood.[61]

BOX 2.
Causes of IUGR

- Intrinsic to the Fetus
  - Aneuploidy
  - Trisomy 13, 18, 21
  - Triploidy
  - Insulin gene VNTR polymorphisms
  - Turner syndrome
  - Extra sex chromosomes (47,XXY)
  - Autosomal deletions
  - 5p- (cri du chat), 5q-, 4p-, 4q-, 18p-, 18q-
  - Uniparental disomy of chromosomes 6, 7, 14, 22
  - Open neural tube disorders
  - Renal agenesis
  - Chondrodystrophies
  - Single umbilical artery
- Extrinsic to the Fetus (Maternal)
  - Medical illnesses
    - Advanced diabetes mellitus (White class C or greater)
    - Collagen vascular disease
    - Systemic lupus erythematosus
    - Polymyositis/dermatomyositis
    - Cyanotic heart disease
    - Hypertension
    - Chronic renal disease
    - Thyrotoxicosis
  - Obstetric Factors
    - Pregnancy-induced hypertension
    - Nulligravida
    - Prior miscarriage, stillborn, or IUGR infant
    - Multiple gestation
    - Medications
    - Chemotherapeutics and antimetabolites
    - Coumadin
    - Phenytoin
    - Steroids
  - Socioeconomic Factors
    - Poor nutritional status
    - Caloric or mineral deficiencies (zinc deficiency)
    - Low prepregnancy weight
    - Low pregnancy weight gain
    - Living at high altitude

(continued)

BOX 2. (continued)

Extrinsic to the Fetus (Maternal)
- Substance Abuse
  - Tobacco
  - Ethanol
  - Street drugs (cocaine, etc)
- Ethnicity
  - Bacterial infection
  - Listeria, syphilis, toxoplasmosis, tuberculosis, malaria
  - Viral infection
  - Cytomegalovirus, rubella, HIV

Abbreviations: IUGR, Intrauterine growth retardation; *VNTR,* variable number of tandem repeats; *HIV,* human immunodeficiency virus.

Abnormal maternal lipoprotein metabolism may contribute to FGR. In healthy pregnancies, maternal cholesterol levels increase 60% between 10 and 35 weeks, but this increase is blunted in gestations with FGR, and low-density lipoprotein (LDL) receptors that bind maternal lipoproteins for placental steroid synthesis are compensatorily increased.[62,63] Placental thrombosis caused by intravascular coagulation, atherosclerotic change, and fibrin deposition in decidual spiral arteries occurs more frequently in placentas from IUGR gestations, prompting investigation of platelet aggregation and vascular function in fetal growth restriction (vide supra).

In utero infections (TORCH) account for 1 of every 10 growth-retarded infants and are often of early onset; fetal viremia inhibits cell mitosis, promotes apoptosis, and reduces cell number.[3,64] In utero exposure to alcohol, carbon monoxide (smoking), heroin, or cocaine may retard fetal growth independently or in association with congenital infection.

Chronic malnutrition is the most common cause of IUGR in developing countries, affecting millions of infants worldwide. Early malnutrition reduces cell size and number, causing proportional growth retardation, whereas later malnutrition reduces cell size, resulting in disproportionate growth with sparing of head circumference.[3] Adequate maternal nutrition reduces the incidence of LBW infants in at-risk populations.[65] Current expert guidelines suggest an optimal gestational weight gain of 25 to 35 lb for women with a BMI of 19.8 to 26 kg/m^2.[66] Further, the incidence of LBW is lower in those who gain in the upper half of the recommended range compared with the lower half.[66]

Maternal hypoxia caused by high altitude, cyanotic heart disease, asthma, or sickle cell anemia compromises fetal growth, as do other maternal systemic diseases such as lupus, hypertension, and thyrotoxicosis, and exposure of the mother to toxic therapeutic agents such as chemotherapy. High parity, prior miscarriage, stillborn, or SGA infant, reduced interpregnancy interval, early menarche, and maternal short stature are also associated with an increased frequency of IUGR.[67]

NEONATAL EFFECTS OF IUGR

The neonate with IUGR is at increased risk for stillbirth or in-hospital death, fetal distress, perinatal asphyxia, metabolic acidosis, hypothermia (high surface area/body weight ratio), hypoglycemia (decreased glycogen stores), hypocalcemia (secondary to asphyxia), polycythemia reflecting chronic hypoxia, and infection (Fig 3). Most perinatal mortality results from peripartum depression, but congenital anomalies in IUGR infants account for one third of deaths.[68] In a population study of congenital malformations, approximately a quarter of 13,000 infants were IUGR, and the frequency of growth retardation was 60% when multiple defects were present.[69] The mortality rate increases with greater severity of growth retardation reflected in disproportionate body growth. The developing central nervous system is at particular risk in IUGR infants, and hypoxic encephalopathy may manifest postnatally with seizures and developmental delay.[44] Hyperviscosity and sludging secondary to hypoxia-induced polycythemia and acidosis occur in about 15% of SGA infants and is 4 times more common than in AGA infants.[71] Reduced fetal size, accelerated lung development, and polycythemia are protective adaptations to reduced fetal nutrient and oxygen supply. A positive consequence is a reduced incidence of hyaline membrane disease in SGA infants, although respiratory distress caused by meconium aspiration, pulmonary hemorrhage, and pneumonia occur more frequently than in gestational age peers.[45,72] Malnutrition alters immune function, resulting in a 9-fold increased risk of (intrauterine and extrauterine) infection in SGA compared with AGA infants.[73]

POSTNATAL GROWTH OF IUGR INFANTS

Most SGA infants, both term and preterm, catch up to their AGA peers in the first 6 to 12 months of life regardless of whether their growth retardation is defined by reduced length or weight at birth.[74] The timing of puberty is normal or slightly earlier in SGA children compared with children of normal heights, and the age of

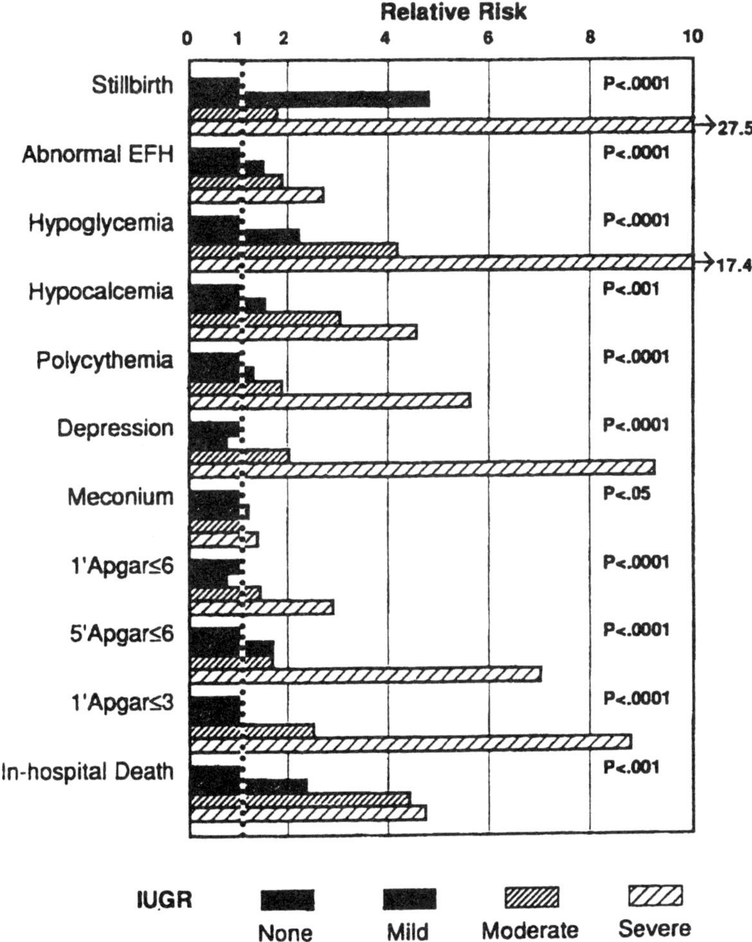

FIGURE 3.
Relative risks of intrauterine growth retardation *(IUGR)* of differing severity in the neonatal period. *EFH* signifies electronic fetal heart pattern. (Courtesy of Kramer MS, Olivieri M, McLean FH, et al: Impact of intrauterine growth retardation and body proportionality on fetal and neonatal outcome. *Pediatrics* 86:711, 1990. Reproduced by permission of *Pediatrics,* vol 86, p 711, copyright 1990.)

menarche is comparable to that in an AGA population.[75] In a cohort of healthy SGA term Swedish infants with birth lengths of less than 2 SD, only 13.4% were below −2 SD by 1 year and less than 8% remained small by 18 years.[76] However, SGA infants have a 7-fold increased risk for short adult stature and represent 20% to

25% of children who are short in later life.[76] Half of the short IUGR children who do not catch up become short adults, an outcome that is primarily influenced by genetics, because adult heights correlate best with maternal heights and birth lengths; women who were themselves SGA at birth have double the risk of delivering an SGA infant.[77] Other risk factors such as infants' weight, length, or head size at birth, maternal weight gain, smoking or toxemia, or placental size are not determinant.[14] The early catch-up growth of the SGA neonate may be stimulated by a transient hypersomatotropism that is manifested in the first days to weeks of life by increased GH pulsatility and an exaggerated GH response to exogenous GHRH.[78,79] In some SGA infants, rapid postnatal weight gain may predispose them to the development of childhood obesity.[80]

POSTNATAL NEURODEVELOPMENT IN IUGR

Infants born with IUGR are reported to be at greater risk for compromised neurodevelopmental outcome characterized by an increased prevalence of minor central nervous system dysfunction, learning difficulties, and behavioral problems, but these morbidities may not be readily manifest in early life.[81] For example, IUGR premature infants have normal brainstem auditory evoked responses in the early neonatal period, and no differences are found in neurodevelopmental outcome at 1 year of age in IUGR infants with impaired uteroplacental circulation (infarcts and accelerated villous maturation) compared with those with normal placentas.[82,83] However, a study of mental health outcome in a large cohort of Australian children aged 4 to 16 years reported that those below the 2nd percentile of percentage of expected birth weight for gestational age (PEBW) had 2 times more mental health problems than those with birth weights above the 90th percentile of PEBW, and were more likely to be rated as academically impaired.[84]

POSTNATAL SEQUELAE OF IUGR

Adaptive responses to nutritional and endocrine stresses during critical periods of intrauterine growth reprogram fetal metabolism in ways that promote in utero survival, but result in increased morbidity and mortality in postnatal life. These "protective" changes include alterations in skeletal muscle and hepatic glucose flux, vascular function, adrenal steroidogenesis, and lipoprotein synthesis that result in insulin resistance and probable resistance to IGF-1. Starvation-induced changes in hepatic periportal and perivenous cell division result in a relative surfeit of glucokinase activity and deficiency of phosphoenolpyruvate carboxykinase.[85] Abnormal hepatic enzyme responses may reflect deficiency of inositolphosphoglycan D-chiro-inositol/galactosamine, a hydrolytic product of cell membrane glycosylphosphatidylinositol that mediates insulin action after insulin binding to its receptor.[86] A significant association has been found between the tandem number of variable repeat locus of the insulin gene III/III genotype and impaired glucose tolerance and type 2 diabetes in patients whose postnatal growth showed little variation in weight standard deviation score between birth and 1 year of age—that is, those infants whose in utero growth would likely have been less influenced by maternal and uterine factors.[60]

Short IUGR children aged 8 to 10 years, without family histories of type 2 diabetes mellitus, already demonstrate insulin resistance compared with normal birth weight controls as assessed by intravenous glucose tolerance testing with tolbutamide infusion, and their insulin sensitivity declines further during puberty.[87] Insulin resistance in adolescents who were fetal growth restricted manifests as increased triglyceride levels and increased ratios of LDL to high-density lipoprotein (HDL).[88] Low birth weight and insulin resistance are also associated with gonadal dysfunction. IUGR adolescent girls may experience exaggerated or premature adrenarche and pubarche and ovarian hyperandrogenism.[88] In IUGR males, low birth weight has been associated with androgen insensitivity, some forms of hypospadius, and an early decrease in Sertoli cell number and function.[89,90]

In adulthood, the insulin-resistant IUGR patient has a hypercoagulable atherogenic state known as syndrome X, characterized by cardiovascular and cerebrovascular disease, hypertension, and impaired glucose tolerance (Table 1).[86] Circulating levels of fibrinogen, factor VII, and apolipoprotein B are increased.[91] Of note, cordocentesis reveals that elevated levels of apolipoprotein B (Apo B) and the ratio of Apo B/A1 are already present in utero in the growth-retarded fetus compared with the normally growing control.[92]

Over time, pancreatic size, ß-cell function, and insulin levels may be reduced in the adult who was IUGR.[87] Impaired glucose tolerance has been documented in adult offspring of mothers exposed to famine in mid to late gestation, and men older than 65 years with birth weights of 5.5 lb or less have a prevalence of type 2 diabetes mellitus which is 2 times that found when birth weights exceeded 9.5 lb (40% vs 14%).[93,94] Insulin resistance occurs independently of lifestyle behaviors such as smoking, but is exacerbat-

TABLE 1.
Percentages of Men in the Hertfordshire Study With Syndrome X According to Birth Weight

Birth Weight (kg)	Total No. of Men	No. (%) With Syndrome X	Odds Ratio* (95% CI)
≤2.50	20	6 (30)	18 (2.6-118)
–2.95	54	10 (19)	8.4 (1.5-49)
–3.41	114	19 (17)	8.5 (1.5-46)
–3.86	123	15 (12)	4.9 (0.9-27)
–4.31	64	4 (6)	2.2 (0.3-14)
>4.31	32	2 (6)	1.0
Total	407	56 (14)	

*Odds ratio adjusted for body mass index (chi-square for trend = 16.0, $P = < .001$).
Abbreviation: CI, Confidence interval.
(Courtesy of Barker DJP, Hales CN, Fall CHO, et al: Type 2 (non-insulin-dependent) diabetes mellitus, hypertension and hyperlipidemia (syndrome X): Relation to reduced fetal growth *Diabetologia* 36:62-67, 1993.)

ed by obesity.[95] Epidemiologic studies demonstrate increased mortality from coronary artery disease in adults who were growth retarded infants. In one population of patients aged 45 years or older, the prevalence of coronary artery disease increased from 4% in those who weighed 3.2 kg or more at birth, to 15% in those weighing 2.5 kg or less at birth.[96]

Glucocorticoids are potent growth inhibitors, and cortisol excess may also play a role in IUGR. Maternal corticosteroid levels significantly exceed fetal values. The fetus is shielded from high cortisol (F) levels by its conversion to cortisone (E) by placental 11β-hydroxysteroid dehydrogenase-2 (11β-HSD2).

The F/E ratio is increased in some IUGR children without catch-up growth, suggesting a partial deficit of 11β-HSD2. Because cortisol also exerts mineralocorticoid effects, and children with IUGR are known to have a nephron deficit, deficiency of 11β-HSD2 may contribute to the hypertension seen in adults with syndrome X.[97]

TREATMENT OF IUGR

PRENATAL

Various studies have addressed the feasibility of stimulating fetal growth in utero by administering amino acids, glucose, oxygen, or growth-promoting hormones to the pregnant mother, into the amniotic fluid (enteral), or directly to the fetus. In normally growing infants in midgestation, active placental transport of amino acids results in a positive fetal to maternal gradient, whereas by late pregnancy amino nitrogen flux favors the placenta.[98] IUGR infants have significantly lower concentrations of branched-chain amino acids than do normally growing infants, suggesting that fetal nitrogen wasting to the placenta is required to sustain placental energy needs and fetoplacental survival during periods of malnutrition.[99] Efforts to reverse this process by feeding mothers a high-protein diet, administering amino acids intravenously, or infusing them into the amniotic fluid to bypass a disordered placenta have generally failed to stimulate fetal growth and may be associated with significant risks. High-protein supplements increase the incidence of preterm delivery and perinatal death if mothers are not protein deficient and have a history of prior SGA infants.[99] Administration of excess amino acids in utero may also inhibit fetal uptake of other essential amino acids. In animal trials, treatment of pregnant sheep with amino acids increased fetal ammonia and urea concentrations and decreased PaO_2 and pH.[100]

The utilization of glucose and oxygen by the IUGR fetus is comparable on a unit weight basis to that of normally growing infants, indicating that deficits of these substrates may impair fetal growth.[98] Normally growing human fetuses whose mothers are infused with glucose, or who receive direct infusion of glucose, experience rapid fetal acidosis, and in experimental animals, increasing blood glucose levels in utero has the potentially harmful effects of increasing oxygen consumption and blood lactate levels.[101]

Energy for growth absorbs 20% to 40% of fetal oxidative metabolism, and insufficient oxygen supply stunts fetal growth.[102] In women living at high altitudes, infant birth weights correlate with maternal oxygen levels in the last trimester; women with cyanotic heart disease have a high incidence of IUGR, which declines after surgical repair of their cardiac lesion.[103,104] Supplementation of maternal oxygen levels increases fetal oxygenation and improves perinatal mortality, but has no effect on fetal growth assessed by ultrasound measurements.[92,105] Late cardiac decelerations have been noted to be increased in IUGR fetuses after discontinuation of maternal hyperoxia. In the hypoglycemic fetus, maternal oxygen administration may potentially shunt blood flow from the brain by increasing cerebral and decreasing peripheral vascular resistance.[106,107] Infusion of the normal ovine fetus with IGF-1 for 10 days increases fetoplacental uptake of glucose and reduces placental lactate release and fetal oxidation of amino acids. Internal organs grow, but there is little increase in overall body size.[108] In contrast, administration of pulses of GH to fetal sheep increases their body weight as well as the size of fetal liver, spleen, and thymus.[109] When GH is given to the mother of a growth-retarded human fetus, there is no increase in fetal growth, but placental urea clearance doubles.[109] Administration of insulin to starved mothers raises fetal IGF-1 levels within 24 hours but fails to increase fetal growth above normal rates.[110]

Low-dose aspirin has been administered during pregnancy in an attempt to prevent FGR, based on the presence of increased thromboxane, a vasoconstrictor and platelet aggregator, and an altered thromboxane/prostacyclin ratio in IUGR.[111] Although some studies have resulted in increased birth weights in treated patients, the overall results have been equivocal.[112]

POSTNATAL

As a group, short children born SGA have reduced GH secretion and an increased incidence of GH deficiency based on provocative testing or assessment of spontaneous GH release.[45] However, as most are neither GH deficient nor resistant, some authors have speculated that their growth delay results from IGF-1 insensitivity.[113] IGF-1 and IGFBP-3 levels are usually normal or low in short SGA children but increase appropriately during GH treatment.[107] As is the case with almost all short patients, SGA children with short stature demonstrate an increased growth velocity in response to treatment with exogenous GH, but higher doses than those usually prescribed to GH-deficient children appear necessary to achieve catch-up growth.[114] An epi-analysis of 6-year growth responses in short, nonclassically GH-deficient, SGA children aged 2 to 8 years used continuous and discontinuous GH treatment protocols.[115] Continuous treatment for 6 years increased mean height by 2.0 to 2.7 SD in a dose-dependent manner, whereas discontinuous therapy of periods averaging 2 years resulted in an increase of mean adjusted height SD to -0.4 ± 0.1 SD with stabilization of posttreatment growth patterns. The authors of this study hypothesized that short-term administration of high-dose GH could restore epiphyseal responsiveness in some short SGA individuals. GH treatment caused no acceleration of pubertal onset, and bone age maturation relative to chronologic age remained minimally delayed. Predictors of growth response to GH in SGA children included cumulative 6-year GH dose, parental-adjusted height SD score, and age at initiation of therapy.[115]

Despite these findings, few studies have yet documented the effects of GH treatment on adult stature of short SGA children, and some data suggest that the increase over predicted height is minimal.[116] GH administration is known to increase insulin resistance. One report found no significant alteration in fasting blood glucose or hemoglobin Alc after 2 years of GH treatment.[114] Other investigators report a significant increase in fasting insulin levels during GH treatment of SGA children and an increase in insulin area under the curve (AUC) during oral glucose tolerance tests after 1 year of GH therapy compared with baseline testing.[114,117] The possible impact of such therapy on the long-term sequelae of IUGR such as type 2 diabetes mellitis and coronary artery disease remains unknown.

NEW DIRECTIONS IN FETAL GROWTH RESEARCH

Future research may elucidate the action of insulin in the pathogenesis of cardiovascular disease, and the mechanisms by which fetal growth restriction programs postnatal insulin resistance and altered sensitivity to endocrine and paracrine growth factors. Safe nutritional, hormonal, and metabolic interventions are needed to treat growth retardation in utero and to reprogram prenatal metabolic pathways that affect adult disease. Continued investigation may help to further elucidate the genetic control of prenatal development, including the role of imprinting on fetal growth.

ACKNOWLEDGMENT

I thank Drs Allen Root and Mark Williams for their helpful review of the manuscript, and Mrs LaRue VanNordstrand for her secretarial assistance.

REFERENCES

1. McIntire DD, Bloom SL, Casey BM, et al: Birth weight in relation to morbidity and mortality among newborn infants. *N Engl J Med* 340:1234-1238, 1999.
2. Campbell S, Thomas A: Ultrasound measurement of the fetal head to abdomen circumferenmce ratio in the assessment of growth retardation. *Br J Obst Gynaecol* 84:165-174, 1977.
3. Botero, D, Lifshitz F: Intrauterine growth retardation and long-term effects on growth. *Curt Opin Pediatr* 11:340-347, 1999.
4. Seeds JW, Peng T: Impaired growth and risk of fetal death: Is the tenth percentile the appropriate standard. *Am J Obstet Gynecol* 178:658-669, 1998.
5. Siber DB, Sung CJ, Wigglesworth JS: Fetal growth and maturation: With standards for body and organ development, in Wigglesworth JS,

Singer DB (ed): *Textbook of Fetal and Perinatal Pathology.* Boston, Blackwell Scientific, 1996, pp 11-47.

6. Sparks JW: Intrauterine growth and nutrition, in Polin RA, Fox WN (eds): *Fetal and Neonatal Physiology,* ed 2. Philadelphia, WB Saunders, 1998, pp 267-289.
7. Brenner WE, Edelman DA, Hendricks CH: A standard for fetal growth for the United States of America. *Am J Obstet Gynecol* 126:555-564, 1976.
8. Lubchenko LO, Hansman C, Dressier, et al: Intrauterine growth as estimated from live born weight data at 24-42 weeks of gestation. *Pediatrics* 32:793-800, 1963.
9. Hobbins J: Morphometry of fetal growth. *Acta Paediatr Suppl* 423:165-168, 1997.
10. Bobrow CS, Soothill PW: Fetal growth velocity: A cautionary tale. *Lancet* 353:1460, 1999.
11. Gardeil F, Greene R, Stuart B, et al: Subcutaneous fat in the fetal abdomen as a predictor of growth restriction. *Obstet Gynecol* 94:209-212, 1999.
12. Lin C-C, Santolaya-Forgas: Current concepts of fetal growth restriction: Part II. Diagnosis and management. *Obstet Gynecol* 93:140-146, 1999.
13. Clapp JF III, Rizk KH, Appleby-Wineberg SK, et al: Second trimester placental volumes predict birth weight at term. *J Soc Gynecol Invest* 2:19-22, 1995.
14. Klebanoff MA, Meirik O, Berendes HW: Second generation consequences of small-for-dates birth. *Pediatrics* 84:343-347, 1989.
15. Gluckman PD: Hormones and fetal growth, in Clarke JR (ed): *Oxford Reviews of Reproductive Biology.* Oxford, England, Clarendon Press, 1986, pp 1-60.
16. Robinson JS, Harwhich KM, Walker SK, et al: Early influences on embryonic and placental growth. *Acta Paediatr Suppl* 423:159-163, 1997.
17. Barker DJP, Bull AR, Osmond C, et al: Fetal and placental size and risk of hypertension in adult life. *BMJ* 301:259-262, 1990.
18. Cetin I, Corbetta C, Sereni LP, et al: Umbilical amino acid concentrations in normal and growth retarded fetuses sampled in utero by cordocentesis. *Am J Obstet Gynecol* 162:253-261, 1990.
19. Sheppard BL, Bonnar J: Uteroplacental hemostasis in intrauterine fetal growth retardation. *Semin Thromb Hemost* 25:443-446, 1999.
20. Schjetlein R, Abdelnoor M, Haugen G, et al: Hemostatic variables as independent predictors for fetal growth retardation in pre-eclampsia. *Acta Obstet Gynecol Scand* 78:191197, 1999.
21. Khaliq A, Dunk C, Jiang J, et al: Hypoxia down-regulates placental growth factor, whereas fetal growth restriction up-regulates placenta growth factor expression: Molecular evidence of placental hyperoxia in intrauterine growth retardation. *Lab Invest* 79:151-170, 1999.
22. Lindquist P, Grennert L, Marsal K: Epidermal growth factor in maternal urine: A predictor of intrauterine growth retardation? *Early Hum Dev* 56:141-150, 1999.

23. de Zegher F, Francois I, van Helvoirt M, et al: Small as a fetus and short as child: From endogenous to exogenous growth hormone. *J Clin Endocrinol Metab* 82:2021-2026, 1997.
24. Massa G, de Zegher F, Vanderschueren-Lodeweyckx M: Serum growth hormone binding protein in the human fetus and infant. *Pediatr Res* 32:69-72, 1992.
25. Gluckman PD: The endocrine regulation of fetal growth in late gestation: The role of insulin-like growth factors. J *Clin Endocrinol Metab* 80:1047-1050, 1995.
26. Palmiter RD, Norstedt G, Gelinas RE, et al: Metallothionein-human GH fusion genes stimulate growth of mice. *Science* 222:809-814, 1983.
27. McIntyre HD, Serek R, Crane DI, et al: Placental growth hormone (GH), GH-binding protein, and insulin-like growth factor axis in normal, growth-retarded, and diabetic pregnancies: Correlations with fetal growth. *J Clin Endocrinol Metab* 85:11431150, 2000.
28. Caufriez A, Frankenne F, Hennen G, et al: Regulation of maternal IGF-1 by placental GH in normal and abnormal human pregnancies. *Am J Physiol* 265:E572-E577, 1993.
29. Barnard R, Chan F-Y, McIntyre HD: Growth hormone-binding protein in normal and pathological gestation: Correlations with maternal diabetes and fetal growth. *J Clin Endocrinol Metab* 82:1879-1884, 1997.
30. Mirlesse V, Frankenne F, Alsat E, et al: Placental growth hormone levels in normal pregnancy and in pregnancies with intrauterine growth retardation. *Pediatr Res* 34:439-442, 1993.
31. Handwerger S, Freemark M: The roles of placental growth hormone and placental lactogen in the regulation of human fetal growth and development. *J Pediatr Endocrinol Metab* 13:343-356, 2000.
32. Lassare C, Hardouin S, Daffos F, et al: Serum insulin-like growth factors and insulin-like growth factor binding proteins in the human fetus: Relationships with growth in normal subjects and in subjects with intrauterine growth retardation. *Pediatr Res* 29:219-225, 1991.
33. Gluckman PD: Endocrine and nutritional regulation of prenatal growth. *Acta Paediatr Suppl* 423:153-157, 1997.
34. Guidice LC, de Zegher F, Gargosky SE, et al: Insulin-like growth factors and their binding proteins in the term and preterm human fetus and neonates with normal and extremes of intrauterine growth. *J Clin Endocrinol Metab* 80:1548-1555, 1995.
35. Vileisis RA, D'Ecole AJ: Tissue and serum concentrations of somatomedin-C/insulin-like growth factor I in fetal rats made growth retarded by uterine artery ligation. *Pediatr Res* 20:126-130, 1986.
36. Beck KD, Powell-Braxton L, Widmer HR, et al: IGF-1 gene disruption results in reduced brain size, CNS hypomyelination, and loss of hippocampal granule and striatal parvalbumin-containing neurons. *Neuron* 14:717-724, 1995.
37. Liu JL, Yakar S, Le Roith D: Conditional knockout of mouse insulin-like growth factor Bi gene using the Cre/lox P system. *Proc Soc Exp Biol Med* 223:344-351, 2000.

38. Gluckman PD, Butler JH, Comline R, et al: The effects of pancreatectomy on the plasma concentrations of insulin-like growth factors 1 and 2 in the sheep fetus. *J Der Physiol* 9:79-88, 1987.
39. Accili D, Nakae J, Kim JJ, et al: Targeted gene mutations define the roles of insulin and IGF-1 receptors in mouse embryonic development. *J Pediatr Endocrinol Metab* 12:475485, 1999.
40. Holmes RP, Holly JMP, Soothill PW: Maternal serum insulin-like growth factor binding protein-2 and B3 and fetal growth. *Hum Reprod* 14:1879-1884, 1999.
41. Zhou J, Bondy CA: Placental glucose transporter gene expression and metabolism in the rat. *J Clin Invest* 91:845-852, 1993.
42. Currie MJ, Bassett NS, Gluckman PD: Ovine glucose transporter-1 and B3 cDNA partial sequences and developmental gene expression in the placenta. *Placenta* 18:393-401, 1997.
43. Holmes RP, Holly JMP, Soothill PW: Maternal insulin-like growth factor binding protein-l, body mass index, and fetal growth. *Arch Dis Child Fetal Neonatal Ed* 82:F113-F117, 2000.
44. Woods KA, Camacho-Hubner C, Savage MO, et al: Intrauterine growth retardation and postnatal growth failure associated with deletion of the insulin-like growth factor I gene. *N Engl J Med* 335:1363-1367, 1996.
45. Rosenfeld RG: Intrauterine growth retardation: Our current understanding and future directions. Acta *Paediatr Suppl* 423:216-217, 1997.
46. Hills FA, English J, Chard T: Circulating levels of IGF-1 and IGF-binding protein-1 throughout pregnancy: Relationship to birthweight and maternal weight. *J Endocrinol* 148:303-309, 1996.
47. Guidice LC, Farrell EM, Pham H, et al: Insulin-like growth factor binding proteins in maternal serum through gestation and in the puerperium: Effects of a pregnancy-associated serum protease activity. *J Clin Endocrinol Metab* 71:806-816, 1990.
48. Diamond F, Eichler D: Leptin: Molecular biology, physiology, and relevance to the pediatrician. *Adv Pediatr* 46:151-187, 19R9.
49. Hassink SG, de Lancey E, Sheslow DV, et al: Placental leptin: An important new growth factor in intrauterine and neonatal development? (on-line) *Pediatrics* 100:124, 1997.
50. Harigaya A, Nagashima K, Nako Y, et al: Relationship between concentration of serum leptin and fetal growth. *J Clin Endocrinol Metab* 82:3281-3284, 1997.
51. Koistinen HA, Koivisto VA, Andersson S, et al: Leptin concentration in cord blood correlates with intrauterine growth. *J Clin Endocrinol Metab* 82:3328-3330, 1997.
52. Ong KKL, Ahmed ML, Dunger DB: The role of leptin in human growth and puberty. *Acta Paediatr Suppl* 433:95-98, 1999.
53. Williams M: Personal communication, 2000.
54. Preece MA, Moore GE: Genomic imprinting, uniparental disomy, and foetal growth. *Trends Endocrinol Metab* 11:270-275, 2000.
55. Spiro RP, Christian SL, Ledbetter DH, et al: Intrauterine growth retar-

dation associated with maternal uniparental disomy for chromosome 6 unmasked by congenital adrenal hyperplasia. *Pediatr Res* 46:510-513, 1999.

56. Fokstuen S, Ginsburg C, Zachman M, Schinzel A: Maternal uniparental disomy 14 as a cause of intrauterine growth retardation and early onset of puberty. *J Pediatr* 134:689-695, 1999.
57. Balmer D, Baumer A, Rothlisberger B, et al: Severe intrauterine growth retardation in a patient with maternal uniparental disomy 22 and a 22-trisomic placenta. *Prenat Diagn* 19:1061-1064, 1999.
58. Price SM, Stanhope R, Garret C, et al: The spectrum of Silver-Russell syndrome: A clinical and molecular genetic study and new diagnostic criteria. *J Med Genet* 36:837-842, 1999.
59. Dunger DB, and the ALSPAC Study Team: Association of the INS VNTR with size at birth. *Nat Genet* 19:98-99, 1998.
60. Ong KKL, Phillips DI, Fall C, et al: The insulin gene VNTR, type 2 diabetes and birth weight. *Nat Genet* 21:262-263, 1999.
61. Al-Mufti R, Lees C, Albaiges G, et al: Fetal cells in maternal blood of pregnancies with severe fetal growth restriction. *Hum Reprod* 15:218-221, 2000.
62. Sattar N, Greer IA, Galloway PJ, et al: Lipid and lipoprotein concentrations in pregnancies complicated by intrauterine growth retardation. *J Clin Endocrinol* Metab 84:128-130, 1999.
63. Stepan H, Faber R, Walther T: Expression of low density lipoprotein receptor messenger ribonucleic acid in placentas from pregnancies with intrauterine growth retardation. *Br J Obstet Gynaecol* 106:1221-1222, 1999.
64. Berge P, Stagno S, Federer W, et al: Impact of asymptomatic congenital cytomegalovirus infection on size at birth and gestational duration. *Pediatr* Infect *Dis* 9:170-175, 1990.
65. Abrams B, Selvin S: Maternal weight gain pattern and birth weight. *Obstet Gynecol* 86:163-169, 1995.
66. Cogswell ME, Serdula MK, Hungerford DW, et al: Gestational weight gain among average-weight and overweight women: What is excessive? *Am J Obstet Gynecol* 172:705-712, 1995.
67. Singer DB, Sung CJ, Wigglesworth JS: Fetal growth and maturation: With standards for body and organ development, in Wigglesworth JS, Singer DB (ed): *Textbook of Fetal and Perinatal Pathology.* Boston, Blackwell Scientific, 1996, pp 11-47.
68. Kramer MS, Olivier M, McLean FH, et al: Impact of intrauterine growth retardation and body proportionality on fetal and neonatal outcome. *Pediatrics* 86:707-713, 1990.
69. Khoury MJ, Erickson JD, Cordero JF, et al: Congenital malformations and intrauterine growth retardation: A population study. *Pediatrics* 82:83-90, 1988.
70. Guaschino S, Spinillo A, Stola E, et al: The significance of ponderal index as a prognostic factor in a low-birth weight population. *Biol Res Pregnancy Perinatol* 7:121-127, 1986.

71. Hakansan DO, Oh W: Hyperviscosity in the small for gestational infants. *Biol Neonate* 37:109-112, 1980.
72. Wennergren M: Perinatal risk factors. With special reference to intrauterine growth retardation and neonatal respiratory adaptation. *Acta Obstet Gynecol Scand Suppl* 135:1-51, 1986.
73. Tudehope DI: Neonatal aspects of intrauterine growth retardation. *Fetal Med Rev* 3:73-85, 1991.
74. Albertsson-Wikland K, Karlberg J: Natural growth in children born small-for-gestational-age (SGA) with and without catch-up growth. *Acta Paediatr Suppl* 399:64-70, 1994.
75. Leger J, Limoni C, Collin D, et al: Prediction factors in the determination of final height in subjects born small for gestational age. *Pediatr Res* 43:808-812, 1998.
76. Karlberg J, Albertsson-Wikland K: Growth in full-term small for gestational age infants: From birth to final height. *Pediatr Res* 38:733-739, 1995.
77. Karlberg J, Albertsson-Wikland K: Spontaneous growth and final height in SGA infants. *Pediatr Res* 33:5(2099):53, 1993.
78. Deiber M, Chatelain P, Naville D, et al: Functional hypersomatotropism in small for gestational age (SGA) newborn infants. *J Clin Endocrinol Metab* 68:232-234, 1989.
79. Job J-C, Chatelain P, Rochiccioli P, et al: Growth hormone response to a bolus injection of 1-44 growth-hormone-releasing hormone in very short children with intrauterine onset of growth failure. *Horm Res* 33:161-165, 1990.
80. Ong KKL, and the ALSPAC Study Team: Postnatal catch-up growth following intrauterine restraint is a major risk factor for childhood obesity. *BMJ* 320:967-971, 2000.
81. Paz I, Gale R, Laor A, et al: The cognitive outcome of full-term small for gestational age infants at late adolescence. *Obsetet Gynecol* 85:452-456, 1995.
82. Kohelet D, Arbel E, Goldberg MN, et al: Intrauterine growth retardation and brainstem auditory-evoked response in preterm infants. *Acta Paediatr* 89:73-76, 2000.
83. Gray PH, O'Callaghan MJ, Harvey JM, et al: Placental pathology and neurodevelopment of the infant with intrauterine growth restriction. *Dev Med Child Neurol* 41:16-20, 1999.
84. Zubrick SR, Kurinczuk JJ, MuDermott BMC, et al: Fetal growth and subsequent mental health problems in children aged 4 to 13 years. *Dev Med Child Neurol* 42:14-20, 2000.
85. Desai M, Crowther NJ, Ozanne SE, et al: Adult glucose and lipid metabolism may be programmed during fetal life. *Biochem Soc Trans* 23:331-335, 1995.
86. Root AW: Editorial overview, endocrine and metabolism. *Curr Opin Pediatr* 11:329-332, 1999.
87. Chiarelli F, di Ricco L, Mohn A, et al: Insulin resistance in short children with intrauterine growth retardation. *Acta Paediatr Suppl* 428:62-65, 1999.

88. Ibanez L, Potau N, Marcos MV, et al: Exaggerated adrenarche and hyperinsulinism in adolescent girls born small for gestational age. *J Clin Endocrinol Metab* 84:4739-4741, 1999.
89. Francois I, van Helvoirt M, de Zegher F: Male pseudohermaphroditism related to complications at conception, in early pregnancy, and in prenatal growth. *Horm Res* 51:91-95, 1999.
90. Francois I, de Zegher F, Spiessens C, et al: Low birth weight and subsequent male subfertility. *Pediatr Res* 42:899-901, 1997.
91. Godfrey KM, Barker DJP: Fetal nutrition and adult disease. *Am J Clin Nutr* 71:1344S-1352S, 2000.
92. Radunovic N, Kuczynski E, Rosen T, et al: Plasma apolipoprotein A-I and B concentrations in growth-retarded fetuses: A link between low birth weight and adult atherosclerosis. *J Clin Endocrinol Metab* 85:85-88, 2000.
93. Lumey LH: Decreased birth weights in infants after maternal in utero exposure to the Dutch famine of 1944-1945. *Paediatr Perinat Epidemiol* 6:240-253, 1992.
94. Hales CN, Barker DJP, Clark PMS, et al: Fetal and infant growth and impaired glucose tolerance at age 64. *BMJ* 303:1019-1022, 1991.
95. Hales CN, Barker DJP: Type 2 (non-insulin dependent) diabetes mellitus: The thrifty phenotype hypothesis. *Diabetologia* 35:595-601, 1992.
96. Stein CE, Fall CHD, Kumaran K, et al: Fetal growth and coronary heart disease in South India. *Lancet* 348:1269-1273, 1996.
97. Houang M, Morineau G, Le Bouc Y, et al: The cortisol-cortisone shuttle in children born with intrauterine growth retardation. *Pediatr Res* 46:189-193, 1999.
98. Harding JE, Charlton V: Treatment of the growth-restricted fetus by augmentation of substrate supply. *Semin Perinatol* 13:211-223, 1989.
99. Stein Z, Susser M, Rush D: Prenatal nutriton and birth weight: Experiments and quasi-experiments in the past decade. *J Reprod Med* 21:287-299, 1978.
100. Charlton V, Johengen M: Effects of intrauterine nutritional supplementation on fetal growth. *Biol Neonate* 48:125142, 1985.
101. Phillips AF, Porte PJ, Stabisksi S, et al: Effects of chronic fetal hyperglycemia upon oxygen consumption in the ovine uterus and conceptus. *J Clin Invest* 74:279-286, 1984.
102. Rudolph A: Oxygenation to the fetus and neonate: A perspective. *Semin Perinatol* 8:158-167, 1984.
103. Moore LG, Rounds SS, Jahnigen D, et al: Infant birth weight is related to maternal arterial oxygenation at high altitude. *J Appl Physiol* 52:695-699, 1982.
104. Shime J, Morcarsky EJM, Hastings D, et al: Congenital heart disease in pregnancy: Short-and long-term implications. *Am J Obstet Gynecol* 156:313-322, 1987.
105. Nicolaides KH, Campbell S, Bradley RJ, et al: Maternal oxygen therapy for intrauterine growth retardation. *Lancet* 1:942-945, 1987.

106. Bekedam DJ, Muller EJH, Snijders RJM, et al: The effects of maternal hyperoxia on fetal breathing movements, body movements and heart rate variation in growth retarded fetuses. *Early Hum Dev* 27:223-232, 1991.
107. Arduini D, Rizzo G, Mancuso S, et al: Short-term effects of maternal oxygen administrationon blood flow velocity waveforms in healthy and growth-retarded fetuses. *Am J Obstet Gynaecol* 159:1077-1080, 1988.
108. Lok F, Owens JA, Mundy L, et al: Insulin-like growth factor I promotes growth selectively in fetal sheep in late gestation. *Am J Physiol* 270:R1148-R1155, 1996.
109. Harding JE, Bauer MK, Kimble RM: Antenatal therapy for intrauterine growth retardation. *Acta Paediatr Suppl* 423:196-200, 1997.
110. Fowden AL, Hughes P, Comline RS: The effects of insulin on the growth rate of the sheep fetus during late gestation. *Q J Exp Physiol* 74:703-714, 1989.
111. McCowan LME, Harding J, Roberts A, et al: Administration of low-dose aspririn to mothers with small for gestational age fetuses and abnormal umbilical Doppler studies to increase birthweight: A randomised double-blind controlled trial. *Br J Obstet Gynaecol* 106:647-651, 1999.
112. Leitch H, Egarter C, Husslein P, et al: A meta-analysis of low-dose aspirin for the prevention of intrauterine growth retardation. *Br J Obstet Gynaecol* 104:450-459, 1997.
113. de Zegher F, Francois I, Ibanez L: Pediatric endocrinopathies related to reduced fetal growth. *Growth Genet Horm* 15:1-5, 1999.
114. de Zegher F, Maes M, Gargosky E, et al: High-dose growth hormone treatment of short children born small for gestational age. *J Clin Endocrinol Metab* 81:1887-1892, 1996.
115. de Zegher F, Albertsson-Wikland K, Wollmann HA, et al: Growth hormone treatment of short children born small for gestational age: Growth responses with continuous and discontinuous regimens over 6 years. *J Clin Endocrinol Metab* 85:2816-2821, 2000.
116. Coutant R, Carel J-C, Letrait M, et al: Short stature associated with intrauterine growth retardation: Final height of untreated and growth hormone-treated children. *J Clin Endocrinol Metab* 83:1070-1074, 1998.
117. Sas T, de Waal W, Mulder P, et al: Growth hormone treatment in children with short stature born small for gestational age: 5-year results of a randomized double-blind, dose-response trial. *J Clin Endocrinol Metab* 84:3064-3070, 1999.

CHAPTER 9

Auditory Development and Hearing Evaluation in Children

Janet E. Stockard-Pope, MS, CCC-A
Instructor, Department of Pediatrics, University of South Florida, Tampa

ABSTRACT

This chapter provides an overview of (1) developmental timetables relevant to hearing, and (2) current pediatric audiological techniques and practices. Structural and functional development of the auditory pathway and the development of primary auditory processing are summarized. These developmental sequences appear to follow similar paths in humans and animals. Speech and music perception involve more complex processing and are strongly influenced by experience. Hearing disorders affect the perception of complex sounds in a variety of ways, depending on the sites of lesions. Early-onset hearing impairment, including conductive loss from chronic otitis media, can seriously impede language development.

Language cannot develop normally without adequate speech stimulation, and deafness is more prevalent than any other handicapping condition for which mandated neonatal screening programs exist. Sensitive and inexpensive techniques are available for performing neonatal hearing screening, and early intervention has a documented positive effect on development of language skills in hearing-impaired children. Thus, the National Institutes of Health has recommended nationwide universal neonatal hearing screening. The rationale for and the methodology of universal screening programs are summarized.

Advances in the genetics of hearing impairment are reviewed. Data from these studies have influenced testing and rehabilitative protocols and have implications for future prevention and treatment of hearing impairment.

Recent advances in the field of auditory physiology, coupled with long-standing concerns about delayed identification of hearing impairment, have precipitated public health initiatives[1] and legislation for neonatal hearing screening programs.[2] Pediatric audiology, once more "art" than science, is now largely based on physiologic methods rather than observed behavior. With current techniques, it is not only possible to detect hearing impairment at birth but also to determine the site of the lesion and to obtain close estimates of hearing threshold at specific frequencies.[3] Habilitative measures, including amplification, can begin within weeks of birth. Protocols for the management of hearing impairment are guided not only by the site of the lesion but by the developmental sequences and interactions among all the child's sensory modalities.

This chapter provides an overview of developmental timetables relevant to hearing and current pediatric audiological techniques and practices.

DEVELOPMENTAL SEQUENCES

PRENATAL STRUCTURAL/PHYSIOLOGIC DEVELOPMENT OF THE AUDITORY SYSTEM

For obvious reasons, most studies of structural and physiologic development of the auditory system have been performed in animals. Fortunately, gross anatomical development of the auditory system in humans appears to follow the same sequence as that of many animal species.[4] Avian species provide particularly useful models because their behavior, including embryonic behavior, has been studied extensively, and their hearing develops similarly to that of humans. Comparative studies show that the relationship between the onset of hearing and time of birth varies among animal species, but the proportion of time between conception and the onset of auditory function (referred to as the *silent period*) is consistent across species. Morey and Carlile[5] demonstrated similarity in this proportion among species by recording the time of onset of the first cochlear response (the cochlear microphonic). Although the time of appearance of the cochlear microphonic is not known in humans, other morphologic and physiologic measures indicate that the silent period in humans is remarkably similar to that of other animals.[4,6]

The otic placode can be identified at approximately 23 days' gestation,[7] and differentiation of the organ of Corti begins about the 10th week of gestation. As in other mammals, structural development follows a base-to-apex gradient, corresponding to the low- and high-frequency regions of the organ of Corti.[6] Differentiation of hair cells, separation of the tectorial membrane from the organ of Corti, and innervation in the human cochlea at 24 weeks' gestation are similar to those of other mammals at the onset of their cochlear function. Action potentials elicited from the eighth cranial nerve at 27 weeks' gestation in preterm infants[8] confirm that the cochlea is functional and the neural connection is present at that time.

DEVELOPMENT OF HEARING FUNCTION

Structurally, the cochlea appears capable of function about 3 months before birth.[9] However, assessing responsivity in utero is complicated by the attenuation of environmental sounds made by the mother's abdomen and amniotic fluid and by the high level of ambient noise in utero. Gross motor responses[10] or heart rate changes[11] can be elicited by intense sound at 26 to 28 weeks' gestational age. Lower intensities are not effective. Response thresholds could be elevated by masking noise, by the lack of air conduction of sound, or by cochlear immaturity. Behavioral studies of preterm infants do not shed much light on the question. There have been no attempts to measure behavioral threshold to sound in preterm infants because behavioral responsivity at this age is not a reliable index of hearing.[12]

Primary auditory processing refers to the extraction and coding of the physical attributes of sound, whereas secondary auditory processing can be thought of as the selection of combinations of both the quantitative and qualitative attributes of sound to accomplish a "perceptual goal,"[13] tasks that might include the detection of sound, discrimination among sounds, and understanding of connected speech. In children, perceptual goals would be revealed by preferential listening tasks. The following sections on the resolution of physical attributes summarize development of primary auditory processing. These fundamental abilities appear to be less influenced by experience than are secondary auditory processing tasks.

Frequency Resolution

Frequency resolution or tuning within the auditory system refers to the specificity with which structures in the auditory system respond to sounds of a particular frequency, a primary function necessary for discrimination of frequencies. In the prenatal period, cochlear and neural maturation are the main contributors to development of frequency resolution. Tuning within the cochlea is mature as early as it has been measured,[14] but within neural structures, it continues to develop until 6 months of age.[15] After that, attention may be the primary factor for the continued improvement in frequency resolution throughout childhood.[16]

Temporal Resolution

Temporal resolution refers to abilities to detect changes in the timing of sound, such as detection of brief gaps in sound, discrimination of sounds of varying duration, and improvement of performance with increasing duration of sound. It has a longer developmental course than intensity or frequency resolution, possibly because it is more dependent on attention and memory.[16] Early in development, factors such as myelination, fiber diameter, and synaptic efficiency are significant contributors to development of temporal resolution.

Intensity Resolution

The dynamic range of auditory neurons is restricted in developing mammals. This might be expected to influence an infant's ability to detect small changes in stimulus intensity or to perceive loudness in a mature fashion. The amplitude of the auditory brainstem response would be a reasonable approach to measuring this ability in infants, but its variability is too large. Thus, the few studies performed to date have relied primarily on behavioral methods, and little is known about the time course of the development of intensity resolution.

Hearing Sensitivity

Developmental studies that use physiologic estimates of hearing threshold reveal that there is a period of rapid improvement from birth to 6 months, followed by a slower phase of development until about 10 years of age.[16] Several mechanisms could explain the improvement in hearing threshold with age.

Maturation of external and middle ear structures is an important contributor. Studies of energy reflectance have shown that the energy transfer through the external and middle ear continues to mature beyond 24 months of age.[17] A caudal to rostral progression of maturation occurs within the auditory pathway: 2 months for the eighth cranial nerve, 2 to 3 years for the auditory brainstem pathway, and the teenage years for cortical pathways.[18]

In children mature enough to understand and cooperate, behavioral measures are used for threshold assessment. These tests are highly dependent on listening strategies, motivation, and attention, which also change with age.

Prenatal factors other than auditory experience may also influence the course of auditory development. Newborns of mothers who smoke are less readily aroused by auditory stimuli than those of nonsmokers.[19] Not surprisingly, maternal undernutrition can result in delayed development of the auditory brainstem pathway. One study suggested more rapid development of brainstem auditory conduction time in breast-fed versus formula-fed newborns.[20]

Complex Sound Perception

The preceding sections have dealt with the most fundamental abilities to distinguish quantitative features of simple sounds. However, the most important properties of hearing function involve the analysis of complex environmental sounds varying in frequency and amplitude over time. Our ability to perceive the qualitative attributes of sound, such as loudness, pitch, and timbre, are more difficult to measure but are essential to the understanding of speech and the perception of music.

The pitch of tones in sequence gives rise to melody, whereas timbre evokes a quality of sharpness or brightness. The vowels in speech can be described as harmonic complexes of different timbres.[16] Although adults can be asked to rate various attributes of complex sound, we can only infer infants' abilities and preferences from discrimination studies based on behavior. From such studies, it appears that infants are particularly responsive to speech stimuli[21] and that a newborn prefers his mother's voice over that of another female.[22] Furthermore, infants are more responsive to "baby talk" or *infant-directed speech*, characterized by high fundamental frequency and unique patterns of intonation.[23] When presented with tonal, nonspeech stimuli mimicking the intonation-contour of infant-directed speech, infants prefer these stimuli over tonal stimuli without the unique contour.[24] Some investigators hypothesize that infant-directed speech facilitates language acquisition either by providing cues to syntactic structure and by segmenting ongoing speech to separate individual words[25] or simply by promoting social interaction.[26] Infants have poor low-frequency discrimination,[27,28] and this ability continues to develop well into childhood.[29] Whether this contributes to their preference for the large intonation contours of infant-directed speech is not known. In contrast, high-frequency discrimination, an important ability for the perception of subtle differences among the consonants of speech, develops quickly during infancy.

Three-month-old infants appear to have an adultlike perception of pitch as it relates to octaves,[30] in that, as one tone approaches an octave above a second tone, the two tones are perceived as similar. When multiple tones are harmonically related, we perceive them as one pitch, which is related to the fundamental or lowest frequency. If the fundamental frequency is removed from the complex, leaving only the harmonics, the perception of pitch is unchanged. This virtual pitch perception appears to be present in infants at least by 7 months of age,[31] but it is not known whether learning and experience play a role. Little is known about the development of musical pattern perception before 6 months of age. It appears that infants are able to process different aspects of music simultaneously. For example, 6-month- old infants are sensitive to changes in rhythm even when melody and tempo are changed simultaneously.[32]

Speech Perception

The smallest segments of speech, which assign or change meaning in words, can be identified by adults regardless of the voice variations among speakers. Therefore, invariant acoustic cues exist, which label these segments or *phonemes*. All the specific abilities relating to intensity, frequency, and timing discussed in previous sections are recruited in the development of detection of these cues for speech perception. For example, the phonemes /b/ and /p/ differ in voice onset time by a matter of milliseconds, but the small timing difference allows us to distinguish the two sounds in words. This example of categorical perception is present in early infancy, but the boundaries between categories in the native language sharpen with development.[33]

Young infants demonstrate the ability to distinguish phonemes that do not exist in their native language.[33,34] They become less sensitive to nonphonemic differences among consonants between 6 and 12 months of age, apparently as a result of linguistic experience.[35] The loss of this ability is permanent. American adults can discriminate the English phonemes /r/ and /l/, but the acoustic difference between these sounds in Japanese does not signal a change in meaning and is not discriminated by mature native Japanese adults.[36]

Similarly, vowels vary greatly in spectral characteristics among speakers, yet adults are able to sort them into equivalent classes based on a general spectral contour, where relative pitch is attended to over absolute pitch. Two-month-old infants are apparently able to categorize at least some vowels.[37]

NORMAL SEQUENCE OF DEVELOPMENT OF SENSORY SYSTEMS

Sensory systems in all animals develop in a predictable order: somatosensory, vestibular, olfactory, auditory, and visual.[38] Animal studies indicate that interactions between auditory structures and the environment are critical to normal development. Knowledge of the effects of abnormal sequencing of sensory events is derived from animal data, but human preterm birth or the absence of auditory stimulation in the deaf infant can approximate those experimental conditions.

It has been proposed that, in immature animals, sensory stimulation that occurs earlier in development than usual can interfere with learning from other sensory modalities.[39] For example, visual structures mature in early intrauterine life, but patterned visual stimuli are not available in that environment. In contrast, auditory structures, which are nearly mature in late intrauterine life, do receive patterned stimulation, primarily from biologic noise and the voice of the mother. Early auditory perception is normally free to develop in the absence of competition from the developing visual system. In the preterm infant, however, patterned visual stimuli are experienced much earlier than usual. Animal studies have clearly demonstrated deficits in auditory learning as a result of improper sequencing of sensory stimulation. Gottlieb et al[40-42] demonstrated that ducklings hatched at a normal time and exposed to mother's vocalizations recognized and "preferred" her vocalizations over other sounds. However, ducklings exposed to light before normal hatching did not learn to recognize the mother's call. Unnatural stimulation of an *earlier* developing system, in this case the visual system, interferes with auditory learning in duck embryos. When embryos and hatchlings were exposed to rapid oscillations of a waterbed, those exposed before hatching were unable to recognize or learn the mother's call, whereas hatchlings exposed to the same stimulation recognized the call.[42] It is not known whether these differences result from changes in neural organization[39] or from altered attention.[41] The normal sequence of patterned stimulation in various modalities is certainly interrupted in infants born prematurely, but the consequences are not known at this time.

The organization of neurons in the auditory areas of the cerebral cortex into clusters occurs in response to stimulation. The period during which the development of sensory areas of the cortex can be compromised by stimulus conditions is referred to as the *sensitive period*. Premature infants at 23 weeks' gestation through the early months of life in the neonatal intensive care unit (NICU) are in the sensitive period for cochlear development. The *critical* period for language development spans the first 2 to 3 years of life, during which adequate speech stimulation is required. Congenitally deaf children who are not provided early amplification should be considered at risk for permanent structural and functional changes in development.

Neuropathologic studies of 7 profoundly deaf humans revealed that cell size in the cochlear nucleus was inversely correlated with the duration of deafness. Similarly, auditory deprivation in animals has been shown to alter functional and structural development in the peripheral and central auditory pathways.[43-46] Deprivation of "meaningful" or patterned sounds results in impaired auditory discrimination and processing in animals. Structural changes in the central auditory pathway can also result from unilateral deafness. All of these findings have implications for global developmental processes in children with hearing impairment.

AUDITORY EXPERIENCE AND LEARNING IN THE FETUS

Although data are limited, it appears that prenatal experience influences auditory development in humans as well as in animals. Although sounds are attenuated by the abdomen and fluid, normal conversation near the pregnant abdomen is probably recognizable in pitch and rhythm and can be appreciated by the term infant.[47] Newborns prefer their mother's voice over other voices. They can be conditioned to suck on a pacifier at a particular rate to initiate the sound of the mother's voice.[22] However, they show no preference for their father's voice—with which they had little or no prenatal experience—over another male voice.[48] Infants exposed for the last 6 weeks in utero to their mothers reading a story with a distinctive cadence preferred hearing it over another story shortly after birth. Newborns who did not have that prenatal experience showed no preference.[49]

HEARING IMPAIRMENT AND DIAGNOSTIC TECHNIQUES

EPIDEMIOLOGY OF HEARING IMPAIRMENT

As estimated by the most recent survey of the prevalence of "serious" hearing impairment in children in this country,[50] the average annual prevalence rate is 1.1 per 1000 children (aged 3-10 years). Two thirds of the children with impairment had a sensorineural loss that did not result from a postnatal cause. Half of those with prenatal or neonatal onset received a diagnosis after the age of 3 years. The survey included only those children with hearing loss of greater than 40 dBHL. However, a loss of 30 to 40 dBHL in the speech frequencies would render most consonants in conversational level speech inaudible to prelingual children. Thus, the reported prevalence from this study is probably not an accurate indication of significant childhood hearing impairment.

Niskar et al[51] tested a sample of 342 children and found that 17% had a hearing loss of at least 25 dBHL at 1, 2, 4, or 6KHz in one or both ears. Other prevalence studies including bilateral hearing impairment of this magnitude have revealed rates of 3 to 5 per 1000.[52,53]

Data from groups of hospitals with universal hearing screening programs have provided specific information on the prevalence of hearing impairment among newborns. In Colorado, more than 41,000 infants were tested, and bilateral congenital hearing loss requiring amplification was found to occur in 2 per 1000 infants.[54] The Rhode Island study of more than 53,000 infants also yielded a rate of 2 per 1000.[55] A study of 54,228 newborns in Texas yielded a rate for bilateral sensorineural hearing loss of 3.14 per 1000.[56]

In Hawaii, 10,372 newborns were screened, and the incidence of bilateral hearing impairment was 1 per 1000 and 5 per 1000 in the well-baby and the NICU populations, respectively.[57] Van Naarden and Decoufle[58] used surveillance data from the Centers for Disease Control and Prevention to estimate that 19% of cases of presumed congenital hearing impairment in the sample were associated with low birth weight. Black infants, particularly boys, had a higher prevalence rate than did other races, even when birth weight was normal.

EARLY IDENTIFICATION OF DEAFNESS

Language cannot develop normally without adequate exposure to speech stimuli during the first 3 years of life. This requirement underscores the urgency of early identification of hearing impairment in children. The prevalence of hearing impairment in infancy exceeds that of all other handicapping conditions for which mandated neonatal screening programs exist.[59] Yet despite the relative frequency of its occurrence, there remains an average delay of 2 to 3 years in the identification of neonatal-onset deafness,[60] because most infants with severe hearing impairment will startle to loud sounds and will laugh and learn to babble at appropriate ages. Less than 10% of parents of infants with moderate-to-severe hearing loss were concerned about the child's hearing at the time of diagnosis.[61] Delayed habilitation throughout the critical period for language development virtually ensures a language deficit in children with early-onset deafness, and that language delay can result in severe learning deficits, including reading problems that are resistant to remediation.

Historical Perspective

In 1982, the release of the position statement of the Joint Committee on Infant Hearing served as the impetus for the development of a number of hearing screening programs for "high-risk" neonates in this country.[62] The methodology for achieving the recommended timetable for identification was not specified, because technology had not yet provided a sensitive, reliable, and efficient tool for identifying infants with hearing impairment. Since the publication of that position statement, the milieu in which screening programs were evolving was altered by the introduction of 2 new techniques: auditory brainstem responses (ABR) and evoked otoacoustic emissions (OAE). The latter offered a rapid, inexpensive screen for hearing impairment,[63] whereas the former provided an estimate of hearing threshold in neonates.[64] With these developments, cost-effective identification and diagnosis became attainable goals.

Once the financial hurdle was lowered, interest shifted toward universal screening rather than screening limited to high-risk neonates. More than half of deaf neonates have no identifiable risk factors for hearing loss and thus would not be detected by a risk-based screening program.[65] This lack of risk factors in many deaf neonates, along with the advent of OAE, prompted the National Institutes of Health to recommend universal neonatal hearing screening with OAE as the first-level screen, with confirmation by ABR.[1]

The wisdom of universal hearing screening was challenged by Bess and Paradise[66] who argued that empirical evidence supporting more favorable outcomes in deaf children identified earlier as compared with those identified later was lacking. However, Yoshinaga-Itano et al[67] have since demonstrated a clear association between age of identification and outcome in hearing-impaired children. Children identified before 6 months of age have expressive and receptive language quotients significantly higher than those of children identified after 6 months. The impact of early identification is present regardless of sex, presence of secondary disability, socioeconomic status, or age at testing. The same group has calculated the actual cost of public services to affected children, the average cost to affected families, and the estimated cost of a screening program in Colorado, thus laying the groundwork for a cost-benefit analysis of universal hearing screening. It was estimated that the direct costs of a screening program in Colorado would be recovered within 10 years of implementation.[54] False negative rates are negligible, and false positive rates in long-standing programs range from 0.3% to 7%.

Appropriate intervention strategies have been outlined by the Joint Committee for Infant Hearing (2000).[68]

Methodology

Equipment with automated "pass/refer" decision-making capability is now commercially available for neonatal screening by OAE and by ABR. In selecting equipment, consideration should be given only to those systems that use a statistically proven algorithm for pass/refer decisions.

Because eustachian tube function is inefficient, reabsorption of middle ear fluid and mesenchymal tissue is incomplete in newborns. Ear canals are typically full of debris in the first days of life. Most "false positive" hearing screens in newborns can be attributed to altered middle ear function or obstruction.[69]

Either OAE or ABR can be used successfully in universal screening programs. OAE equipment is less expensive, easier to operate, and faster. It is unaffected by electrical noise. On the negative side, referral rates are higher because of the sensitivity of OAE to middle ear dysfunction. High levels of ambient noise (as in the NICU) can interfere with testing.

Infants in the NICU are at increased risk of eighth cranial nerve and brainstem dysfunction, which would not alter OAE. ABR can detect such lesions. This test is also less affected by transient middle ear dysfunction and ambient noise, so referral rates are lower than those of OAE-based programs. However, start-up costs are higher, screening requires more time, and electrical noise can interfere with the test. When the nursing staff is responsible for screening, the time factor becomes critical.

The ideal model is a 2-level inpatient screen with an OAE screen followed by ABR in those infants failing the OAE. Babies who fail the second-level screen are referred to a physician for medical management, an audiologist for diagnosis and aural rehabilitation, and an early intervention program, if available in the community.

Training

Reimbursement rates for screening are low (or nonexistent in some states). For that reason, existing hospital staff, low pay-scale employees, or volunteers usually serve as screeners. Nurses may be resentful of additional responsibilities, turnover rates are high for poorly paid employees, and volunteers may not be sufficiently committed to the screening program. Efficient and effective training programs are therefore essential to a national implementation plan.

Data Management

Tracking of children who were discharged without a screen or who failed the screen is a critical component of an effective program. It is not sufficient to inform a parent of the possibility of deafness. In mass screening programs, data management must be computer-based. Software packages designed specifically for universal hearing screening are available, the most commonly used being Oz Screening Information Management Solution and HI*TRACK. Most automated OAE or ABR systems are compatible with one or both of these database programs.

TYPES OF HEARING IMPAIRMENT

Encoding of acoustic information occurs at multiple levels of the auditory pathway, and lesions from the end organ upward can disrupt the processing of auditory information. Consequently, the nature and severity of symptoms vary widely as a function of the site of the lesion in the auditory pathway.

Conductive Hearing Impairment

Normally, low- to moderate-intensity sound reaches the cochlea via air conduction through the external auditory canal, where it impinges sequentially on the tympanic membrane, the ossicular chain, and the oval window of the cochlea. The middle ear normally serves as a mechanical amplifier. Any condition that impedes the flow of air in the canal or the movement of the structures of the middle ear will reduce the efficiency of this amplifier and result in attenuation of sound intensity with less distortion of quality than with other types of hearing impairment. Higher-intensity sounds (>60 dB) will still reach the cochlea via vibration of the bones of the skull, bypassing the middle ear system. Mild, transient conductive hearing impairment is relatively inconsequential in an older child or adult. In a young child, mild to moderate conductive loss may render imperceptible many of the consonants in conversational-level speech, thus interfering with speech and language development. If the loss persists over long periods during the critical period for language acquisition, it can have serious structural and functional consequences for language development. For example, 4- to 5-year-old children with histories of chronic otitis media are less able to distinguish words signaled by different voice onset times, regardless of intelligence or hearing sensitivity on the day of testing.[70]

Hearing loss associated with chronic otitis media is usually fluctuating in nature, interfering with the normal binaural hearing experience. This could result in impaired sound localization ability and speech processing in noisy environments. Binaural function has been shown to be abnormal in 5- to 7-year-old children with past histories of chronic otitis media.[71] Breier and Gray[72] were unable to demonstrate any improvement in sound localization or speech processing abilities after surgical correction of unilateral atresia in children, suggesting that the effects were permanent.

Sensory (Cochlear) Hearing Impairment

The fluid within the cochlea can be set into motion either by vibration of the skull (bone conduction) or by movement of the stapes in the oval window of the cochlea (air conduction via the middle ear). The fluid motion results in shearing of the stereocilia of the sensory cells (hair cells), which, in turn, initiates the firing of single nerve fibers terminating in the eighth cranial nerve (Fig 1). Coding of frequency information begins in the cochlea. Injuries at this level are irreversible and can have devastating effects on both the loudness and quality of sound. Even unilateral hearing loss in children affects speech perception, learning, self-image, and social skills.

Hearing aids are usually effective in cases of pure cochlear hearing loss if there is residual hearing in the speech frequencies. Unfortunately, in many cases, neurons within the cochlea begin to deteriorate, and eighth nerve dysfunction complicates rehabilitation.

Neural Hearing Impairment

Axons of the single nerve fibers of the cochlea assemble to form the auditory portion of the eighth cranial nerve. Their concentric organization by frequency provides evidence of the nerve's function as a second-level coding device for acoustic information. Complex analyses of the intensity, frequency, and temporal information

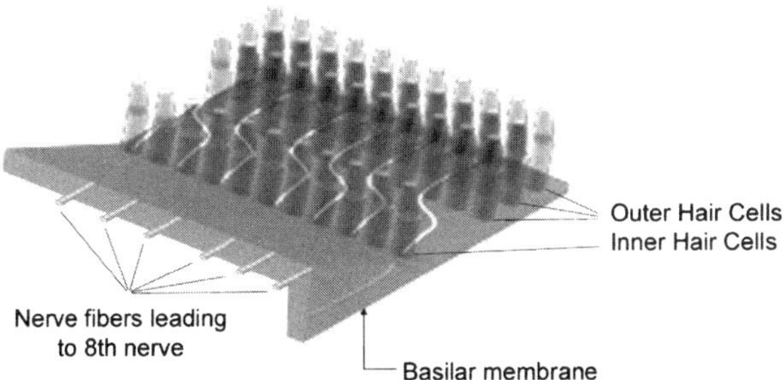

FIGURE 1.
Schematic representation of the inner and outer hair cells of the organ of Corti on the basilar membrane with nerve fibers leading to the eighth nerve. Relative motion of the membranes encasing the organ of Corti causes shearing of the stereocilia of the hair calls, which initiates firing of the nerve fibers.

in speech are based in part on firing patterns of the eighth nerve. Auditory nerve pathology can lead to total deafness or to such severe distortion that speech sounds cannot be discriminated. Extraction of meaningful sounds from background noise becomes extremely difficult. Hearing aids are less effective or ineffective.

Sensory hearing loss may progress to sensorineural hearing loss when neurons within the cochlea begin to degenerate. This progression helps to explain the variability in reported efficacy of hearing aids among individuals with similar audiograms. In fact, hearing thresholds to pure tones are extremely poor predictors of the success of amplification devices.

Until recently, sensory and neural hearing impairments were not distinguishable by objective testing techniques; thus, the term sensorineural hearing impairment was applied to virtually all permanent hearing disorders. Since the development of techniques for separate assessment of the eighth nerve and the hair cells of the cochlea, auditory neuropathy has been recognized as a distinct auditory disorder. It is characterized by poor speech discrimination out of proportion to the pure tone hearing thresholds,[73] which may be within normal limits. Binaural processing of sound, frequency discrimination, and intensity discrimination are impaired. Ambient noise severely alters speech intelligibility. Temporal aspects of auditory perception are compromised in these patients.[74] They are unable to detect brief gaps in sounds normally. The symptoms are attributed to abnormal neural synchrony, which is important for the perception of acoustic cues in speech. They may act behaviorally deaf as infants and then demonstrate responsivity at later ages, despite the fact that responses cannot be recorded from the eighth nerve or auditory brainstem pathway. Cochlear responses (OAE and cochlear microphonics) are present but may deteriorate with age, possibly as a result of retrograde degeneration of the cochlea. Auditory neuropathy is frequently associated with severe neonatal hyperbilirubinemia, which tends to affect structures above the level of the cochlea. Hearing aids are not helpful in these patients.

GENETICS OF DEAFNESS

Inherited syndromic deafness does not present the same identification dilemma as that of nonsyndromic deafness because related anomalies usually lead to early testing. New techniques in molecular genetics have greatly increased our understanding of monogenic inherited disorders. Linking to a single gene requires analysis in large affected families, and long-term studies of several families are currently underway. Based on the symptoms of a disorder in a family and existing knowledge about the function of specific genes, a candidate gene is first analyzed in the family for abnormal sequencing. Genes serve as templates for the creation and regulation of proteins, guiding development, providing for renewal of tissues, and regulating the function of organs at the biochemical level. Fifteen genes with various mutations responsible for nonsyndromic hearing loss have been identified. The inheritance of monogenic congenital hearing loss is autosomal recessive in 75%, autosomal dominant in 20%, X-linked in 5%, and mitochondrial in less than 1%.[75]

The *POU* family of genes is responsible for encoding transcription factors. Mutations on chromosome Xq21 in or around the nuclear gene POU3F4 are responsible for X-linked deafness type 3 (DFN3), with progressive hearing loss and fixation of the stapes. DFN15, an autosomal dominant form of progressive hearing loss, is related to the POU4F3 gene on chromosome 5q, which is responsible for transcription of target genes important for the survival of cells in the organ of Corti. Table 1 lists all the known loci for nonsyndromic hearing loss.

A cross-section of the cochlea and sites where genetic defects can occur is shown in Figure 2. The 2 ducts flanking the cochlear duct are filled with perilymph. Potassium-rich endolymph fills the cochlear duct housing the organ of Corti between the basilar and the tectorial membranes, which serve as resonators. The relative movement of these membranes leads to the influx of potassium ions through channels on the myosin-controlled filaments linking the tips of the stereocilia of the hair cells. Depolarization of the hair cells results in an electrical signal, which is transmitted to the eighth cranial nerve. Potassium ions probably then flow out through potassium channels in the lateral wall of the hair cells to surrounding support cells, to cochlear fibrocytes and the stria vascularis via connexin channels where they are secreted back into endolymph through another potassium channel.

Mutations have been identified in genes affecting middle ear and cochlear bone development, structural characteristics of the tectorial membrane, myosin (present in the stereocilia), diaphanous (involved in maintenance of the actin-filled stereocilia of the hair cells), fibrocytes (associated with ion channels), and connexin.[75] Connexins are channel-forming proteins in membranes, fibrocytes, and supporting cells of the cochlea. Mutations in the gene for connexin-26 account for as much as 50% of autosomal recessive hearing loss.[75]

TABLE 1.
Nuclear Gene Loci for Nonsyndromic Hearing Loss

Locus	Gene	Chromosomal Location
Autosomal dominant (DFNA)		
DFNA1	Diaphanous	5q31
DFNA2	Connexin 31 and KCNQ4	1p34
DFNA3	Connexin 26	13q12
DFNA4		19q13
DFNA5	ICERE-1	7p15
DFNA6		4p16
DFNA7		1q21-23
DFNA8	a-Tectorin	11q22-24
DFNA9	COCH	14q11-13
DFNA10		6q22-23
DFNA11	Myosin 7A	11q12-21
DFNA12	a-Tectorin	11q22-24
DFNA13		6p21
DFNA14		4p16
DFNA15	POU4F3	5q31
DFNA16		2q24
DFNA17		22q
DFNA18		3q22
DFNA19		10
Autosomal recessive (DFNB)		
DFNB1	Connexin 26	13q12
DFNB2	Myosin 7A	11q13
DFNB3	Myosin 15	17p11
DFNB4	Pendrin	7q31
DFNB5		14q12
DFNB6		3p14-21
DFNB7		9q13-21
DFNB8		21q22
DFNB9	Otoferlin	2p22-23
DFNB10		21q22
DFNB11		9q13-21
DFNB12		10q21-22
DFNB13		7q34-36
DFNB14		7q31 and 19p13
DFNB15		3q21-25
DFNB16		15q21-22
DFNB17		7q31
DFNB18		11p14-15
DFNB19		18p11
DFNB20		11q25-ter
DFNB21	a-Tectorin	11q

(continued)

TABLE 1. (continued)

Locus	Gene	Chromosomal Location
X-linked recessive (DFN)		
DFN 1	DDP	Xq22
DFN 2		Xq22
DFN 3	POU3F4	Xq21
DFN 4		Xp21
DFN 5		Withdrawn
DFN6		Xp22

(Reprinted with permission, from Willems PJ: Genetic causes of hearing loss. *N Engl J Med* 342:1101-1109.

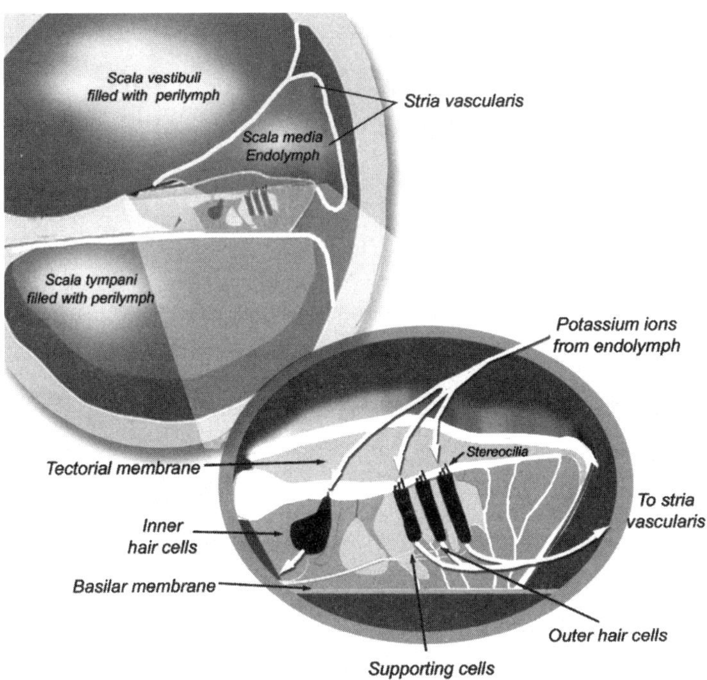

FIGURE 2.

Cross-section of the cochlea showing the position of the organ of Corti between the basilar membrane and the tectorial membrane. When these membranes are set into motion, the actin-filled stereocilia tilt, opening potassium channels. The tips of the stereocilia are linked by myosin-controlled filaments. Potassium from endolymph flows in the tips and out through the lateral wall of the hair cells to support cells and fibrocytes. It then flows to the stria vasclaris via connexin channels and back into endolymph through potassium channels. Genetic mutations can interrupt this normal process at multiple sites within the cochlea.

The mechanism by which the mutation results in a disorder may be investigated by developing a mutant strain of animal.[76] Several animal models of genetic deafness have been developed, contributing greatly to our understanding of variability in the type, severity, and time-course of inherited hearing disorders. For example, one X-linked mouse model produced profoundly deaf mice with no gross cochlear anatomical defects but with a marked reduction in the endocochlear potential. Fibrocytes, which play a role in the regulation of cochlear potassium homeostasis, are severely affected by the mutation. Another mutant strain has been developed that blocks the normal development of the bony labyrinth and the ossicles.

Data from both humans and animals may lead to gene therapies for preventing or reversing hearing loss.

CONTRIBUTIONS OF GENETIC STUDIES TO REHABILITATION

Studies in families with progressive hearing loss have been particularly useful in revealing patterns of destruction of the cochlea and neurons within the cochlea and their relationship to speech intelligibility, the effects of noise, and the efficacy of hearing aids and cochlear implants. Temporal bone studies have been performed in many cases.[77] As mentioned earlier, pure tone thresholds do not correlate well with hearing aid efficacy, probably because the detection of simple sounds does not require as many functional channels of intact hair cells, single nerve cells, and functional connections among auditory structures as are required for speech perception and extraction of signals from noise. When speech intelligibility deteriorates after depopulation of neurons within the cochlea, hearing aids become less effective, and cochlear implants or sign language must be considered.

Disorders of Central Auditory Processing

Structural organization by frequency, or *tonotopic organization,* is characteristic of every level of the auditory pathway. Functionally diverse fibers of the eighth cranial nerve branch to the separate frequency regions of the cochlear nuclei of the brainstem. These structures—the first way stations in the brainstem auditory pathway—demonstrate selective vulnerability to bilirubin toxicity[78] and perinatal hypoxic/ischemic injury,[79] thus representing a common site of lesion in perinatally acquired auditory dysfunction. In many cases, children with lesions of the brainstem auditory pathway will demonstrate deficiencies in the processing of auditory stimuli rather than reduced sensitivity to sound in a quiet environment, and learning disabilities are common in these children.

Cortical deafness is a clinical rarity not readily diagnosed because patients tend to show inconsistent responsivity to sound with poor speech production and understanding, in spite of normal physiologic responses from the peripheral and brainstem auditory pathways. In behavioral audiometric testing with pure tones in a sound room, patients may exhibit normal "hearing" thresholds. Bilateral temporal lesions and cortical deafness have been noted to result from fever,[80] congenital malformation,[81] meningitis,[82] or cerebral infarcts.[83] Amplification in such patients is ineffective and inappropriate. Rather, training in sign language should begin immediately upon diagnosis.

HEARING SCREENING AND DIAGNOSTIC METHODS

Assessment of Middle Ear Status

Tympanometry and acoustic reflex (stapedius muscle) testing are collectively known as *immittance audiometry.* The probe of the tympanogram contains a miniature microphone to measure the intensity of a tone which, when introduced into the ear canal, reflects off the tympanic membrane and travels back to the probe. The air pressure in the ear canal is systematically changed from positive to negative to alter the compliance of the tympanic membrane which, in part, determines the amount of sound energy that will be reflected versus absorbed (Fig 3).

Tympanometry is a sensitive test for the presence of fluid in the middle ear, retraction of the tympanic membrane (negative pressure), disarticulation of the ossicles, or perforation of the tympanic membrane in children aged 7 months or older. Before that age, the walls of the ear canal are cartilaginous and may expand when air pressure is increased in the canal, resulting in a falsely normal reading.

Acoustic reflexes are absent or elevated in threshold when there is sensorineural hearing loss or middle ear dysfunction. The acoustic reflex was at one time used to assess brainstem integrity, but more sensitive tests have since replaced it.

Tests of Cochlear Integrity

Before the discovery of evoked OAE, no direct physiologic test of cochlear integrity existed. Clinical application of this hair cell response, in combination with the ABR, now permits the separate functional assessment of the cochlea and the eighth cranial nerve. The OAE is rapid (4-5 minutes), inexpensive, reliable, and objec-

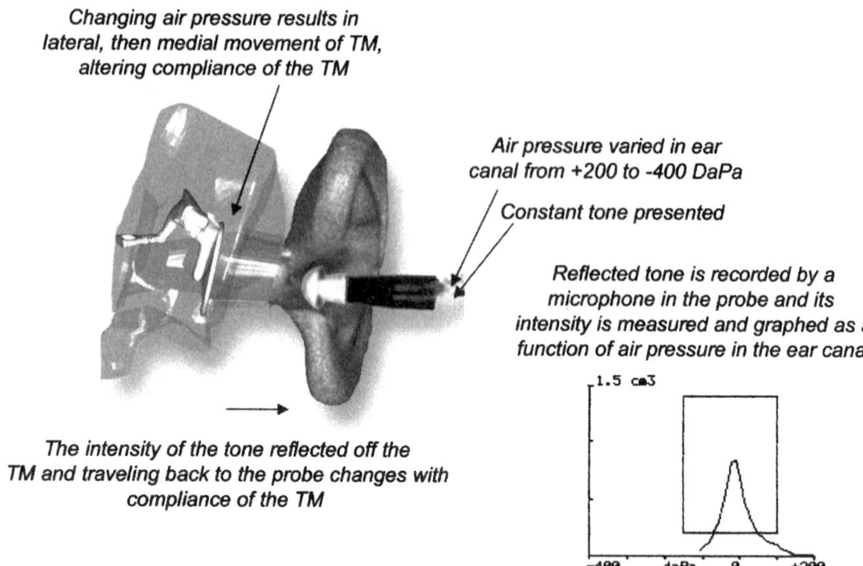

FIGURE 3.
Schematic representation of tympanometry. Air pressure in the ear canal is gradually changed from +200 to –400 daPa to apply lateral and medial pressure to the tympanic membrane *(TM)*. A constant tone is presented during the pressure change, and the intensity of the tone reflected off the TM is measured by a microphone in the probe. The intensity of the reflected tone is partially a function of compliance of the TM.

tive. It can be recorded in the preterm and term newborn (awake or asleep) and is highly sensitive to moderate hearing impairment of either conductive or sensory (cochlear) origin. The evoked OAE is thought to be generated by the elongation and contraction of the outer hair cells of the cochlea in response to either repetitive clicks (transient evoked OAE) or 2-tone stimulation (distortion product OAE). The distortion product OAE can be elicited at specific frequencies to assess cochlear function at specific locations along the basilar membrane on which the hair cells are situated. A small probe placed at the entrance to the ear canal presents the tones and delivers the response to a microphone (Fig 4). Computer software generates either a series of clicks or a "sweep" of 2 tones across a wide range of frequencies. The same software generates a graph of the spectrum of the emissions recorded in response to the stimuli. These tests do not provide an estimate of hearing threshold.

Tests of Neural Function

The action potential of the eighth cranial nerve can be recorded noninvasively from the early preterm period onward. It is usually recorded in combination with the ABR, by using the same electrode configuration and signal-averaging equipment.

Tests of Central Auditory Function

ABR is used both for the objective assessment of the brainstem auditory pathway (Fig 5) and for the estimation of hearing threshold. The latter permits the selection of appropriate amplification at an early age. Electrodes are taped to the scalp, and repetitive clicks or brief tones are presented through an earphone. Brief samples of the electroencephalogram are collected after the presentation of each stimulus, stored in a computer, and then summated by a signal-averaging system. The noise is nulled through averaging, leaving only the response, which is time-locked to the stimulus. The patient must be sleeping during threshold estimation.

Sensitive, objective, and simple tests of function of higher levels of the auditory pathway have not been developed at this time.

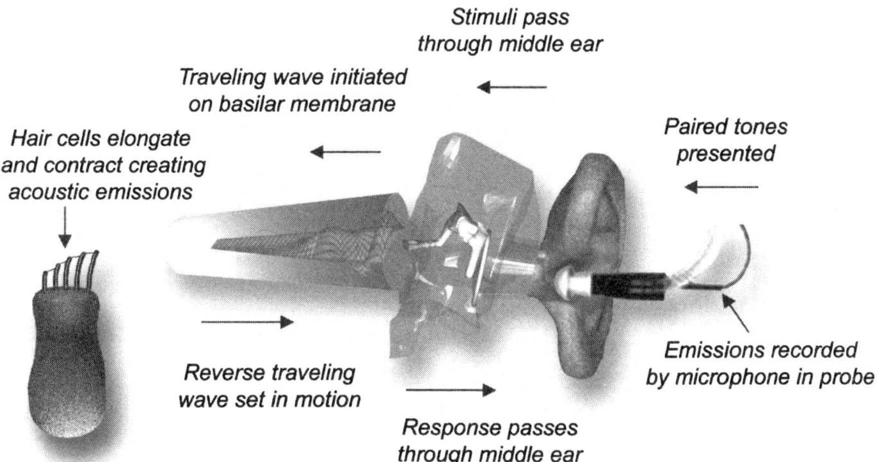

FIGURE 4.
Schematic representation of the measurement of distortion product otoacoustic emissions. Paired tones sweeping from low to high frequencies are presented. This stimulation results in elongation and contraction of the outer hair cells of the cochlea, producing an acoustic signal (emission) that can be measured by the microphone in the probe.

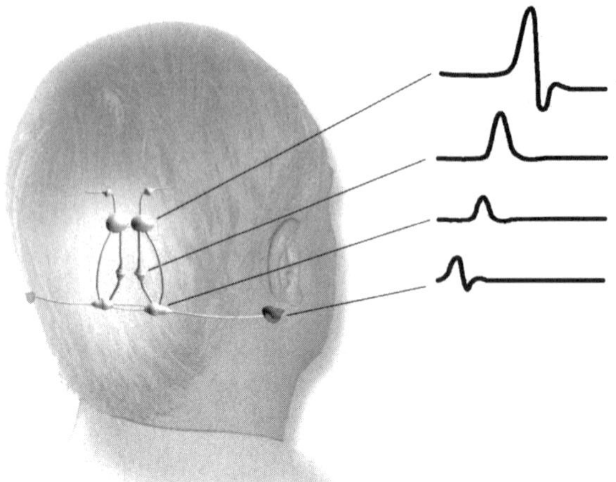

FIGURE 5.
Schematic representation of the origin of the auditory brainstem response. The first peak is generated by the eighth nerve action potential, and the subsequent peaks are produced by the sequential activation of the auditory nuclei of the brainstem.

Behavioral batteries of tests of central auditory processing have not proved to be sensitive or specific.[84]

SUMMARY

Hearing impairment of any type in early childhood can have serious permanent effects on development. It can be detected and diagnosed in the newborn period, and early intervention significantly improves language development and reading abilities. Chronic otitis media during the critical period for language development may result in altered production and perception of consonants of speech. An aggressive approach to identification, diagnosis, and prompt treatment of all types of auditory disorders is recommended.

REFERENCES

1. National Institutes of Health: Early identification of hearing impairment in infants and young children. *NIH Consensus Statement* 11:1-24, 1993.
2. Blake PE, Hall JW: The status of statewide policies for neonatal hearing screening. *J Am Acad Audiol* 1:67-74, 1990.
3. Werner LA, Folsom RC, Mancel LR: The relationship between auditory brainstem response and behavioral thresholds in normal hearing infants and adults. *Hear Res* 68:131-141, 1993.

4. Pujol R, Lavigne-Rebillard M, Uziel A: Physiological correlates of development in the human cochlea. *Semin Perinatol* 14:275-280, 1990.
5. Morey AL, Carlile S: Auditory brainstem of the ferret: Maturation of the brainstem auditory evoked response. *Dev Brain Res* 52:279-288, 1990.
6. Bredberg G: Cellular pattern and nerve supply of the human organ of Corti. *Acta Otolaryngol Suppl* 236:1-135, 1968.
7. Streeter L: The development of the scala tympani and perioticular cistern in the human embryo. *Am J Anat* 21:299-320, 1917.
8. Stockard JE, Stockard JJ, Coen RW: Auditory brain stem response variability in infants. *Ear Hear* 4:11-23, 1983.
9. Lavigne-Rebillard M, Pujol R: Hair cell innervation in the fetal human cochlea. *Acta Otolaryngol* 105:398-402, 1988.
10. Wedenberg E: Prenatal tests of hearing. *Acta Otolaryngol* 206:27-31, 1965.
11. Tanaka Y, Arayama T: Fetal responses to acoustic stimuli. *Practica Oto-Rhino-Laryngol* 31:269-273, 1969.
12. Gerber SE, Lima CG, Copriviza KL: Auditory arousal in peterm infants. *Scand Audiol Suppl* 17:88-93, 1983.
13. Werner LA: The development of auditory behavior (or what the anatomists and physiologists have to explain) *Ear Hear* 17:438-446, 1996.
14. Abdala C, Sininger Y: The development of cochlear frequency resolution in the human auditory system. *Ear Hear* 17:374-385, 1996.
15. Folsom RC, Wynne MK: Auditory brainstem responses from human adults and infants: Wave V tuning curves. *J Acoust Soc Am* 81:412-417, 1987.
16. Werner LA, Marean GC: *Human Auditory Development.* Boulder, Colo, Westview Press, 1996.
17. Keefe DH, Ling R, Bulen JC: Method to measure acoustic impedance and reflection coefficient. *J Acoust Soc Am* 91:470-485, 1992.
18. Ponton CW, Don M, Eggermont JJ, et al: Maturation of human cortical auditory function: Differences between normal-hearing children and children with cochlear implants. *Ear Hear* 17:430-437, 1996.
19. Franco P, Groswasser J, Hassid S, et al: Prenatal exposure to cigarette smoking is associated with a decrease in arousal in infants. *J Pediatr* 135:34-38, 1999.
20. Amin SB, Merle KS, Orlando MS, et al: Brainstem maturation in premature infants as a function of enteral feeding type. *Pediatrics* 106:318-322, 2000.
21. Hutt SJ, Hutt C, Lenard HG, et al: Auditory responsivity in the human neonate. *Nature* 218:888-890, 1968.
22. DeCasper AJ, Fifer WP: Of human bonding: Newborns prefer their mothers' voices. *Science* 208:1174-1176, 1980.
23. Fernald A: Four-month-old infants prefer to listen to motherese. *Infant Behav Dev* 8:181-195, 1985.
24. Fernald A, Kuhl P: Acoustic determinants of infant perception for motherese speech. *Infant Behav Dev* 10:279-293, 1987.

25. Morgan JL, Meier RP, Newport EL: Structural packaging in the input to language learning: Contributions of prosodic and morphological marking of phrases to the acquisition of language. *Cogn Psychol* 19:498-550, 1987.
26. Snow CE: Understanding social interaction and language development: Sentences are not enough, in Bornstein M, Bruner J (eds): *Interaction in Human Development*. Hillsdale, NJ, Erlbaum, 1993.
27. Olsho LW: Infant frequency discrimination. *Infant Behav Dev* 7:27-35, 1984.
28. Olsho LW, Koch EG, Halpin CF: Level and age effects in infant frequency discrimination. *J Acoust Soc Am* 82:454-464, 1987.
29. Maxon AB, Hochberg I: Development of psychoacoustic behavior: Sensitivity and discrimination. *Ear Hear* 3:301-308, 1982.
30. Demany L, Armand F: The perceptual reality of tone chroma in early infancy. *J Acoust Soc Am* 76:57-66, 1984.
31. Clarkson MG, Clifton RK: Infant pitch perception: Evidence for responding to pitch categories and the missing fundamental. *J Acoust Soc Am* 77:1521-1528, 1985.
32. Trehub SE, Thorpe LA: Infants' perception of rhythm. Categorization of auditory sequences by temporal structure. *Can J Psychol* 43:217-229, 1989.
33. Aslin RN: Experiential influences and sensitive periods in perceptual development: A unified model, in Aslin RN, Alberts JR, Petersen MR (eds): *Development of Perception: Psychological Perspectives*. New York, Academic Press, 1981, pp 45-94.
34. Lasky R, Syrdal-Lasky A, Klein RE: VOT discrimination by four to six and a half month olds from Spanish environments. *J Exp Child Psychol* 20:215-225, 1975.
35. Werker JF, Lalone CE: Cross-language speech perception: Initial capabilities and developmental change. *Dev Psychol* 24:672-683, 1988.
36. Miyakawa K, Strange W, Verbrugge R, et al: An effect of linguistic experience: The discrimination of /r/ and /l/ by native speakers of Japanese and English. *Perception Psychophys* 18:331-340, 1975.
37. Marean GC, Werner LA, Kuhl PK: Vowel categorization by very young infants. *Dev Psychol* 28:396-405, 1992.
38. Gottleib G: Otogenesis of sensory function in birds and mammals, in Tobach E, Aronson LR, Shaw E (eds): *The Biopsychology of Development*. New York, Academic Press, 1971, pp 67-128.
39. Turkewitz G, Kenny PA: Limitations on input as a basis for neural organization and perceptual development: A preliminary theoretical statement. *Dev Psychobiol* 15:357-368, 1982.
40. Gottleib G: Development of species identification in ducklings: VII. Highly specific early experience fosters species-specific perception in wood ducklings. *J Comp Physiol* 94:1019-1027, 1980.
41. Gottleib G, Tomlinson TW, Radell PL: Developmental intersensory interference: Premature visual experience suppresses auditory learning in ducklings. *Infant Behav Dev* 12:1-12, 1989.

42. Radell PL, Gottleib G: Developmental intersensory interference: Augmented prenatal sensory experience interferes with auditory learning in duck embryos. *Dev Psychol* 28:795-803, 1992.
43. Batkin S, Groth H, Watson JR, et al: Effects of auditory deprivation on the development of auditory sensitivity in albino rats. *Electroencephalogr Clin Neurophysiol* 28:351-359, 1970.
44. Webster DB, Webster M: Neonatal sound deprivation affects brain stem auditory nuclei. *Arch Otolaryngol* 103:392-396, 1977.
45. Moore DR: Auditory brainstem of the ferret: Early cessation of developmental sensitivity of neurons in the cochlear nucleus to removal of the cochlea. *J Comp Neurol* 302:810-823, 1990.
46. Tierney TS, Russell FA, Moore DR: Susceptibility of developing cochlear nucleus neurons to deafferentation-induced death abruptly ends just before the onset of hearing. *J Comp Neurol* 378:295-306, 1997.
47. Stern DN, Spieker S, MacKain K: Intonation contours as signals in maternal speech to prelinguistic infants. *Dev Psychol* 18:727-735, 1982.
48. DeCasper AJ, Prescott PA: Human newborns' perception of male voices: Preference, discrimination, and reinforcing value. *Dev Psychobiol* 17:481-491, 1984.
49. DeCasper AJ, Spence MJ: Prenatal maternal speech influences newborns' perception of speech sounds. *Infant Behav Dev* 6:19-25, 1986.
50. CDC: Serious hearing impairment among children aged 3-10 years: Atlanta, Georgia, 1991-1993. *MMWR* 46:1073-1076, 1997.
51. Niskar AS, Kieszak SM, Holmes A, et al: Prevalence of hearing loss among children 6 to 19 years of age: The Third National Health and Nutrition Examination survey. *JAMA* 279:1071-1075, 1998.
52. Sorri M, Rantakallio P: Prevalence of hearing loss at the age of 15 in a birth cohort of 12,000 children from northern Finland. *Scand Audiol* 14:203-207, 1985.
53. Watkin PM, Baldwin M, Laoide S: Parental suspicion and identification of hearing impairment. *Arch Dis Child* 65:846-850, 1990.
54. Mehl AL, Thompson V: Newborn hearing screening: The great omission. *Pediatrics* 101:4-14, 1998.
55. Vohr BR, Carty LM, Moore PE, et al: The Rhode Island Assessment program: Experience with statewide hearing screening (1993-1996). *J Pediatr* 133:353-358, 1998.
56. Finitzo T, Albright K, O'Neal J: The newborn with hearing loss: Detection in the nursery. *Pediatrics* 102:1452-1460, 1998.
57. Mason JA, Herrman KR: Universal hearing screening by automated auditory brainstem response measurement. *Pediatrics* 101:221-228, 1998.
58. Van Naarden K, Decoufle P: Relative and attributable risks for moderate to profound bilateral sensorineural hearing impairment associated with lower birth weight in children 3 to 10 years old. *Pediatrics* 104:905-910, 1999.
59. Johnson JL, Mauk GW, Takakawa KM, et al: Implementing a statewide system of services for infants and toddlers with hearing disabilities. *Semin Hear* 14:105-119, 1993.

60. Harrison M, Roush J: Age of suspicion, identification, and intervention for infants and young children with hearing loss: A national study. *Ear Hear* 17:55-62, 1996.
61. Garganta C, Seashore MR: Universal hearing screening for hearing loss. *Pediatr Ann* 29:302-308, 2000.
62. Joint Committee on Infant Hearing: Joint Committee on Infant Hearing Position Statement. *Pediatrics* 70:496-497, 1982.
63. Kemp DT, Ryan S: The use of transient evoked otoacoustic emissions in neonatal hearing screening programs. *Semin Hear* 14:30-45, 1993.
64. Picton TW, Ouellette J, Hamel G, et al: Brainstem evoked potentials to tonepips in notched noise. *J Otolaryngol* 8:289-314, 1979.
65. American Speech and Hearing Association Committee on Infant Hearing: Audiologic screening of infants who are at risk for hearing impairment. *ASHA* 31:61-64, 1989.
66. Bess FH, Paradise JL: Universal screening for infant hearing impairment: Not simple, not risk-free, not necessarily beneficial, and not presently justified. *Pediatrics* 93:330-334, 1994.
67. Yoshinaga-Itano C, Sedey AL, Coulter DK, et al: Language of early- and later-identified children with hearing loss. *Pediatrics* 102:1161-1171, 1998.
68. Joint Committee on Infant Hearing: Year 2000 position statement: Principles and guidelines for early hearing detection and intervention programs. *Pediatrics* 106:798-817, 2000.
69. Stockard JJ, Curran JS: Transient elevation of threshold of the neonatal auditory brain stem response. *Ear Hear* 11:21-28, 1990.
70. Clarkson RL, Eimas PD, Marean GC: Speech perception in children with histories of recurrent otitis media. *J Acoust Soc Am* 85:926-933, 1989.
71. Gunnarson AD, Finitzo T: Conductive hearing loss during infancy: Effects on later auditory brainstem electrophysiology. *J Speech Hear Res* 34:1207-1215, 1991.
72. Breier JI, Gray L: Pre- and postnatal postoperative source localization in patients with unilateral atresia. *Assoc for Res in Otolaryngol Abstracts* 16:40, 1993.
73. Starr A, Picton TW, Sininger Y, et al: Auditory neuropathy. *Brain* 11:741-753, 1996.
74. Sininger YS, Doyle KJ, Moore JK: The case for early identification of hearing loss in children: Auditory system development, experimental auditory deprivation and development of speech and hearing. *Pediatr Clin North Am* 46:1-14, 1999.
75. Willems PJ: Genetic causes of hearing loss. *N Engl J Med* 342:1101-1108, 2000.
76. Anderson J, Herrup K, Breakfield X: Creation of transgenic mice that over-express MAO-B neuronally. *Ann Am Acad Sci* 648:178-188, 1992.
77. Halpin C, Herrmann B, Wheaty M: A family with autosomal dominant progressive sensorineural hearing loss: Rehabilitation and counseling. *Am J Audiol* 5:23-32, 1996.

78. Gerrard J: Nuclear jaundice and deafness. *J Laryngol* 66:387-397, 1952.
79. Hall JG: On the neuropathological changes in the central nervous system following neonatal asphyxia. *Acta Otolaryngol Suppl* 188:331-338, 1964.
80. Hood LJ, Berlin CI, Allen P: Cortical deafness: A longitudinal study. *J Am Acad Audiol* 5:330-342, 1994.
81. Landau WM, Goldstein R, Kleffner FR: Congenital aphasia: A clinicopathologic study. *Neurology* 7:915-921, 1957.
82. Lechevalier B, Rosaa Y, Eustache F, et al: Case of cortical deafness sparing the music area. *Rev Neurol (Paris)* 140: 190-201, 1984.
83. Jerger J, Weikers N, Sharbrough FW, et al: Bilateral lesions of the temporal lobe. *Acta Otolaryngol* 258:5-51, 1969.
84. Singer J, Hurley RM, Preece JP: Effectiveness of central auditory processing tests with children. *Am J Audiol* 7:1-11, 1998.

CHAPTER 10

Gastroesophageal Reflux in Infants and Children

Peter Lee, MD
Fellow, Division of Pediatric Gastroenterology and Nutrition, Children's Hospital Medical Center, Cincinnati, Ohio

Colin Rudolph, MD, PhD
Professor of Pediatrics, Chief, Pediatric Gastroenterology, Hepatology and Nutrition, Medical College of Wisconsin, Milwaukee

Gastroesophageal reflux (GER) is defined as the retrograde movement of gastric contents through the lower esophageal sphincter and into the esophagus. GER is extremely common in infancy, with approximately half of all infants up to 3 months, and two thirds of infants between 4 and 6 months of age having symptoms of recurrent vomiting.[1] The vast majority of these infants have effortless regurgitation with no apparent GER-associated complications and spontaneous resolution of their symptoms by 9 to 12 months of age.[2] Nonetheless, a small proportion of infants and children will develop symptoms of GER, described as gastroesophageal reflux disease (GERD). These include esophagitis, poor weight gain, reactive airway disease, recurrent pneumonia, laryngitis, and apparent life-threatening events.

The approach to evaluation of the infant or child with suspected GER-related disease varies depending on the presenting symptoms, but certain principles apply in all cases. First, other causes of the presenting symptom need to be considered. For example, the infant with vomiting may have an anatomical abnormality or an underlying metabolic disorder. Second, a cause-and-effect relationship between GER and the symptom must be established. Third, appropriate treatment is selected based on the expected natural history and severity of disease.

PHYSIOLOGY OF GER AND PROTECTIVE MECHANISMS

GER is a normal physiologic event that occurs in all infants, children, and adults. Caustic gastric contents enter the esophagus many times each day in the adult. In infants, passage of gastric contents through the pharynx, with regurgitation from the mouth, is common. A series of protective mechanisms prevent damage to the esophagus and airway when GER occurs, whereas failures of these mechanisms account for GER-associated disorders.

The barrier between the stomach and the esophagus is known as the lower esophageal sphincter (LES). It consists of the intrinsic lower esophageal sphincter, which is a specialized smooth muscle in the distal esophagus, the abdominal crura, and the intra-abdominal portion of the esophagus (Fig 1). The LES is composed of smooth muscle and is normally tonically contracted, with a resting pressure between 10 and 30 mm Hg in the adult.[3] The infant LES has a resting tone of 18 mm Hg at term and reaches adult tone by 6 weeks of age.[4] In the premature infant, the LES pressure is 5 to 10 mm Hg at 25 to 30 weeks' gestation, and appears to correlate with postconceptual rather than postnatal age.[5] Most infants with GER have normal LES pressure,[6,7] and therefore, the increased fre-

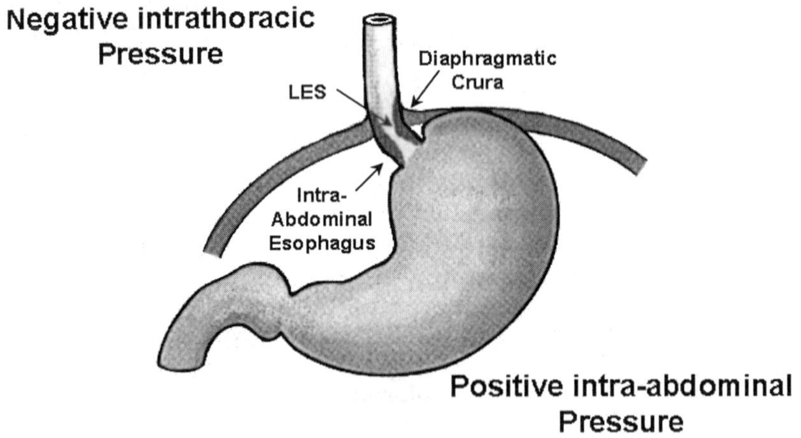

FIGURE 1.
Anatomy of the gastroesophageal junction. Gastroesophageal reflux is prevented during inspiration by several mechanisms: (1) intrinsic lower esophageal sphincter *(LES)* tone, (2) compression of the gastroesophageal junction by the diaphragmatic crura, and (3) closure of the intra-abdominal portion of the esophagus.

quency of regurgitation in infants cannot be explained by a "weak sphincter." The pressure barrier between the stomach and esophagus is also generated by the diaphragmatic crura that wrap around the lower sphincter region[8,9] and the intra-abdominal segment of the esophagus. During inspiration and straining, when the intra-abdominal pressure relative to intrathoracic pressure is increased, the diaphragmatic crura contract around the esophagus, preventing GER. In addition, during straining the intra-abdominal segment of the esophagus is compressed. These latter mechanisms may be ineffective in infants because the LES is located 2 cm above the diaphragm for the first 6 months of life.[10] The descent of the LES into the abdominal cavity results in an intra-abdominal segment of the esophagus. This mechanism is absent in the presence of a hiatal hernia in older children and adults, who are more prone to GER complications.

Most episodes of GER occur during transient lower esophageal sphincter relaxations (TLESRs).[11] TLESRs have been observed in premature and term infants, children, and adults, and are believed to be a mechanism to allow the venting of air from the stomach.[12,13] They occur throughout the day but are seen primarily after meals when the stomach is distended, and rarely occur during sleep.[14] Omari et al[13] studied the etiology of 193 reflux events in 24 infants and found that 82% of reflux episodes were associated with TLESRs, compared with 13% that occurred during swallow-associated LES relaxation, and only 2 episodes that were associated with straining.

In the normal infant or adult, refluxed gastric contents are rapidly cleared from the distal esophagus with no apparent sequelae. Both mechanoreceptors and acid receptors mediate esophageal clearance. Distention or acidification of the esophagus triggers a secondary peristaltic wave that pushes any gastric refluxate back into the stomach.[15] Any residual acid within the esophagus is usually buffered by subsequent swallows of saliva.[16] In infants, GER reaches the upper esophagus more frequently because infants tend to be recumbent and the length and capacity of their esophagus is smaller than in adults. Therefore, after an episode of GER, infants are more prone to distend the upper esophagus and then expel gastric contents out of the mouth.

The upper esophageal sphincter (UES) is the primary barrier to refluxed material entering the hypopharynx from the upper esophagus. The cricopharyngeus muscle is the major component of the UES, and similar to the LES, it also maintains a state of tonic contraction. UES pressure increases with small volumes of GER, preventing passage of refluxate into the pharynx. However, larger volume episodes of GER that rapidly distend the upper esophagus will result in UES relaxation[17] and the likely expulsion of gastric contents from the mouth. This reflex relaxation is likely a protective mechanism to prevent esophageal perforation during vomiting. UES pressure also decreases during sleep[18] and would therefore predispose sleeping infants to vomiting or regurgitation during episodes of GER to the upper esophagus.

To protect the respiratory tract from harmful gastric contents, a series of complex protective reflexes have evolved to close off the airway to further exposure. Unfortunately, these reflex responses can also result in apnea, stridor, or wheezing. Distention of the upper esophagus by an episode of GER triggers the esophagoglottal closure reflex.[19] This reflex mimics the laryngeal protective mechanisms of swallowing, with anterior displacement of the larynx, apnea, and vocal cord closure. Direct exposure of the larynx to liquids results in the temporary cessation of breathing, vocal cord closure, and the initiation of swallowing.[20] Any liquid that does manage to enter the airway is cleared by the cough reflex and may be associated with a reflex bronchoconstriction. This reflex is presumably an attempt to prevent liquids from reaching the alveoli and impairing proper gas exchange. Similarly, esophageal acid exposure alone may also trigger reflex bronchoconstriction,[21] especially in the premature infant. The nature of the reflex response may also be age dependent. Studies in puppies demonstrated that water stimulation of the larynx causes prolonged apnea, whereas in older dogs it causes cough.[22,23] This apparent age-dependent variation in response has been attributed to differences in central nervous system integrative processing[22] and may reflect a maturational effect. This may explain the propensity of infants to have obstructive apneic events associated with episodes of GER (see discussion of apnea below).

Any disruption of the normal protective reflexes will predispose the infant or child to possible esophageal or respiratory complications from GER. Poor esophageal clearance will cause esophagitis. Inadequate airway protective mechanisms may result in laryngitis, asthma, or recurrent pneumonia. Patients with neurologic disease often have poor esophageal motility and reduced esophageal acid clearance, which increases the risk of GER-associated esophagitis. A similar risk of esophagitis caused by poor motility occurs with rheumatologic disorders and with anatomical abnormalities of the esophagus, such as tracheoesophageal fistula.[24] Both anatomical defects of the larynx or impaired laryngeal protective reflexes may predispose patients to aspiration during episodes of GER.

The pathogenesis of GERD involves multiple interacting elements where a single event or combination of events can easily disrupt the balance between physiologic GER and GERD. Researchers have identified a gene on chromosome 13q14 in a group of families with severe pediatric GERD.[25] The resultant physiologic defect has yet to be defined. Because these individuals are a small subset of patients with severe familial GERD, it is likely that the genetic abnormality associated with this locus will not be present in all patients with GERD.

DIAGNOSTIC EVALUATION

Demonstration of a causal relationship between GER and a particular symptom is often challenging. Each diagnostic test may be useful in specific clinical scenarios but may be of little value in others (Table 1). For example, esophageal pH monitoring can establish that there is increased esophageal acid exposure, and this likely provides an explanation for GER causing esophagitis. However, a normal esophageal pH monitoring study does not exclude the possibility that recurrent pneumonia is caused by GER because even one brief episode of pharyngeal reflux could cause pneumonia if airway protective mechanisms are inadequate. Furthermore, esophageal inflammation from another cause such as eosinophilic/allergic esophagitis may alter esophageal clearance mechanisms, and treatment of the underlying disorder may improve esophageal clearance. Therefore, it is important that each test be interpreted carefully, with a clear understanding of what physiologic mechanisms the test evaluates and of the pathogenesis of the GER-related symptom being studied. Although many of these tests are able to detect the presence of GER, they are best used to address specific clinical situations rather than for routine use in the evaluation and treatment of GERD.

HISTORY AND PHYSICAL EXAMINATION

The history and physical examination remain the cornerstone for the diagnosis of GER, and have yet to be supplanted by the numerous tests now available to the clinician. Signs and symptoms commonly attributed to GERD in infants and children are listed in Table 2. Recurrent vomiting in the infant requires careful evaluation to exclude any infectious, anatomical, neurologic, or metabolic conditions. A history of bilious vomiting, abdominal distention, lethargy, hypotonia, convulsions, fever, or hepatosplenomegaly should prompt an evaluation for other etiologies besides GER.

TABLE 1.
Diagnostic Tests Used for Evaluation of GERD

Diagnostic Test	Esophageal Disorders	Respiratory Disorders
Upper GI contrast study	Can identify other etiologies such as malrotation, pyloric stenosis, antral webs, achalasia Can detect stricture formation	Can identify TEF, laryngeal cleft, vascular rings May detect aspiration but has poor sensitivity
Nuclear scintigraphy	Not useful	May detect episodes of aspiration and nonacidic GER
Esophageal pH monitoring	Risk of esophagitis correlates with degree of acid exposure Calculation of symptom index may be helpful to correlate symptoms with episodes of GER	Prolonged acid exposure may increase risk of GER-related asthma May be helpful in asthmatic patients without symptoms of GER to select potential responders to therapy
Esophageal pH monitoring with pneumogram	Not useful	May establish relationship between episodes of GER and apnea
Esophagoscopy with biopsy	Best tool for evaluating the presence and severity of esophagitis Can detect other causes of esophagitis such as infectious, allergic, or Crohn disease	Presence of esophagitis may increase risk of GER-related airway disorders

Bronchoscopy with lipid-laden macrophages	Not useful	High numbers of lipid-laden macrophages may be associated with chronic aspiration
Laryngoscopy	Not useful	Presence of laryngeal erythema or edema may be associated with upper airway symptoms caused by GER
Swallowing studies (videofluoroscopic or fiberendoscopic)	Not useful	Absent or impaired airway protective mechanisms may increase the risk of aspiration with GER
Empirical medical therapy	Reasonable approach in patients with pain as their presenting symptom	May use a 3-month trial of aggressive antisecretory medications in asthmatic patients if clear end points are set Can also use in suspected laryngeal inflammation

Abbreviations: GERD, Gastroesophageal reflux disease; *GI,* gastrointestinal; *TEF,* tracheoesophageal fistula.

TABLE 2.
Signs and Symptoms of GERD in Infants and Children

Infants	Children
Recurrent vomiting	Intermittent vomiting
Irritability	Regurgitation
Anorexia	Heartburn
Dysphagia	Dysphagia
Back-arching	Chest pain
Hematemesis	Hematemesis
Anemia	Anemia
Cough	Cough
Wheezing	Wheezing
Choking	Hoarseness
Gagging	Sandifer posturing
Stridor	
Apnea	

Abbreviation: GERD, Gastroesophageal reflux disease.

Although there is some overlap in symptoms between infants and preschool-age children, the older child will tend to have more adultlike complaints with intermittent vomiting, regurgitation, and heartburn. Because it is the natural history of GER to improve by 1 year of age, symptoms persisting or appearing after 18 months also require careful evaluation for other etiologies.

RADIOGRAPHIC CONTRAST STUDIES

Radiographic contrast studies of the upper gastrointestinal tract have not been shown to be useful in accurately determining the presence of GERD.[26-28] GER often occurs in normal infants so it is not surprising that GER may occur during an upper gastrointestinal examination in a normal infant. Rather, the upper gastrointestinal examination is useful to exclude other conditions that may be mistaken for GER. Anatomical abnormalities such as pyloric stenosis, malrotation, antral web, or tracheoesophageal fistula can be excluded. It is also useful in the detection of other esophageal disorders that may cause vomiting, chest pain, or both, including achalasia and esophageal strictures.

NUCLEAR SCINTIGRAPHY

Nuclear scintigraphy is another imaging tool available for the detection of GER. It involves labeling food or formula with a radioactive isotope and measuring the number of postprandial episodes of GER and any aspiration events. Its major advantages include the detection of postprandial nonacid GER events, assessment of gastric emptying, and the detection of aspiration events up to 24 hours after the initial feeding.[29] The primary drawbacks with nuclear scintigraphy are the lack of normative data in the pediatric age group and the absence of any data regarding the value of these studies to predict response to therapy for GERD.

ESOPHAGEAL PH MONITORING

Esophageal pH monitoring measures the frequency and duration of episodes of esophageal acidification over an extended period, typically 18 to 24 hours. Multiple study variables can affect the accuracy and validity of the test including position, activity level, mode of feeding, and the type of pH electrode used. Modification of the study protocol depends on the specific clinical question asked. Risk assessment for the development of esophagitis can be determined by using a standard pH probe with the patient on a normal diet and level of activity. The reflux index is used as a measure of esophageal acid exposure. It is the percentage of time that the esophageal pH is less than 4. A reflux index of greater than 11% in infants up to 1 year, and greater than 6% in children and adults is considered abnormal and is associated with an increased risk of esophagitis.[30-34]

Correlation of airway symptoms with esophageal acidification requires the use of an electrode with quick response times and accurate recording of each event in question. In infants with suspected apnea caused by GER, the combination of pH recording, oxygen saturation, nasal airflow, and chest wall movement provides the most meaningful data. However, this type of study is rarely conclusive, in part because of a significant number of missed postprandial nonacidic GER events[35] that have been buffered by breast milk or standard formula.

Symptom correlation with esophageal acidification can also be assessed by using a symptom index, because some patients will have a normal amount of esophageal acid exposure but still exhibit reproducible symptoms with brief episodes of GER. The symptom index is the percentage of symptoms associated with esophageal acidification. In adult studies evaluating heartburn and GER, patients with a symptom index of more than 0.5 responded well to acid-suppressive therapy.[36] The symptom index has been reported to be useful in children to demonstrate an association of GER and abdominal pain.[37] Esophageal pH monitoring can also be used to determine the efficacy of acid-suppressive therapy before airway surgery or the evaluation of new or breakthrough symptoms while receiving therapy.

Measurement of intraluminal electrical impedance with a specialized catheter is a new technique for the detection of GER and is particularly useful to assess the relationship of nonacidic GER to symptoms such as apnea.[38] One study that used esophageal pH monitoring combined with pneumogram data in 22 infants with regurgitation or pulmonary symptoms found 49 GER-related apneic events, of which 78% were detected by electrical impedance but not by esophageal pH monitoring.[39] Electrical impedance study is still in the experimental stage and should only be performed as part of a research protocol.

Esophagoscopy enables both visualization and biopsy of the esophageal epithelium. It is the best test to evaluate for esophageal complications of GER including esophagitis and Barrett esophagus. It also allows exclusion of other disorders, such as Crohn disease, webs, and eosinophilic or infectious esophagitis as a cause of symptoms. A normal appearance of the esophagus during endoscopy does not exclude histopathologic esophagitis, and subtle mucosal changes of erythema and pallor may be observed in the absence of esophagitis.[40-42] Esophageal friability, erosions, and ulcers indicate more severe disease. Because of poor correlation between endoscopic appearance and histopathology, esophageal biopsy should be performed to diagnose esophagitis.

In healthy infants and children, eosinophils and neutrophils are not present in the esophageal epithelium.[43,44] Basal zone hyperplasia (>20%-25% of total epithelial thickness) and increased papillary length (>50%-75% of epithelial thickness) correlate with increased acid exposure.[44,45] If there are large numbers of eosinophils (>20 per high-power field), the diagnosis of eosinophilic esophagitis, instead of GERD, should be considered.[46,47]

GERD EVALUATION AND MANAGEMENT

Clinical, radiographic, or pH probe evidence of GER does not necessarily imply that GERD is also present. Complications of GER can be divided into nutritional, esophageal, and respiratory disorders. In the otherwise healthy infant with recurrent vomiting, a thorough history and physical examination allow the clinician to establish a diagnosis of uncomplicated GER without any other diagnostic tests. Warning signs such as forceful, bilious, or blood-tinged vomiting, hematochezia, anemia, poor weight gain, associated diarrhea or constipation, fever, lethargy, abdominal distension or tenderness, hepatosplenomegaly, seizures, or other chronic diseases suggest that other causes of vomiting need to be considered. In these cases, other diagnostic tests such as an upper gastrointestinal series or a metabolic evaluation may be warranted. The approach to GERD evaluation and treatment will depend on the presenting symptom and suspected complication in question.

MALNUTRITION AND FAILURE TO THRIVE

The major nutritional complication associated with GER is malnutrition or failure to thrive. Inadequate weight gain in the patient with GER rarely stems from excessive vomiting and the loss of potential calories. Most patients have inadequate caloric consumption secondary to restricted intake. Oftentimes, parents (or physicians) will limit the volume of formula per feed in an attempt to reduce the amount or frequency of vomiting. Parental reassurance, education, and anticipatory guidance on monitoring for other potential complications are usually all that is needed in this situation. A careful dietary history generally provides an indication of whether adequate calories are being offered or ingested. Although some infants refuse feedings because of pain from esophagitis,[48] other causes of feeding disorders should not be ignored. Mistakenly blaming GER for poor feeding may result in overlooking other causes of feeding difficulties.[49]

Rarely, an infant may be unable to gain weight despite ingesting adequate calories. In these cases, it is important to consider other causes of vomiting, including metabolic disorders, infections, renal or urinary tract disease, malabsorptive disorders, and anatomical obstruction. If no abnormalities are found, then therapeutic options include thickening of the formula, a trial of hypoallergenic formula to exclude cow milk allergy as a cause of vomiting, prone positioning, and acid suppression therapy. Prokinetic therapy is also useful, but no effective agent is easily available in the United States. Occasionally, infants may benefit from either nasogastric or transpyloric continuous feeding to improve their nutritional status.[50] Hospitalization for observation and endoscopy with biopsy may be necessary to clarify the cause of vomiting and poor growth. Careful follow-up is necessary to ensure adequate weight gain. Most infants will be able to maintain weight gain without continued interventions by 4 to 6 months of age.

ESOPHAGEAL COMPLICATIONS OF GER

GER-associated esophagitis results from poor acid clearance and therefore exposure of the esophageal mucosa to caustic gastric material. Esophagitis in infancy often manifests as irritability or feeding refusal, whereas in children and adolescents the symptoms are heartburn, chest pain, or dysphagia. Severe esophagitis can present with hematemesis, melena, and anemia, whereas chronic inflammation may cause stricture formation with resulting dysphagia. One unusual presentation of esophageal pain from GER is Sandifer syndrome. It is characterized by repetitive stretching movements of the neck and can be easily mistaken for atypical seizures.

A trial of empirical medical therapy in patients with milder symptoms is a reasonable alternative to initial endoscopic evaluation. Moreover, in infants where it is difficult to discriminate whether vomiting is caused by GERD or formula allergy, a 2-week trial of a hypoallergenic formula is also reasonable.[51,52] Failure of empirical therapy or serious presenting symptoms often warrant more definitive diagnostic evaluation. Evaluation for esophageal complications is best achieved with esophagoscopy. Biopsy specimens should always be obtained to assess the severity of GER-associated esophagitis or potentially diagnose other causes of esophageal inflammation, as discussed above. Untreated severe esophagitis may result in stricture formation or Barrett esophagus. True Barrett epithelium always shows intestinal metaplasia on biopsy. Because Barrett epithelium is a premalignant condition, either antireflux surgery or long- term, high-dose antisecretory therapy is required. Neither therapy is completely effective at inducing regression of Barrett mucosa,[53,54] making regular endoscopic surveillance for dysplasia or malignancy mandatory after diagnosis of Barrett esophagitis.

At the other end of the spectrum of esophageal disease is a subset of patients with typical symptoms of heartburn but no evidence of esophageal inflammation on endoscopy. Esophageal pH monitoring reveals a normal reflux (% time esophageal pH < 4), but pain is associated with episodes of GER.[55] These patients with a "hypersensitive esophagus" presumably have altered visceral sensitivity with decreased pain thresholds.[56] Acid-suppressive therapy has been shown to be effective for treatment in this situation.[57] Thus, normal endoscopic findings and a normal esophageal pH manometry study cannot exclude GER as a cause of esophageal symptoms.

In most instances, the esophageal complications of GER will respond to conventional pharmacologic therapy. The advent of proton pump inhibitors (PPIs) has dramatically improved the efficacy of medical therapy for esophagitis. However, in one long-term follow-up study of adults treated with omeprazole for a mean of 6.5 years (range, 1.4-11.2 years), 12% developed Barrett metaplasia during the treatment period, raising some doubts about the ability of PPI therapy to prevent serious sequelae of GERD.[58] Antireflux surgery is currently only recommended when maximum medical therapy proves to be ineffective, but no long term studies in pediatric patients have compared the risks, benefits, or costs of prolonged medical therapy with a PPI with laparoscopic surgical therapy.

RESPIRATORY COMPLICATIONS OF GER

The respiratory complications of GER can be subdivided into inflammatory or reflex-associated disorders. They frequently pose both a diagnostic and treatment challenge to the clinician.

Obstructive apnea or an apparent life-threatening event (ALTE) can be associated with episodes of GER (Fig 2).[59-61] A careful review of the circumstances surrounding the event can help to determine whether GER is contributory. Infants will often be awake during an episode and because of reflex laryngospasm, they may become cyanotic despite apparent respiratory effort.[62] Most episodes resolve without intervention and with no apparent sequelae. This exaggerated airway protective response diminishes as the infant matures, and by 6 to 8 months of age it is uncommon.[63] A subset of patients exhibit severe manifestations including prolonged apnea or cardiac arrest.[64,65] Exclusion of other potential causes of apnea, such as seizure disorder or innominate artery airway compression, is essential during diagnostic evaluation. Standard medical therapy for this complication is usually sufficient and can include a combination of conservative measures and pharmacologic medications. Life-threatening manifestations obviously warrant surgical intervention.

GER-associated reactive airway disease is a frequent concern in asthmatic patients. Between 25% and 75% of children with persistent asthma have evidence of increased esophageal acidification by pH monitoring,[66-69] and approximately half of these patients will not have any apparent symptoms of GER.[66,70] Despite this increased prevalence, it is unlikely that GER has a direct causal relationship with asthma but may have an impact on disease severity. Experimentally, esophageal acid infusion has been shown to increase airway resistance in humans.[71-74] The mechanism of exacerbation is controversial but likely involves vagal-mediated airway hyperresponsiveness from either microaspiration of acid or stimulation of esophageal acid receptors during episodes of GER.[71,72,75]

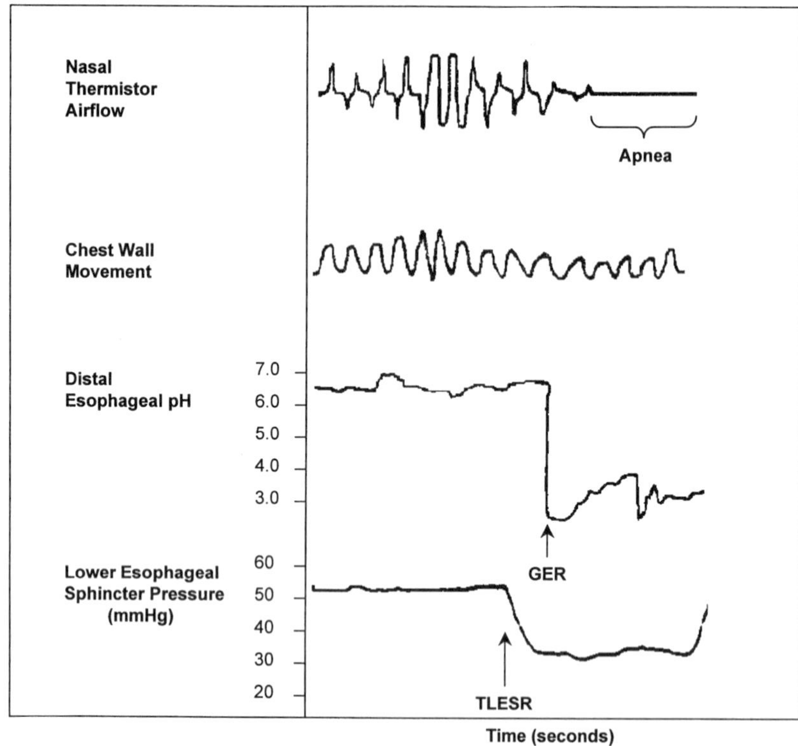

FIGURE 2.
Simultaneous pH monitoring, pneumogram, and manometry that show a period of obstructive apnea occurring shortly after a transient lower esophageal sphincter relaxation *(TLESR)* and an episode of esophageal acidification *(GER)*. Note that there is no airflow despite persistent respiratory effort with chest wall movements.

Prolonged medical therapy has been shown to improve respiratory symptoms and reduce the need for bronchodilator and anti-inflammatory medications in approximately 60% of patients with persistent asthma.[68,70,76] In patients with coexistent GER and asthma, aggressive acid-suppressive therapy for at least 3 months may be required before a significant improvement in respiratory symptoms is observed.[77] The seasonal variation in asthma symptoms makes it difficult to be certain that any improvement is the result of GER treatment. Selection of those patients most likely to benefit from medical or surgical therapy remains problematic, so that often therapy is initiated and the response is monitored. If this strategy is chosen, clear end points on and off therapy must be established and monitored for several months. These may include the frequency and severity of gastrointestinal or respiratory symptoms, the results of pulmonary function testing, and the amount of antiasthmatic medication required. In asthmatic patients without symptoms of GER, pH monitoring may be useful to select potential responders to medical or surgical therapy. Surgical therapy has also been reported to be highly effective in patients with steroid-dependent asthma and evidence of other GER-associated complications.[78-80] Patients demonstrated both symptomatic improvement and a reduction in the amount of bronchodilator and anti-inflammatory medication usage. Because there are no tests to accurately predict which patients will respond to antireflux therapy, careful patient selection is recommended. Fundoplication should be considered in asthmatic patients with abnormal esophageal pH monitoring studies, severe exacerbations, steroid dependency, or other coexistent complications of GER including recurrent pneumonia, erosive esophagitis, and failure to thrive.

Airway inflammation from direct acid exposure is another potential complication of GER. Refluxate penetrating the laryngeal inlet can produce laryngeal inflammation and symptoms of hoarseness, stridor, or chronic cough.[81-83] These symptoms can occur in the absence of esophageal symptoms or inflammation.[84] Laryngoscopy may show evidence of laryngeal erythema or edema, but there are large interobserver variations in the interpretation of findings, and it is likely that similar findings may be observed with other disease etiologies such as allergy. GER-associated laryngeal inflammation will respond to aggressive medical management, but recurrence is common off therapy.[85]

Recurrent pneumonia from aspiration of gastric contents is a serious complication of GER that also can occur without any evidence of esophageal disease.[86,87] Results of esophageal pH monitoring may be normal because even infrequent episodes of GER can result in aspiration if the normal laryngeal protective mechanisms are absent. GER-associated aspiration is rare in normal infants and children, but is seen more commonly among patients with previous esophageal or laryngeal anatomical abnormalities or neuromuscular disease.[88]

The assessment of the contribution of GER to recurrent pneumonia usually begins with a chest radiograph or computerized tomography to evaluate for the typical changes seen with aspiration. Bronchoscopy can also be performed to look for lipid-laden macrophages as additional supportive evidence of chronic aspiration.[89] Some lipid-laden macrophages may be present in normal individuals, but a large percentage of lipid-laden macrophages increases the probability that the lung disease is caused by aspiration.[90-92] This does not, of course, exclude direct aspiration from above. A barium contrast video swallowing study can be used to evaluate the adequacy of laryngeal protective mechanisms. However, evidence of laryngeal penetration with contrast during swallowing does not exclude episodes of aspiration with GER to the upper esophagus.[93] In fact, those patients who have inadequate airway protection during swallowing are much more likely to aspirate during episodes of pharyngeal reflux.

The effectiveness of medical therapy in preventing GER-related pneumonia is unclear, but it may be considered in patients with mild or infrequent complications. The most logical therapy would be a prokinetic that would reduce the amount and frequency of GER, but no effective prokinetic is readily available in the United States. The efficacy of antisecretory therapy (histamine$_2$-receptor antagonists [H_2RAs] or PPIs) has not been evaluated in this setting. Patients with significant pulmonary disease will require antireflux surgery, which has been shown to be effective for prevention of GER-related pneumonia.[80,94]

TREATMENT OPTIONS

CONSERVATIVE THERAPY

Conservative measures such as positioning or the alteration of formula consistency are often used in infants with GER. The addition of thickening agents such as rice cereal to formula will decrease the frequency of vomiting but not necessarily the degree of esophageal acidification during pH monitoring.[95-97] The addition of rice cereal will increase the caloric density of the formula and likely benefit the infant with GER and poor weight gain. Any improvement in weight gain may not entirely result from the increased caloric density but from an increase in the amount consumed as well. Other newer formulas containing agents that thicken on contact with gastric acid also appear to be effective in the treatment of symptomatic GER.[98] Unlike rice cereal–thickened formula, these formulas have a normal consistency before administration and do not require crosscutting of the nipple to facilitate flow.

Several esophageal pH studies have shown a significant decrease in GER when infants are placed in the prone position when compared with supine.[99,100] Moreover, the frequency of GER actually increases in the semisupine position, as seen with infant seat placement.[101] Left lateral positioning has also been advocated based on one study that demonstrated a similar decrease in GER when compared with prone positioning.[102] Despite the apparent advantages of prone positioning, the increased risk of sudden infant death syndrome (SIDS) precludes its use during sleeping,[103,104] and should only be recommended when the risk of complications from GER clearly outweigh the increased risk of SIDS. One example of the reasonable use of prone positioning therapy would be a hospitalized patient with a laryngeal cleft before either airway repair or antireflux surgery. The decision to use prone positioning should be accompanied by the removal of any soft bedding that may further increase the risk of SIDS.[105]

In children and adolescents, elevation of the head of the bed during sleep and maintenance of an upright position after meals will likely reduce the frequency of GER. Other lifestyle changes have been investigated, and there is some evidence that limiting caffeine and alcohol consumption and possibly tobacco smoke exposure is beneficial.[109]

PHARMACOLOGIC THERAPY

Acid-suppressive and prokinetic medication are the major pharmacologic agents available for the treatment of GERD. Acid-suppressive agents such as antacids, H_2RAs, or PPIs reduce gastric acid exposure of the esophagus and airway by either acid neutralization or inhibition of acid secretion. In contrast, prokinetic agents have no effect on acid secretion. These agents reduce acid exposure by enhancing gastrointestinal motility and thus improving acid clearance.[110]

Acid Suppressives

Antacid therapy is frequently used in the short-term relief of GER-associated symptoms in children, adolescents, and adults. Although the efficacy of high-dose antacids has been shown to be equivalent to that of H_2RAs in the treatment of esophagitis in infants and children, there is a potential risk of aluminum toxicity in infants.[111,112] With the advent of antisecretory agents that have a longer duration of effect and better side effect profile, long-term antacid therapy should not be used. Intermittent antacid therapy for symptom relief in older children and adolescents is reasonable, but the requirement for frequent use indicates more severe disease requiring evaluation.

H_2RAs inhibit histamine-mediated acid secretion. They have been shown to significantly reduce esophageal acid exposure and improve both symptoms and esophageal histology.[111,113] In general, there are no significant differences in efficacy among the various H_2RAs, which include cimetidine, ranitidine, famotidine, and nizatidine. There are minor differences in side effect profiles, with increased drug interactions and gynecomastia being observed with cimetidine therapy compared with the other agents. PPIs are generally more effective than H_2RAs in acid suppression. However, one study of adults who had persistent nocturnal acid breakthrough despite receiving twice-a-day PPI therapy showed that a nighttime dose of ranitidine was more effective than an additional dose of omeprazole.[114]

PPIs prevent acid secretion by blocking the H^+/K^+ ATPase pump in the gastric parietal cell. Simultaneous administration of an H_2RA may reduce the effectiveness of PPI therapy because the presence of acid in the parietal cell cannilicul us is required for the PPI to bind and deactivate the pump.[115] The need for cannilicular secretion also explains why PPIs are most effective when given about 20 to 30 minutes before a meal, allowing absorption into the bloodstream with peak serum levels coincident with meal-stimulated acid secretion. Several reported studies in adults have demonstrated greater efficacy of PPIs when compared with H_2RAs in the treatment and maintenance of remission of esophagitis.[116,117] Although no randomized controlled trials of PPI therapy have been conducted in pediatric patients, several case series reports show resolution of esophagitis in patients previously refractory to high-dose H_2RA therapy.[118,119] The few studies done to evaluate proper dosage regimens for infants and children suggest a starting dosage of 0.5 to 0.7 mg/kg per day and range up to 3.3 mg/kg per day.[120]

Traditionally, clinicians have prescribed acid-suppressive therapy in a step-up approach by using H_2RAs as first-line therapy, followed by PPIs at increasing doses to achieve adequate acid suppression. In adults, there is increasing evidence that suggests the use of initial and maintenance PPI therapy because it is more cost-effective, and that a step-down approach is more appropriate.[58] Patients are started on high-dose PPI therapy until symptomatic improvement is achieved. This is followed by normal doses of PPIs for maintenance and then, if possible, H_2RAs.

Prokinetic Agents

Of all the pharmacologic therapies available, prokinetic agents would seem to be an ideal therapy for GER because they tend to improve gastrointestinal motility. The combination of enhanced esophageal motility, accelerated gastric emptying, and possibly reduced TLESRs should theoretically improve acid clearance and reduce the risk of GERD development. Various prokinetic agents have been used in the treatment of GERD including bethanechol, metoclopramide and cisapride. Bethanechol is a direct cholinergic agonist that is seldom used because of its limited efficacy and high incidence of cholinergic side effects.[121] Metoclopramide is an antidopaminergic agent that has not been shown to be effective as GER therapy and has the potential for significant central nervous system side effects.[122-124] Cisapride is the only prokinetic agent that has demonstrated some efficacy in the treatment of GERD. Several pediatric trials have shown a decrease in both the frequency and volume of vomiting as well as improvement in several objective measures, such as esophageal acid exposure and histopathology.[125-128] Unfortunately, because of an increased risk of serious cardiac arrhythmias, cisapride has been withdrawn from the US market and is now only available through a limited access protocol that requires strict monitoring with frequent electrocardiograms and blood studies. To minimize the risk of cardiac arrhythmias, the use of cisapride should be combined with careful patient selection, restriction of the dosage to a maximum of 0.8 mg/kg per day, and the avoidance of medications known to inhibit cisapride metabolism.

SURGICAL THERAPY

Severe GERD that is unresponsive to aggressive medical management often warrants surgical intervention. GER-associated respiratory complications such as recurrent pneumonia, life-threatening reactive airway disease, or ALTE are the most common indications for surgical therapy. Less common indications include prevention of postoperative laryngeal injury after airway reconstruction, esophageal stricture formation secondary to erosive esophagitis, or Barrett esophagus.

Nissen fundoplication is the most common antireflux procedure used, and success rates ranging from 60% to 90% have been reported.[129-131] Operative mortality is approximately 1%, but ranges from 0% to 4.9% in several case series.[129,132,133] The potential complications associated with the procedure are listed in Box 1. Gas bloat and dysphagia are relatively common complications but tend to resolve with time. One of the more discouraging complications is postfundoplication gagging and retching, which can occur in up to 10% to 15% of patients.[134,135] Complication rates also tend to be higher in patients with neurologic dysfunction or altered esophageal motility.[136] The Thal procedure, which is a partial fundoplication, has been advocated for patients with

BOX 1.
Complications of Antireflux Surgery

Breakdown of the fundoplication
Intrathoracic herniation
Bowel obstruction
Dysphagia
Gas bloat
Dumping syndrome
Gagging
Retching

impaired esophageal motility. However, the overall complication rates compared with Nissen fundoplication appear to be the same.[137] An increasing number of fundoplications are now being performed laparoscopically. Complication rates with laparoscopic therapy are similar or less than those with open surgical procedures, and the immediate postoperative morbidity is dramatically decreased with a significant reduction in recovery time.[138]

Newer endoscopic therapies for GERD are now available for use in adults. One method uses an endoscopic sewing device to achieve an internal plication. Another device uses electrodes to cause localized coagulation and swelling at the LES region. These procedures are poorly validated even in adult trials. No pediatric data are available for either device, and questions remain regarding their accommodation to esophageal growth in the pediatric population. Any of these newer procedures should be considered only in clinical trials, especially in children.

CONCLUSION

GER is a normal physiologic event in infants, children, and adults. Abnormalities of the normal protective mechanisms result in disease. Poor esophageal clearance results in esophagitis with sequelae including pain, dysphagia, hematemesis, anemia, stricture formation, or a Barrett esophagus. GER combined with inadequate airway protective mechanisms may cause recurrent pneumonia or laryngeal inflammation, or may exacerbate asthma. Infant obstructive apnea may represent an inappropriately robust GER-triggered airway protective reflex. In all presentations of GERD, other potential causes of the presenting symptom or sign must be excluded. Diagnostic and treatment options must be selected based on the presentation and severity of disease.

REFERENCES

1. Nelson SP, Chen EH, Syniar GM, et al: Prevalence of symptoms of gastroesophageal reflux during infancy. A pediatric practice-based survey. Pediatric Practice Research Group. *Arch Pediatr Adolesc Med* 151:569-572, 1997.
2. Nelson SP, Chen EH, Syniar GM, and Christoffel KK: One-year follow-up of symptoms of gastroesophageal reflux during infancy. Pediatric Practice Research Group. *Pediatrics* 102:E67, 1998.
3. Kahrilas PJ: Functional anatomy and physiology of the esophagus, in Castell DO (ed): *The esophagus.* Boston, Little, Brown and Co, 1992.
4. Boix-Ochoa J, Canals J: Maturation of the lower esophagus. *J Pediatr Surg* 11:749-756, 1976.
5. Novak DA: Gastroesophageal reflux in the preterm infant. *Clin Perinatol* 23:305-320, 1996.
6. Werlin SL, Dodds WJ, Hogan WJ, et al: Mechanisms of gastroesophageal reflux in children. *J Pediatr* 97:244-249, 1980.
7. Kawahara H, Dent J, Davidson G: Mechanisms responsible for gastroesophageal reflux in children [see comments]. *Gastroenterology* 113:399-408, 1997.
8. Boyle JT, Altschuler SM, Nixon TE, et al: Role of the diaphragm in the genesis of lower esophageal sphincter pressure in the cat. *Gastroenterology* 88:723-730, 1985.
9. Mittal RK, Rochester DF, McCallum RW: Effect of the diaphragmatic contraction on lower oesophageal sphincter pressure in man. *Gut* 28:1564-1568, 1987.
10. Moroz SP, Espinoza J, Cumming WA, et al: Lower esophageal sphincter function in children with and without gastroesophageal reflux. *Gastroenterology* 71:236-241, 1976.
11. Dent J, Dodds WJ, Friedman RH, et al: Mechanism of gastroesophageal reflux in recumbent asymptomatic human subjects. *J Clin Invest* 65:256-267, 1980.
12. Cucchiara S, Staiano A, Di Lorenzo C, et al: Pathophysiology of gastroesophageal reflux and distal esophageal motility in children with gastroesophageal reflux disease. *J Pediatr Gastroenterol Nutr* 7:830-836, 1988.
13. Omari TI, Barnett C, Snel A, et al: Mechanisms of gastroesophageal reflux in healthy premature infants. *J Pediatr* 133:650-654, 1998.
14. Mittal RK, McCallum RW: Characteristics and frequency of transient relaxations of the lower esophageal sphincter in patients with reflux esophagitis. *Gastroenterology* 95:593-599, 1988.
15. Helm JF, Dodds WJ, Riedel DR, et al: Determinants of esophageal acid clearance in normal subjects. *Gastroenterology* 85:607-612, 1983.
16. Helm JF, Dodds WJ, Pelc LR, et al: Effect of esophageal emptying and saliva on clearance of acid from the esophagus. *N Engl J Med* 310:284-288, 1984.
17. Kahrilas PJ, Dodds WJ, Dent J, et al: Upper esophageal sphincter function during belching. *Gastroenterology* 91:133-140, 1986.

18. Davidson GP, Dent J, Willing J: Monitoring of upper oesophageal sphincter pressure in children. *Gut* 32:607-611, 1991.
19. Shaker R, Dodds WJ, Ren J, et al: Esophagoglottal closure reflex: A mechanism of airway protection. *Gastroenterology* 102:857-861, 1992.
20. Harding R, Johnson P, McClelland ME: Liquid-sensitive laryngeal receptors in the developing sheep, cat and monkey. *J Physiol (Lond)* 277:409-422, 1978.
21. Boyle JT, Tuchman DN, Altschuler SM, et al: Mechanisms for the association of gastroesophageal reflux and bronchospasm. *Am Rev Respir Dis* 131:S16-S20, 1985.
22. Boggs DF, Bartlett D Jr: Chemical specificity of a laryngeal apneic reflex in puppies. *J Appl Physiol* 53:455-462, 1982.
23. Johnson P, Salisbury D, Storey A: Apnea induced by stimulation of sensory receptors in the larynx, in Bosma JF (ed): *Development of Upper Respiratory Anatomy and Function*. Washington, DC, US Government Printing Office, 1975.
24. Dudley NE, Phelan PD: Respiratory complications in long-term survivors of oesophageal atresia. *Arch Dis Child* 51:279-282, 1976.
25. Hu FZ, Post JC, Johnson S, et al: Mapping of a gene for severe pediatric gastroesophageal reflux to chromosome 13q14. *JAMA* 284:325-334, 2000.
26. Stephen TC, Younoszai MK, Massey MP, et al: Diagnosis of gastroesophageal reflux in pediatrics. *J Ky Med Assoc* 92:188- 191, 1994.
27. Meyers WF, Roberts CC, Johnson DG, et al: Value of tests for evaluation of gastroesophageal reflux in children. *J Pediatr Surg* 20:515-520, 1985.
28. Thompson JK, Koehler RE, Richter JE: Detection of gastroesophageal reflux: Value of barium studies compared with 24-hr pH monitoring [see comments]. *AJR Am J Roentgenol* 162:621- 626, 1994.
29. McVeagh P, Howman-Giles R, Kemp A: Pulmonary aspiration studied by radionuclide milk scanning and barium swallow roentgenography. *Am J Dis Child* 141:917-921, 1987.
30. Vandenplas Y, Goyvaerts H, Helven R, et al: Gastroesophageal reflux, as measured by 24-hour pH monitoring, in 509 healthy infants screened for risk of sudden infant death syndrome. *Pediatrics* 88:834-840, 1991.
31. Euler AR, Byrne WJ: Twenty-four-hour esophageal intraluminal pH probe testing: A comparative analysis. *Gastroenterology* 80:957-961, 1981.
32. Sondheimer JM: Continuous monitoring of distal esophageal pH: A diagnostic test for gastroesophageal reflux in infants. *J Pediatr* 96:804-807, 1980.
33. Boix-Ochoa J, Lafuenta JM, Gil-Vernet JM: Twenty-four hour esophageal pH monitoring in gastroesophageal reflux. *J Pediatr Surg* 15:74-78, 1980.
34. Quigley EM: 24-h pH monitoring for gastroesophageal reflux disease:

Already standard but not yet gold (editorial)? *Am J Gastroenterol* 87:1071-1075, 1992.
35. Schwartz DJ, Wynne JW, Gibbs CP, et al: The pulmonary consequences of aspiration of gastric contents at pH values greater than 2.5. *Am Rev Respir Dis* 121:119-126, 1980.
36. Katzka DA, Paoletti V, Leite L, et al: Prolonged ambulatory pH monitoring in patients with persistent gastroesophageal reflux disease symptoms: Testing while on therapy identifies the need for more aggressive anti-reflux therapy [see comments]. *Am J Gastroenterol* 91:2110-2113, 1996.
37. Corrado G, Cavaliere M, Frandina G, et al: Primary gastro-oesophageal reflux disease and irritable oesophagus syndrome as causes of recurrent abdominal pain in children. *Ital J Gastroenterol* 28:462-469, 1996.
38. Wenzl TG, Skopnik H: Intraluminal impedance: An ideal technique for evaluation of pediatric gastroesophageal reflux disease. *Curr Gastroenterol Rep* 2:259-264, 2000.
39. Wenzl TG, Silny J, Schenke S, et al: Gastroesophageal reflux and respiratory phenomena in infants: Status of the intraluminal impedance technique. *J Pediatr Gastroenterol Nutr* 28:423-428, 1999.
40. Leape LL, Ramenofsky ML: Surgical treatment of gastroesophageal reflux in children. Results of Nissen's fundoplication in 100 children. *Am J Dis Child* 134:935-938, 1980.
41. Chadwick LM, Kurinczuk JJ, Hallam LA, et al: Clinical and endoscopic predictors of histological oesophagitis in infants. *J Paediatr Child Health* 33:388-393, 1997.
42. Biller JA, Winter HS, Grand RJ, et al: Are endoscopic changes predictive of histologic esophagitis in children? *J Pediatr* 103:215-218, 1983.
43. Shub MD, Ulshen MH, Hargrove CB, et al: Esophagitis: A frequent consequence of gastroesophageal reflux in infancy. *J Pediatr* 107:881-884, 1985.
44. Black DD, Haggitt RC, Orenstein SR, et al: Esophagitis in infants. Morphometric histological diagnosis and correlation with measures of gastroesophageal reflux. *Gastroenterology* 98:1408-1414, 1990.
45. Winter HS, Madara JL, Stafford RJ, et al: Intraepithelial eosinophils: A new diagnostic criterion for reflux esophagitis. *Gastroenterology* 83:818-823, 1982.
46. Liacouras CA, Wenner WJ, Brown K, et al: Primary eosinophilic esophagitis in children: Successful treatment with oral corticosteroids [see comments]. *J Pediatr Gastroenterol Nutr* 26:380-385, 1998.
47. Ruchelli E, Wenner W, Voytek T, et al: Severity of esophageal eosinophilia predicts response to conventional gastroesophageal reflux therapy. *Pediatr Dev Pathol* 2:15-18, 1999.
48. Mathisen B, Worrall L, Masel J, et al: Feeding problems in infants with gastro-oesophageal reflux disease: A controlled study. *J Paediatr Child Health* 35:163-169, 1999.

49. Rudolph CD: Feeding disorders in infants and children. *J Pediatr* 125:S116-124, 1994.
50. Ferry GD, Selby M, Pietro TJ: Clinical response to short-term nasogastric feeding in infants with gastroesophageal reflux and growth failure. *J Pediatr Gastroenterol Nutr* 2:57-61, 1983.
51. Cavataio F, Iacono G, Montalto G, et al: Gastroesophageal reflux associated with cow's milk allergy in infants: Which diagnostic examinations are useful? *Am J Gastroenterol* 91:1215-1220, 1996.
52. Iacono G, Carroccio A, Cavataio F, et al: Gastroesophageal reflux and cow's milk allergy in infants: A prospective study. *J Allergy Clin Immunol* 97:822-227, 1996.
53. Bozymski EM, Shaheen NJ: Barrett's esophagus: Acid suppression, but no regression (editorial). *Am J Gastroenterol* 92:556-558, 1997.
54. Hassall E, Weinstein WM: Partial regression of childhood Barrett's esophagus after fundoplication. *Am J Gastroenterol* 87:1506-1512, 1992.
55. Shi G, Bruley des Varannes S, Scarpignato C, et al: Reflux related symptoms in patients with normal oesophageal exposure to acid [see comments]. *Gut* 37:457-464, 1995.
56. Trimble KC, Pryde A, Heading RC: Lowered oesophageal sensory thresholds in patients with symptomatic but not excess gastro-oesophageal reflux: Evidence for a spectrum of visceral sensitivity in GORD. *Gut* 37:7-12, 1995.
57. Watson RG, Tham TC, Johnston BT, et al: Double blind cross-over placebo controlled study of omeprazole in the treatment of patients with reflux symptoms and physiological levels of acid reflux: The "sensitive oesophagus." *Gut* 40:587-590, 1997.
58. Klinkenberg-Knol EC, Nelis F, Dent J, et al: Long-term omeprazole treatment in resistant gastroesophageal reflux disease: Efficacy, safety, and influence on gastric mucosa [see comments]. *Gastroenterology* 118:661-669, 2000.
59. Herbst JJ, Minton SD, Book LS: Gastroesophageal reflux causing respiratory distress and apnea in newborn infants. *J Pediatr* 95:763-768, 1979.
60. Menon AP, Schefft GL, Thach BT: Apnea associated with regurgitation in infants. *J Pediatr* 106:625-629, 1985.
61. Walsh JK, Farrell MK, Keenan WJ, et al: Gastroesophageal reflux in infants: Relation to apnea. *J Pediatr* 99:197-201, 1981.
62. Spitzer AR, Boyle JT, Tuchman DN, et al: Awake apnea associated with gastroesophageal reflux: A specific clinical syndrome. *J Pediatr* 104:200-205, 1984.
63. Tirosh E, Kessel A, Jaffe M, et al: Outcome of idiopathic apparent life-threatening events: Infant and mother perspectives. *Pediatr Pulmonol* 28:47-52, 1999.
64. See CC, Newman LJ, Berezin S, et al: Gastroesophageal reflux-induced hypoxemia in infants with apparent life-threatening event(s). *Am J Dis Child* 143:951-954, 1989.

65. Jolley SG, Halpern LM, Tunell WP, et al: The risk of sudden infant death from gastroesophageal reflux [see comments]. *J Pediatr Surg* 26:691-696, 1991.
66. Buts JP, Barudi C, Moulin D, et al: Prevalence and treatment of silent gastro-oesophageal reflux in children with recurrent respiratory disorders. *Eur J Pediatr* 145:396-400, 1986.
67. Malfroot A, Vandenplas Y, Verlinden M, et al: Gastroesophageal reflux and unexplained chronic respiratory disease in infants and children. *Pediatr Pulmonol* 3:208-213, 1987.
68. Tucci F, Resti M, Fontana R, et al: Gastroesophageal reflux and bronchial asthma: Prevalence and effect of cisapride therapy [see comments]. *J Pediatr Gastroenterol Nutr* 17:265-270, 1993.
69. Balson BM, Kravitz EK, McGeady SJ: Diagnosis and treatment of gastroesophageal reflux in children and adolescents with severe asthma. *Ann Allergy Asthma Immunol* 81:159-164, 1998.
70. Andze GO, Brandt ML, St Vil D, et al: Diagnosis and treatment of gastroesophageal reflux in 500 children with respiratory symptoms: The value of pH monitoring. *J Pediatr Surg* 26:295-300, 1991.
71. Mansfield LE Stein MR: Gastroesophageal reflux and asthma: A possible reflex mechanism. *Ann Allergy* 41:224-226, 1978.
72. Spaulding HS Jr, Mansfield LE, Stein MR, et al: Further investigation of the association between gastroesophageal reflux and bronchoconstriction. *J Allergy Clin Immunol* 69:516-521, 1982.
73. Davis RS, Larsen GL, Grunstein MM: Respiratory response to intraesophageal acid infusion in asthmatic children during sleep. *J Allergy Clin Immunol* 72:393-398, 1983.
74. Hoyoux C, Forget P, Lambrechts L, et al: Chronic bronchopulmonary disease and gastroesophageal reflux in children. *Pediatr Pulmonol* 1:149-153, 1985.
75. Pellegrini CA, DeMeester TR, Johnson LF, et al: Gastroesophageal reflux and pulmonary aspiration: Incidence, functional abnormality, and results of surgical therapy. *Surgery* 86:110-119, 1979.
76. Berquist WE, Rachelefsky GS, Kadden M, et al: Gastroesophageal reflux-associated recurrent pneumonia and chronic asthma in children. *Pediatrics* 68:29-35, 1981.
77. Harding SM, Richter JE, Guzzo MR, et al: Asthma and gastroesophageal reflux: Acid suppressive therapy improves asthma outcome. *Am J Med* 100:395-405, 1996.
78. Ahrens P, Heller K, Beyer P, et al: Antireflux surgery in children suffering from reflux-associated respiratory diseases. *Pediatr Pulmonol* 28:89-93, 1999.
79. Rothenberg SS: Laparoscopic anti-reflux procedures and gastrostomy tubes in infants and children. *Int Surg* 79:328-331, 1994.
80. Foglia RP, Fonkalsrud EW, Ament ME, et al: Gastroesophageal fundoplication for the management of chronic pulmonary disease in children. *Am J Surg* 140:72-79, 1980.
81. Irwin RS, Corrao WM, Pratter MR: Chronic persistent cough in the

adult: The spectrum and frequency of causes and successful outcome of specific therapy. *Am Rev Respir Dis* 123:413-417, 1981.
82. Fitzgerald JM, Allen CJ, Craven MA, et al: Chronic cough and gastroesophageal reflux. *CMAJ* 140:520-524, 1989.
83. Katz PO: Ambulatory esophageal and hypopharyngeal pH monitoring in patients with hoarseness. *Am J Gastroenterol* 85:38- 40, 1990.
84. Gumpert L, Kalach N, Dupont C, et al: Hoarseness and gastroesophageal reflux in children. *J Laryngol Otol* 112:49-54, 1998.
85. Wo JM, Grist WJ, Gussack G, et al: Empiric trial of high-dose omeprazole in patients with posterior laryngitis: A prospective study [see comments]. *Am J Gastroenterol* 92:2160-2165, 1997.
86. Blecker U, de Pont SM, Hauser B, et al: The role of "occult" gastroesophageal reflux in chronic pulmonary disease in children. *Acta Gastroenterol Belg* 58:348-352, 1995.
87. Tovar JA, Angulo JA, Gorostiaga L, et al: Surgery for gastroesophageal reflux in children with normal pH studies. *J Pediatr Surg* 26: 541-545, 1991.
88. Wilkinson JD, Dudgeon DL, Sondheimer JM: A comparison of medical and surgical treatment of gastroesophageal reflux in severely retarded children. *J Pediatr* 99:202-205, 1981.
89. Colombo JL, Hallberg TK: Pulmonary aspiration and lipid-laden macrophages: In search of gold (standards) (editorial). *Pediatr Pulmonol* 28:79-82, 1999.
90. Ahrens P, Noll C, Kitz R, et al: Lipid-laden alveolar macrophages (LLAM): A useful marker of silent aspiration in children [see comments]. *Pediatr Pulmonol* 28:83-88, 1999.
91. Collins KA, Geisinger KR, Wagner PH, et al: The cytologic evaluation of lipid-laden alveolar macrophages as an indicator of aspiration pneumonia in young children [see comments]. *Arch Pathol Lab Med* 119:229-231, 1995.
92. Knauer-Fischer S, Ratjen F: Lipid-laden macrophages in bronchoalveolar lavage fluid as a marker for pulmonary aspiration. *Pediatr Pulmonol* 27:419-422, 1999.
93. Morton RE, Wheatley R, Minford J: Respiratory tract infections due to direct and reflux aspiration in children with severe neurodisability. *Dev Med Child Neurol* 41:329-334, 1999.
94. Chen PH, Chang MH, Hsu SC: Gastroesophageal reflux in children with chronic recurrent bronchopulmonary infection. *J Pediatr Gastroenterol Nutr* 13:16-22, 1991.
95. Vandenplas Y, Sacre L: Milk-thickening agents as a treatment for gastroesophageal reflux [published erratum appears in *Clin Pediatr (Phila)* 26:148, 1987.]. *Clin Pediatr (Phila)* 26:66-68, 1987.
96. Orenstein SR, Magill HL, Brooks P: Thickening of infant feedings for therapy of gastroesophageal reflux. *J Pediatr* 110:181-186, 1987.
97. Bailey DJ, Andres JM, Danek GD, et al: Lack of efficacy of thickened feeding as treatment for gastroesophageal reflux. *J Pediatr* 110:187-189, 1987.

98. Borrelli O, Salvia G, Campanozzi A, et al: Use of a new thickened formula for treatment of symptomatic gastrooesophageal reflux in infants. *Ital J Gastroenterol Hepatol* 29:237-242, 1997.
99. Meyers WF, Herbst JJ: Effectiveness of positioning therapy for gastroesophageal reflux. *Pediatrics* 69:768-772, 1982.
100. Vandenplas Y, Sacre-Smits L: Seventeen-hour continuous esophageal pH monitoring in the newborn: Evaluation of the influence of position in asymptomatic and symptomatic babies. *J Pediatr Gastroenterol Nutr* 4:356-361, 1985.
101. Orenstein SR, Whitington PF, Orenstein DM: The infant seat as treatment for gastroesophageal reflux. *N Engl J Med* 309:760-763, 1983.
102. Tobin JM, McCloud P, Cameron DJ: Posture and gastro-oesophageal reflux: A case for left lateral positioning. *Arch Dis Child* 76:254-258, 1997.
103. Oyen N, Markestad T, Skaerven R, et al: Combined effects of sleeping position and prenatal risk factors in sudden infant death syndrome: The Nordic Epidemiological SIDS Study. *Pediatrics* 100:613-621, 1997.
104. Mitchell EA, Thach BT, Thompson JM, Williams S: Changing infants' sleep position increases risk of sudden infant death syndrome: New Zealand Cot Death Study. *Arch Pediatr Adolesc Med* 153:1136-1141, 1999.
105. Mitchell EA, Thompson JM, Ford RP, et al: Sheepskin bedding and the sudden infant death syndrome. New Zealand Cot Death Study Group. *J Pediatr* 133:701-704, 1998.
106. Pehl C, Pfeiffer A, Wendl B, et al: The effect of decaffeination of coffee on gastro-oesophageal reflux in patients with reflux disease. *Aliment Pharmacol Ther* 11:483-486, 1997.
107. Murphy DW, Castell DO: Chocolate and heartburn: Evidence of increased esophageal acid exposure after chocolate ingestion. *Am J Gastroenterol* 83:633-636, 1988.
108. Vitale GC, Cheadle WG, Patel B, et al: The effect of alcohol on nocturnal gastroesophageal reflux. *JAMA* 258:2077-2079, 1987.
109. Alaswad B, Toubas PL, Grunow JE: Environmental tobacco smoke exposure and gastroesophageal reflux in infants with apparent life-threatening events. *J Okla State Med Assoc* 89:233- 237, 1996.
110. Ramirez B, Richter JE: Review article: Promotility drugs in the treatment of gastro-oesophageal reflux disease. *Aliment Pharmacol Ther* 7:5-20, 1993.
111. Cucchiara S, Staiano A, Romaniello G, et al: Antacids and cimetidine treatment for gastro-oesophageal reflux and peptic oesophagitis. *Arch Dis Child* 59:842-847, 1984.
112. Sedman A: Aluminum toxicity in childhood. *Pediatr Nephrol* 6:383-393, 1992.
113. Simeone D, Caria MC, Miele E, et al: Treatment of childhood peptic esophagitis: A double-blind placebo-controlled trial of nizatidine. *J Pediatr Gastroenterol Nutr* 25:51-55, 1997.

114. Peghini PL, Katz PO, Castell DO: Ranitidine controls nocturnal gastric acid breakthrough on omeprazole: A controlled study in normal subjects. *Gastroenterology* 115:1335-1339, 1998.
115. Wolfe MM, Sachs G: Acid suppression: Optimizing therapy for gastroduodenal ulcer healing, gastroesophageal reflux disease, and stress-related erosive syndrome. *Gastroenterology* 118:S9-S31, 2000.
116. Klinkenberg-Knol EC, Jansen JM, Festen HP, et al: Double-blind multicentre comparison of omeprazole and ranitidine in the treatment of reflux oesophagitis. *Lancet* 1:349-351, 1987.
117. Vigneri S, Termini R, Leandro G, et al: A comparison of five maintenance therapies for reflux esophagitis [see comments]. *N Engl J Med* 333:1106-1110, 1995.
118. De Giacomo C, Bawa P, Franceschi M, et al: Omeprazole for severe reflux esophagitis in children. *J Pediatr Gastroenterol Nutr* 24:528-532, 1997.
119. Alliet P, Raes M, Bruneel E, et al: Omeprazole in infants with cimetidine-resistant peptic esophagitis. *J Pediatr* 132:352-354, 1998.
120. Gunasekaran TS, Hassall EG: Efficacy and safety of omeprazole for severe gastroesophageal reflux in children [see comments]. *J Pediatr* 123:148-154, 1993.
121. Levi P, Marmo F, Saluzzo C, et al: Bethanechol versus antacids in the treatment of gastroesophageal reflux. *Helv Paediatr Acta* 40:349-359, 1985.
122. Leung C, Lai W: Use of metoclopramide for the treatment of gastroesophageal reflux in infants and children. *Curr Ther Res* 36:911-915, 1984.
123. Machida HM, Forbes DA, Gall DG, et al: Metoclopramide in gastroesophageal reflux of infancy. *J Pediatr* 112:483-487, 1988.
124. Putnam PE, Orenstein SR, Wessel HB, et al: Tardive dyskinesia associated with use of metoclopramide in a child. *J Pediatr* 121:983-985, 1992.
125. Van Eygen M, Van Ravensteyn H: Effect of cisapride on excessive regurgitation in infants. *Clin Ther* 11:669-677, 1989.
126. Cohen RC, O'Loughlin EV, Davidson GP, et al: Cisapride in the control of symptoms in infants with gastroesophageal reflux: A randomized, double-blind, placebo-controlled trial [see comments]. *J Pediatr* 134:287-292, 1999.
127. Cucchiara S, Staiano A, Boccieri A, et al: Effects of cisapride on parameters of oesophageal motility and on the prolonged intraoesophageal pH test in infants with gastro-oesophageal reflux disease. *Gut* 31:21-25, 1990.
128. Vandenplas Y, de Roy C, Sacre L: Cisapride decreases prolonged episodes of reflux in infants. *J Pediatr Gastroenterol Nutr* 12:44-47, 1991.
129. Dalla Vecchia LK, Grosfeld JL, West KW, et al: Reoperation after Nissen fundoplication in children with gastroesophageal reflux: Experience with 130 patients. *Ann Surg* 226:315-323, 1997.

130. Randolph J: Experience with the Nissen fundoplication for correction of gastroesophageal reflux in infants. *Ann Surg* 198:579-584, 1983.
131. Blane CE, Turnage RH, Oldham KT, et al: Long-term radiographic follow-up of the Nissen fundoplication in children. *Pediatr Radiol* 19:523-526, 1989.
132. Caniano DA, Ginn-Pease ME, King DR: The failed antireflux procedure: Analysis of risk factors and morbidity. *J Pediatr Surg* 25:1022-1026, 1990.
133. Fonkalsrud EW, Ashcraft KW, Coran AG, et al: Surgical treatment of gastroesophageal reflux in children: A combined hospital study of 7467 patients [see comments]. *Pediatrics* 101:419-422, 1998.
134. Jolley SG, Tunell WP, Leonard JC, et al: Gastric emptying in children with gastroesophageal reflux: II. The relationship to retching symptoms following antireflux surgery. *J Pediatr Surg* 22:927-930, 1987.
135. Borowitz SM, Borowitz KC: Oral dysfunction following Nissen fundoplication. *Dysphagia* 7:234-237, 1992.
136. Pearl RH, Robie DK, Ein SH, et al: Complications of gastroesophageal antireflux surgery in neurologically impaired versus neurologically normal children. *J Pediatr Surg* 25:1169-1173, 1990.
137. Ceriati E, Guarino N, Zaccara A, et al: Gastroesophageal reflux in neurologically impaired children: Partial or total fundoplication? *Langenbecks Arch Surg* 383:317- 319, 1998.
138. Rothenberg SS: Experience with 220 consecutive laparoscopic Nissen fundoplications in infants and children. *J Pediatr Surg* 33:274-278, 1998.

CHAPTER 11

Fatal Child Neglect

Carol D. Berkowitz, MD
Professor of Clinical Pediatrics, University of California Los Angeles School of Medicine; Executive Vice Chair, Department of Pediatrics, Harbor-University of California Los Angeles Medical Center, Torrance, Calif

ABSTRACT
Child neglect results from either acts of omission or of commission. Fatalities from neglect account for 30% to 40% of deaths caused by child maltreatment. Deaths may occur from failure to provide the basic needs of infancy such as food or medical care. Medical care may also be withheld because of parental religious beliefs. Inadequate supervision may contribute to a child's injury or death through adverse events involving drowning, fires, and firearms. Recognizing the factors contributing to a child's death is facilitated by the action of multidisciplinary child death review teams. As with other forms of child maltreatment, prevention and early intervention strategies are needed to minimize the risk of injury and death to children.

The issue of child homicide conjures up images of bruised, battered, and assaulted children. Yet at least one third of child maltreatment fatalities are a consequence of neglect, a determination that may be difficult to make, even after autopsy.[1,2] Child neglect is diagnosed when care required to meet the basic needs of children is omitted. Such needs include food, shelter, clothing, health care including dental care, and education.[3] Insufficient supervision is often responsible for a child's death or serious injury, although sometimes these cases are misclassified as accidental or undetermined. The omission of love and nurturing, also important human needs, is the most difficult to document, yet may have fatal consequences, as when an unloved child commits suicide. Neglect is usually recognized when an adverse event occurs or when the child's physical condition reflects some problems such as malnutrition, rampant dental caries, or poor hygiene.[4]

Like other forms of child maltreatment, child neglect has a legal definition that involves the neglect of a child (failure to provide the basic needs) or the exposure of the child to a harmful situation (potential or actual) by an individual responsible (custody, charge, or care) for that child.[3] Yet even the legal definition varies from state to state, and sometimes between different counties within the state.[5]

Other conditions are related to neglect. Failure to thrive, although sometimes diagnosed in a neglected child, is a separate condition from neglect.[6] In its narrowest definition, failure to thrive involves growth impairment without an organic basis. A more expansive definition includes impaired interactional and developmental skills in a child who has received inadequate nurturing. Child endangerment, related to neglect, occurs when the actions of the caretaker, either acts of omission or commission, place the child in a precarious position.[3,7] Child abandonment, another related condition, is differentiated into a number of categories.[3] The most "benign" category occurs when parents leave their children in the care of another for a defined period but then fail to reappear. Inadequate parental supervision can be deemed abandonment. The consequence of such inadequate supervision may be harm, injury, or even death to the child. Emotional abandonment is particularly difficult to quantify or document but is a factor in the lives of teens who, although disparagingly called runaways, are more appropriately termed throwaways, having been rejected or abandoned by their families. At its worst, abandonment has fatal or near-fatal consequences.[3]

EPIDEMIOLOGY

Data from the National Incidence Surveillance for 1996 reported 949,001 cases of neglect. Educational neglect (chronic truancy, failure to enroll, failure to provide remedial services) accounted for 397,300 cases, physical neglect accounted for 338,901 cases, and emotional neglect accounted for 212,800 cases.[8] Because these figures are based on a surveillance mechanism, where suspected cases are noted, the figures do not reflect actual reported cases or cases substantiated in a court of law.

Figures from the National Committee to Prevent Child Abuse (NCPCA) note approximately 1 million children ("confirmed or indicated") as victims of abuse or neglect. More than half the children (55%) were neglected: general neglect 52%, medical neglect 3%. An additional 14% had been abandoned.[9]

Approximately 2000 children die each year as a result of child maltreatment.[2] Many of these cases are dramatic and receive much in the way of media publicity. On the other hand, deaths as a result of neglect may go unrecognized, mistakenly ruled accidental.[10] Neglectful deaths may also go unreported as such, in part because standards of neglect vary from community to community, and sometimes parental culpability is defined only when legislation is enacted, such as responsibility for loaded firearms or unprotected swimming pools.[11] The investigation by multidisciplinary child fatality review boards has assisted in the evaluation of the death of children when the circumstances surrounding the death are less than straightforward.[12]

FATAL CHILD NEGLECT

MODE OF DEATH

There are many circumstances in which the neglectful actions of caregivers may contribute to a child's death. Assessing the degree that caregiver actions contributed to the child's death often involves input from a number of disciplines.[13] One of the key investigators is the medical examiner who may perform an autopsy and do a death scene investigation.[14]

The purpose of an autopsy is to determine both a cause and a mode or manner of death. The cause of death is the condition that led to the individual's demise. Massive head injury, overwhelming sepsis, multiple gunshot wounds, or disseminated carcinoma are causes of death. The mode of death relates to the mechanism behind the cause and is the official category that is assigned for the death certificate. The mode of death may be natural (a child with leukemia dies from disseminated candidemia); accidental (a child dies from massive head injury sustained in a motor vehicle collision); suicide (a child dies from a self-inflicted gunshot wound); homicide (a child dies from gunshot wounds sustained during a drive-by shooting); or undetermined. The mode of death may be considered undetermined if there are conflicting factors that preclude assigning the death to any other category. For instance, a 4-month-old girl is found in full cardiac arrest after being placed in her crib. The autopsy does not reveal a cause of death. Thymic petechiae are present, consistent with a diagnosis of sudden infant death syndrome (SIDS). However, there are 2 old rib fractures (estimated age, 2-4 weeks) and a subdural neomembrane. Although these findings cannot account for the infant's death, their presence precludes the death from being ruled natural.

Homicide is death at the hands of another. The coroner makes no assessment as to the intent of the responsible individual. It is usually the district attorney who will determine whether a charge of murder is appropriate. Murder includes the notion of malice aforethought. Other possibilities include manslaughter both voluntary (in the heat of passion or in self-defense) and involuntary.

INFANT ABANDONMENT

CASE 1

A dead abandoned newborn infant was found in a temporary waste dumpster as the trash was being loaded onto a garbage truck. The placenta and umbilical cord were found attached to the body of the infant, but the head was decapitated and had been crushed. The assessment was that the decapitation was a postmortem event. The death was ruled a homicide. However, the mother was never located, and no charges were filed.

CASE 2

A 19-year-old unmarried college student, accompanied by her mother, presented to the emergency department complaining of heavy vaginal bleeding after having collapsed at home. She initially denied being pregnant, but after being medically stabilized and reinterviewed she disclosed that she had delivered an infant at home and placed the infant in a trash can. Law enforcement was dispensed to the scene where they found the infant along with soiled clothing and rags.

At autopsy, the infant, a boy, weighed 2570 g and had an estimated gestational age of 37 to 38 weeks. There were no congenital anomalies or defects. A wad of tissue was found in the infant's mouth, and there was a 1 × ⅛-inch bruise on the infant's neck that extended down to the deep muscle layers involving the sternocleidomastoid and sternohyoid muscles. The lungs floated when placed in water, and there was microscopic evidence of aeration. In contrast, the liver did not float, evidence that the aeration of the lungs was not a postmortem event.

A determination was made that the infant would have lived had he received appropriate basic care after his birth. The death was ruled a homicide, and the 19-year-old mother was tried for murder. She was found guilty of involuntary manslaughter and sentenced to 4 years in state prison.

Infant abandonment has been practiced throughout the world as a means of gender and population control. Sometimes economic hardship is the motivating force. At other times, shame associated with out-of-wedlock birth is the key factor. In its most benign form, the mother fantasizes that another family will find and care for the infant. Such practices were not uncommon in mid 19th century Japan, brought on by economic difficulties after the rapid industrial modernization of the country.[15] Infants were left at temples or shrines, or even sold to other families. In the 1970s, Japan experienced a resurgence of this phenomenon, a problem that became referred to as "coin-operated locker babies." Dead infants were discovered in lockers located in railroad stations. Most were boys and because they had been in the lockers for several months before they were discovered, locating their mothers was virtually impossible.

Infant abandonment also occurs in the United States. The actual figures related to infant abandonment outside the hospital setting are difficult to obtain. With information gathered from newspaper articles, the Department of Health and Human Services reported that 1005 infants were abandoned in 1998, and 33 of the infants were found dead.[16] These mothers are often adolescents or young adults who had become pregnant out of wedlock. The pregnancy is not only hidden from the family, but the mother may be in such strong denial that she does not even acknowledge the pregnancy to herself. Most often the baby is born, unattended, at home, sometimes delivered precipitously into the toilet bowl because the mother mistakes her labor pains as a need to defecate. If the infant cries, there may be efforts to quiet the infant by stuffing paper or a towel in the infant's mouth. Frequently, the infant is wrapped in a towel and placed in a trash bag along with other evidence of the birth, including the placenta.

Many issues are related to cases of fatal infant abandonment. These include the assessment by the coroner as to the viability of the infant, and whether the death was related to acts of omission, acts of commission, or both. Can the parents (particularly the mother) be located? If the mother is known, what action should be taken against her? What factors influence the latter decision? For instance, if the mother has previous infants, does that make it less likely that she would "fail" to recognize her pregnancy? What can be done on a societal level to prevent infant abandonment?

One challenge for the coroner in the assessment of these infants is to determine whether the baby was born alive and was potentially viable. Although the presence of pulmonary aeration suggests that the infant breathed after birth, decomposition of tissues can produce air in the lungs as well as in other organs. A preterm infant born at home may be deemed nonviable. The presence of injuries to the baby, or evidence that the baby's airway was occluded supports the fact that acts of commission contributed to the baby's death. Acts of commission suggest "malice aforethought" and the potential for a charge of murder.

What are the appropriate charges to bring against a young mother whose newborn infant dies after being abandoned?[17] The answer to this question is not easy. Certainly there is stronger sentiment against the older mother or one who has a prior pregnancy that she should have been aware of alternative actions to manage her pregnancy. Community resources are a consideration. Are there programs for unwed mothers?

In recent years, interest has arisen about legislation that would allow a mother to leave her infant in a designated place (usually a hospital, or with law enforcement or social service agencies), no questions asked, and for her not to be prosecuted for infant abandonment. Some states refer to this as an amnesty program. Legislation usually provides an upper limit on the age of the infant, often 30 days. Some counties in the United States have enacted similar measures without formal legislation. It is unclear whether such programs have an impact on fatal infant abandonment. Texas, in the first months after enactment of the legislation, failed to find any change in the number of abandoned infants.[16] Obviously, publicizing the program is important. Opponents to such legislation criticize the plan for facilitating teens to engage in sexual activities without accepting the consequences and responsibilities of their actions.

DEATH FROM STARVATION

Case 1

A 14-year-old girl with muscular disease died. At autopsy, her weight was 44 lb, the weight of an average 6-year-old child. The case had been referred to the Department of Children and Family Services on several occasions, but the accusations were never sustained because medical evidence was provided that the girl had a medical condition that led to her malnutrition. The parents were convicted of involuntary manslaughter, felony child abuse, and conspiracy to commit child abuse.

Case 2

A 6-week-old male infant was brought by paramedics to the emergency department in full cardiac arrest. His temperature was 90°F, and his blood glucose was 16 mg/dL. He had been born after a full-term pregnancy to a 34-year-old, 220 lb, 5 ft 7 inch, Gravida 10, Para 7, Ab 2 mother. His measurements at birth were as follows: weight, 1975 g (small for gestational age); length, 44½ cm; and head circumference, 28½ cm. Apgar scores were 8 at 1 minute and 9 at 5 minutes. The infant was noted to be jittery at birth, to have increased muscle tone, and to nipple poorly. Illicit drug exposure was suspected, but a drug screen was negative. The infant was discharged home with his mother.

He was taken for an acute care visit at 1 month of age because of congestion, but care was not provided because the infant was not enrolled in the medical plan. At the time of his death, the infant weighed 1770 g (205 g below his birth weight), measured 46 cm, and had a head circumference of 31 cm (Fig 1). His weight should have been 3235 g if weight gain had progressed normally. Autopsy revealed only 0.1 cm of subcutaneous tissue.

Case 3

An infant was born to a 14½-year-old mother who resided with her 33-year-old mother, the infant's maternal grandmother. Birth weight was 3655 g, and length was 49.5 cm. The infant was seen in a private physician's office at 15 days of age. The weight at that time was 3300 g, 10% below birth weight. The infant was diagnosed with thrush and failure to thrive, which was attributed to the thrush. They were advised to return in 72 hours.

The infant was next seen at 22 days (1 week later). His weight was still 3300 g. He was said to be eating 3 oz every 3 hours. Thrush was noted to be improving. They were told to return in 2 weeks.

The infant was brought into the emergency department at 40 days of age in full cardiopulmonary arrest. His weight was 2950 g (Fig 2). The autopsy revealed severe emaciation and a healing injury to the labial frenulum.

Death from starvation usually involves infants younger than 1 year but can occur in older, chronically ill or neurodevelopmentally disabled children. Even when children are receiving medical care and intervention, their care may be episodic or their parents may not be compliant with medical recommendations. Some of these children receive a diagnosis of failure to thrive that is attributed to an underlying medical condition, and felt to be nonremedial.

Failure to thrive is a separate clinical diagnosis made in a *living* child who is not growing or gaining weight in an appropriate manner.[6] If a child dies as a result of "failure to thrive," the pathologic findings relate to the presence of severe malnutrition. The cachectic appearance of the child may be readily apparent (Fig 3). Findings related to malnutrition include greatly diminished subcutaneous tissue and a lack of Bichat's fat-pad normally present in the buccal area (Box 1). There may be fatty infiltration of the liver. There is often atrophy of the thymus gland as well as of the muscles and other organs. Edema may develop from hypoproteinemia. There

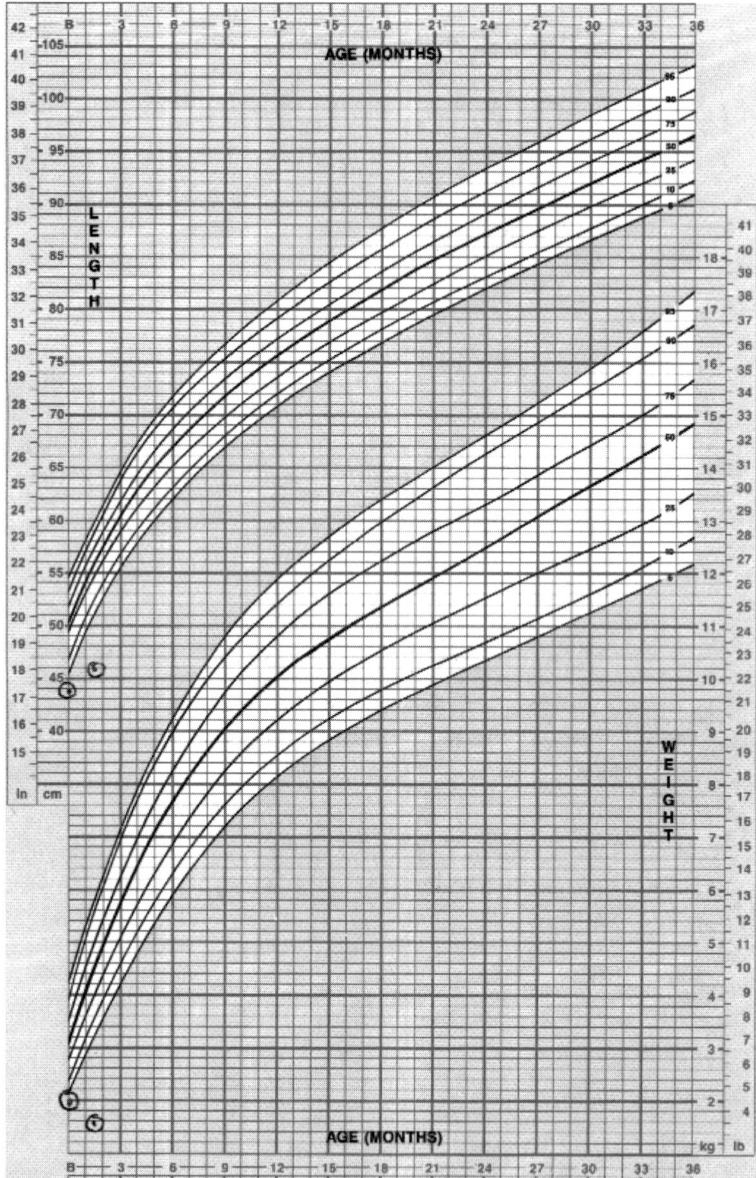

FIGURE 1.

Case 2: Death from starvation. Growth curve showing continued linear growth but loss of weight. (Adapted from National Center for Health Statistics: *NCHS Growth Charts, 1976. Monthly Vital Statistics Report*, vol 25, No 3, suppl [HRA] 76-1120, Health Resources Administration, Rockville, Md, June 1976. Data from the National Center for Health Statistics.)

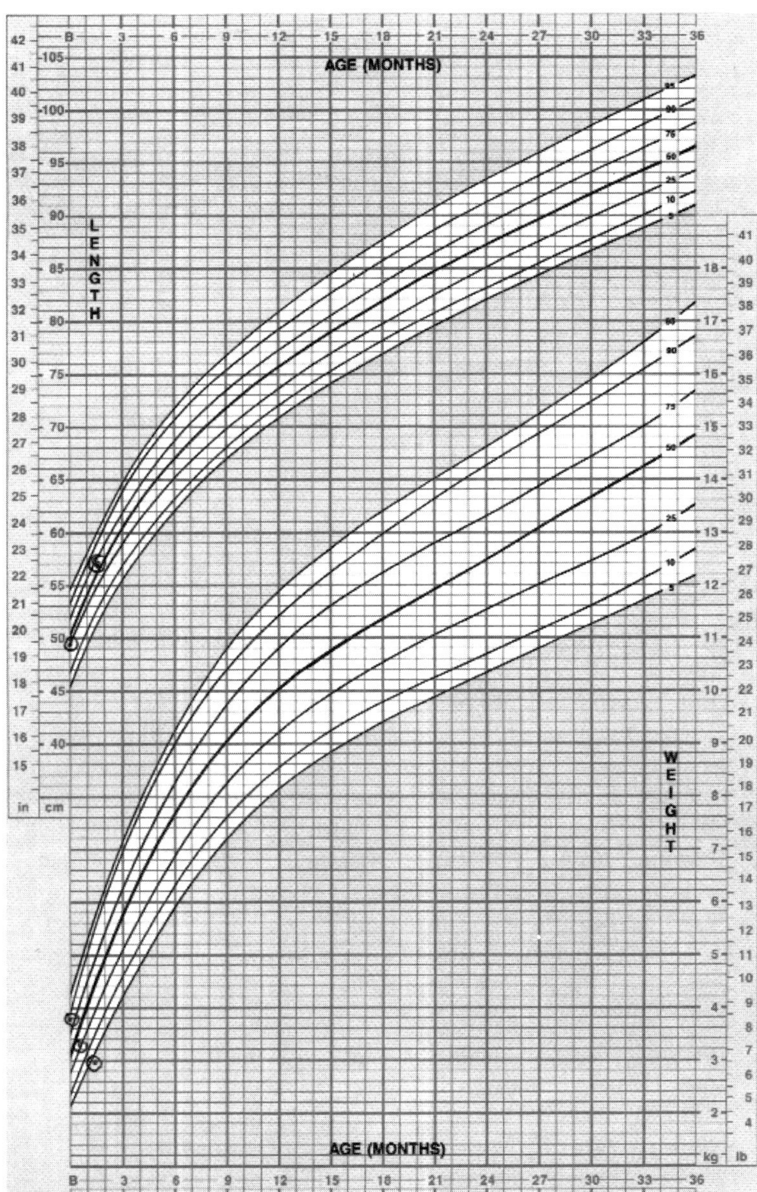

FIGURE 2.
Case 3: Death from starvation. Growth curve showing continued linear growth but loss of weight. (Adapted from National Center for Health Statistics: *NCHS Growth Charts, 1976. Monthly Vital Statistics Report*, vol 25, No 3, suppl [HRA] 76-1120, Health Resources Administration, Rockville, Md, June 1976. Data from the National Center for Health Statistics.)

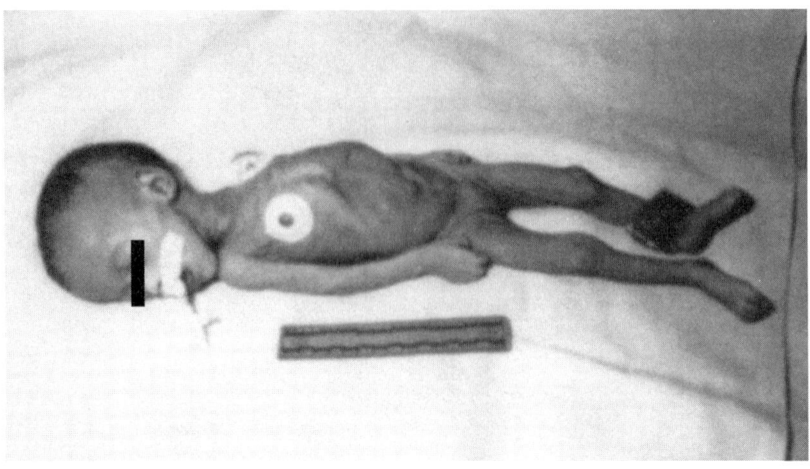

FIGURE 3.
Baby died of starvation. Note severe cachectic appearance.

may be ulcerations or swelling of the intestinal lining. Perforated duodenal (stress) ulcers may also be noted. Absence of any food in the stomach supports the conclusion that the infant was starved.[18-20] Sometimes there are oral injuries, evidence of an attempt at forced feedings. Electrolyte disturbances are difficult to determine in postmortem serum specimens, although examination of the vitreous may reveal elevated sodium, chloride, and blood urea nitrogen (BUN) levels as evidence of dehydrating events before death. Often there are no findings other than severe inanition.

When assessing whether a death may be attributable to starvation, reviewing as many previous weights and lengths as are available is helpful. In the face of malnutrition, linear growth continues for a while after weight gain has ceased. Linear growth may continue even when the infant is losing weight. Estimating the duration of starvation can be accomplished by knowing the infant's previous growth parameters and understanding the normal rate of weight gain for an infant that age. Meade and Brissie[21] demonstrate this methodology by computing the expected weight (based on prior measurements), subtracting the actual weight, and assessing the degree of dehydration (by estimating or using vitreal electrolytes). Caloric deficit can be calculated, or one can use expected daily weight gain to determine the number of days without adequate nutrition. This information is often key during judicial determinations about starvation-related deaths in young infants.

Another factor to examine when assessing the circumstances surrounding the death of a child from starvation is the home environment (Fig 4). Some environments are overtly filthy. There are piles of unwashed dishes, human and animal excrement, and hazards such as broken glass and exposed electrical wires.[7,20] Other environments may hold more subtle clues to their neglectful components, such as the absence of infant formula or other necessities such as diapers or clothing.

The exact mechanism of death as related to starvation is unclear. Bronchopneumonia is a common nonspecific finding that does not represent the actual cause of death. Although reduced resistance to infection is usually cited, cultures taken at the time of autopsy are frequently unrevealing and yield multiple organisms, consistent with postmortem tissue breakdown.

Who shoulders the responsibility for the death of a child from starvation when there have been visits to a physician or in-home visitation? What happens when a parent tries to access care for a child but is turned away because of the lack of medical insurance? How can such interactions be substantiated if the encounter is never recorded, but the parent maintains that medical care was sought? All infants and children must be guaranteed access to medical care. Growth parameters must be obtained at each health care encounter, and measurements must be plotted on age- and gender-appropriate curves. Interventional strategies including home assessment need to be implemented for children who are not growing at their expected rate. Home visitation is incomplete, however, if an infant is not completely undressed.

BOX 1.

Pathologic Findings Associated With Death From Starvation

- Paucity of subcutaneous tissue
- Absent Bichat's fat pad
- Hepatic steatosis
- Thymic atrophy
- Skeletal muscle atrophy
- Intestinal ulceration
- Swelling of intestinal lining
- Absence of food in stomach
- Elevated sodium, chloride, blood urea nitrogen in vitreous

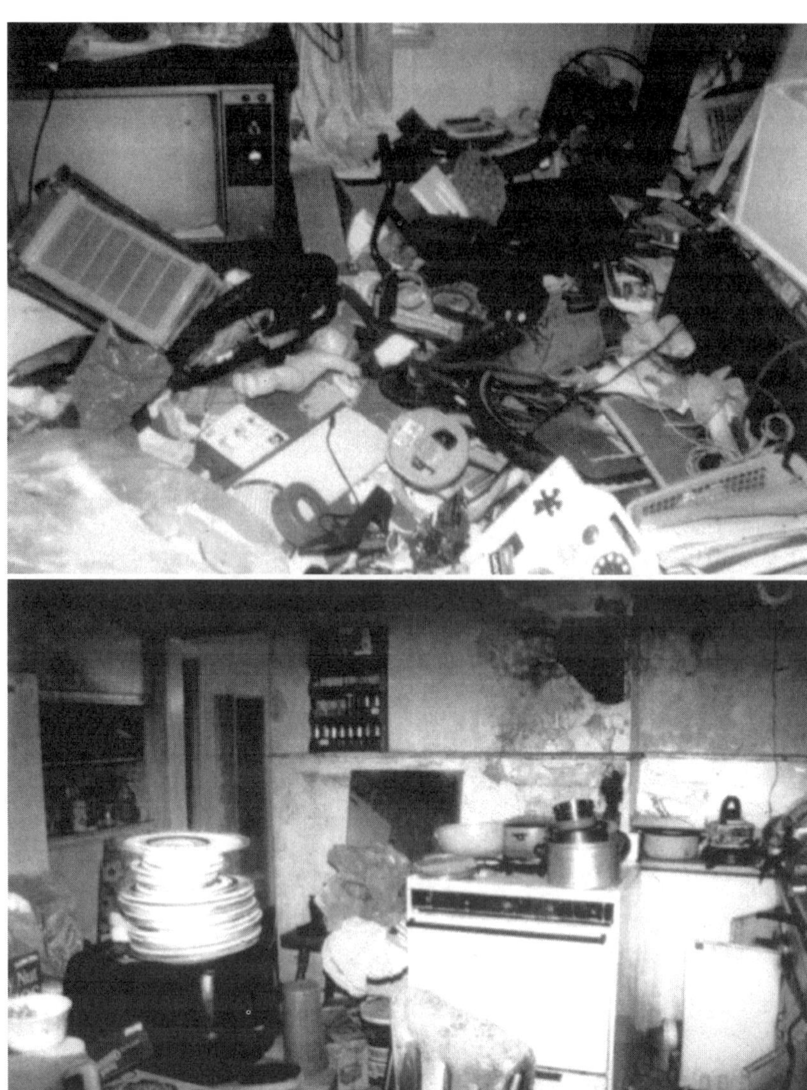

FIGURE 4.
Cluttered, dirty, unkempt home environment of infant in Figure 3.

An infant wrapped in a sleeper and blankets may appear healthy and fat.[4,22]

Home visitation is particularly helpful for developmentally disabled adults who are caring for their own offspring. Some developmentally disabled adults are very concrete in their thinking. If they are told to feed their infant every 3 hours, they may not have the flexibility to alter the schedule if the infant is sleeping at the feeding time, or if the infant wants to eat sooner. Careful assessment of the growth of infants of developmentally disabled adults is critical for the success of this dyad. Additionally, parenting programs geared for individuals with limited skills should be implemented.[23,24]

Starvation may also lead to death in older children, especially those with neurodevelopmental disabilities. Caring for such children may drain a family's energies and resources. A simple feeding interaction may require an extended period. Children who are receiving medications including anticonvulsants may be drowsy and disinterested in feeding. Calorie-dense foods as well as the use of nasogastric tubes, or gastrostomies, may significantly improve the child's nutrition. Unfortunately, some well-meaning parents resist the use of gastrostomy tubes. They view oral feeding as a sign (perhaps the only one) of their child's normalcy. A neurodevelopmentally disabled child who dies of malnutrition, and who has not benefited from a program of augmented nutrition, has been a victim of medical neglect on the part of the parent or the medical practitioners caring for the child.

DEATH RELATED TO MEDICAL NEGLECT

Case 1

A 6-month-old Hispanic infant had been smuggled across the border along with his 3-year-old brother. He did well for 2 days but then developed fever, cough, and diarrhea. He was treated with acetaminophen and initially improved, but 3 days later he experienced shortness of breath and increasing temperature. At 6 AM on Sunday he was taken to a "Clinica." A physician did not arrive until 10:20 AM. The family was advised the Clinica could not care for the infant and was referred to a local hospital. The infant experienced a cardiorespiratory arrest *en route*. At the hospital, the temperature was 103.2°R, and the infant could not be resuscitated.

Case 2

A 2-year old child aspirated a piece of banana. His parents were present, and they summoned members of their religious group who engaged in prayer for about an hour. The child died of asphyxia.[25]

There are various forms of medical neglect.[7] Sometimes medical care is delayed, and the effect on the child is minimal. Other times the outcome is fatal, as in case 1. Delay may result from various factors including parental and societal ones. Parents may fail to recognize the significance or seriousness of their child's injury or illness. When a child has been injured, delays in accessing medical care may raise concern that the injuries have been inflicted. Parents may also delay care because of inadequate access, either perceived or real. They may be concerned about the cost of care, or notification of the authorities about one's status as an immigrant.[26]

Medical care may be received in a sporadic manner. A child may miss multiple appointments only to return to the emergency department in severe distress, often with intractable asthma or diabetic ketoacidosis. The medical community is responsible for monitoring compliance with appointments as well as adherence to medical recommendations.

However, it is not appropriate to assume that parents must follow all medical recommendations blindly and without question. Although failure to follow medical directions may contribute to an adverse outcome, the precise causality between the noncompliance and the outcome may be unproven. For instance, an infant is discharged from the neonatal intensive care unit on an apnea monitor, which is discontinued by the mother who claims that after 2 months, the only time the monitor sounded was for false alarms. The baby subsequently dies of SIDS. Is that mother responsible for her infant's death?[27] What if a mother has failed to follow her pediatrician's advice to place the infant in a supine position, and her infant dies of SIDS? Does this constitute medical neglect, and is the mother responsible for the child's death? What if the physician never advised the mother to place the infant on his back for sleep?[28] Is the physician responsible? What about cosleeping? There are some studies that suggest a higher incidence of SIDS in families where infants sleep with their parents. What about cosleeping with an inebriated parent, or one under the influence of drugs? There is an increased risk of rolling over and suffocating an infant when a parent is inebriated.[11]

The answers to these questions are not easy or straightforward. How compliant with physician recommendations should parents be? Most laws require that a parent acts as a "reasonable" or "prudent" caregiver.[7,19] How important is the medical evidence that the recommendations really do make a difference? For instance, what is the evidence that apnea monitors prevent death from SIDS?

The strength of the scientific evidence supporting a medical intervention is critical when evaluating decisions of parents to withhold medical care on religious grounds. The United States

Constitution guarantees freedom of religion. Under this protection, an individual can choose to follow certain practices, including those involved with personal health care decisions. The decision to impose those beliefs on another, particularly a dependent child when the life of the child is in danger, is more controversial.[29,30] Many instances have occurred when the court has intervened on behalf of a child, such as with the administration of blood to a hemorrhaging child of Jehovah's Witnesses. However, the laws surrounding religious exemptions from adjudicating a parent as negligent are complicated and involve issues as diverse as immunizations and cancer therapy. Asser and Swan[25] reviewed 172 children who had died between 1975 and 1995 where the death was believed to be related to "religion-motivated medical neglect." They concluded that for 140 children, medical intervention would have resulted in survival rates of more than 90%. Survival rates would have reached 50% for an additional 18 children. Conditions affecting children included food aspiration, bacterial meningitis, acute appendicitis, intussusception, diabetes, leukemia, solid tumors, and congenital heart disease. Interestingly, 59 perinatal deaths were related to religion-motivated medical neglect. The report notes 23 different denominations from 34 different states, linked together in the belief that prayer alone was sufficient to treat children's medical problems. Obviously, scientific evidence would not support such a conclusion.

The use of nontraditional medicine, including that of non-Western origin, may affect a child's health care in several ways. Certain practices such as coining, cupping, spooning, and cao gai do not harm a child but, because they may be mistaken for inflicted trauma, may disrupt the integrity of a family reported for physical abuse.[31] The right of parents to utilize these modalities is sanctioned by most legal and medical communities as long as the medical needs of the child are also being attended to. A problem arises if appropriate, definitive medical care is delayed or omitted because of the practice of nontraditional medicine. For instance, oil rubbed on the sunken fontanelle of a Latino child by a curandero (healer) will not restore the vascular volume of a dehydrated child.[32] Spinal manipulation by a chiropractor will not treat meningitis. Lastly, the treatment itself may prove harmful. A well-meaning grandmother, trying to relieve colicky symptoms, added baking soda to her grandchild's bottle, and the 6-week-old infant died of hypernatremic alkalosis. Culturally aware and sensitive medical care should be available to all children. Such care demands that all physicians receive adequate training in this area, and be prepared to care for children from the diverse cultural and ethnic backgrounds that make up the population of the United States.[24,33]

CHILD FATALITIES RELATED TO INADEQUATE SUPERVISION

Parents have an obligation to ensure the safety and well-being of their children through adequate supervision, either by themselves or suitably designated caregivers such as baby-sitters. Parents must act in a prudent and reasonable manner, recognizing that adverse events may happen with even the most vigilant parents.[7,19]

CHILD FATALITIES THROUGH DROWNING

CASE 1

A 3-year-old boy was picked up from day care by his biologic father at 4:00 PM during January in southern California. They arrived home at 4:05 PM. The father went to fold some laundry, then noticed his son was missing, and found him floating in the backyard pool at 4:40 PM. Cardiopulmonary resuscitation (CPR) was initiated and paramedics were summoned. The child was taken to the emergency department where his temperature on arrival was 86°F and his pH was 6.18. He could not be resuscitated. The autopsy findings were consistent with drowning.

CASE 2

A 2½-year-old boy was pulled from a backyard Jacuzzi. Allegedly his mother and her boyfriend had been watching television for about 10 minutes when they noticed him missing. CPR was initiated, but he could not be resuscitated. The autopsy revealed a few petechiae on the thymus and a red-purple contusion on the knee, findings that were felt to be consistent with a drowning. The death was ruled accidental.

CASE 3

An 11-month-old boy drowned while taking a bath with his 2-year-old sibling. The story the mother provided the police changed with 3 different interviewers, but this may have reflected language differences. In the final version, both boys were being bathed in a tub that was one-third to one-half filled with water plus toys. The mother left the room briefly (1 minute by her report) to get soap and lower the volume on the stereo set. When she returned, she found the 11-month-old boy submerged and blue/purple. She pulled the infant from the tub, pushed on his chest, water came out of his mouth, but he was still blue. Her sister called 911. Paramedics arrived on the scene within 10 minutes. Water was draining from the infant's mouth. The infant was in full cardiorespiratory arrest, and despite advanced pediatric life support measures, could not be resuscitated. An autopsy showed scattered petechiae on the visceral pleura and petechial hemorrhages on the thymus.

Drowning ranks as the second leading cause of accidental death in childhood after motor vehicle and auto-pedestrian collisions.[34] The incidence and epidemiology of drowning varies with geographic location. For instance, the swimming pool as the location of drowning was reported in 89% of Los Angeles fatal submersions, but in only 59% of Seattle drownings.[35] In Oregon, in 1998, 16 children younger than 17 years drowned. Eleven of the submersions occurred in rivers and lakes when strong currents and cold water contributed to the deaths.[11]

Although this report focuses on neglect, it is important to recognize that there are 3 potential questions to be answered when assessing a drowning: was the drowning intentional or nonintentional, and if nonintentional, was parental supervision inadequate (ie, did neglect play a role)? Studies to help differentiate intentional from nonintentional drowning have focused on the circumstances surrounding drowning.[36] Some authors have noted that up to two thirds of bathtub drowning are either abuse or neglect.[37] Other factors suggestive of intentional drowning are bucket and toilet drowning; unusual time of day for bathing; "child abuser" profile of caregiver; prior history of domestic violence; and older infant (15-30 months) as opposed to a younger infant (9-15 months). The presence of an older sibling in the tub (case 3 above) was a negative correlate to intentional drowning.[38]

Although drowning in a bathtub may be intentional, accidental bathtub drowning does occur. Margolin[39] reported that 4 of 11 infants who drowned in a bathtub had been left unattended for what parents perceived was a brief period. Parental distraction by another child, or parents leaving the room to get soap, shampoo, or a towel, or to answer the phone or doorbell, may have fatal consequences. In that instant, the infant slips below the water. The parent returns to find a cyanotic, apneic baby who has sustained significant asphyxia, with subsequent irreversible brain damage or death. Although it is unclear exactly how long an infant must be submerged in warm bathtub water before brain damage occurs, studies suggest that the amount of time may be brief, probably only several minutes. Schmidt and Madea[40] report that consciousness is lost after only 3 minutes because of cerebral hypoxia. Most caregivers underestimate the length of time they are absent from the room, believing only several seconds rather than several minutes have passed.

Bathtub drowning, which accounts for 10% of submersions, raises the issue of what is reasonable and prudent parental supervision.[41] Physicians and parents alike concur that children, especially infants, should never be left in a bathtub unsupervised. This is the standard of care.[40] Unfortunately, the standard that is practiced is often different. In informal surveys, many caregivers admit to having, on occasion, left young children unattended while they are bathing. Sometimes they are left with older preschool children who are incapable of providing necessary supervision.[41] Although it is reasonable not to prosecute a mother for a momentary lapse in supervision, it is incumbent on the medical community to ensure that the standard of care is advertised and promoted. Safe bathing should be incorporated into anticipatory guidance at all health maintenance visits. On the other hand, there are blatant cases where caregivers placed children in bathtubs as a means to amuse the children, and then went to sleep or became intoxicated, leaving the children totally unsupervised. Such cases mandate prosecution for neglect with a fatal outcome.

Pool drowning may occur because of neglect or inadequate supervision. Older children may be given the responsibility for supervising younger children in a pool, but the older children are engaged in their own play and do not notice when one of the younger children becomes submerged. Some children drown because they wander into the yard and fall into an unprotected pool when adult attention is diverted elsewhere. Often the adult does not realize the child has left the house. In some areas where many homes have pools, legislation has been enacted to mandate that residential pools be enclosed with what is referred to as "perimetry" fencing. Such fencing completely encircles the pool within the owner's property, reaches a minimum of 5 ft, has self-latching gates, and is entirely separate from fencing that may separate one's property from one's neighbor. The effectiveness of such fencing has not been fully studied.[42] Often legislation is enacted but covers only newly built pools. Other times the legislation is retroactive, but there are no agencies to enforce the law's implementation. Additional measures include placing alarm systems on any door leading to the pool area, so that a noise is heard when anyone exits the back of the house. Safeguarding children against drowning, as against all injuries, demands a combined effort of parents, physicians, the community, and legislators.[43]

CHILD FATALITIES IN HOME FIRES

CASE 1

Law enforcement and firefighters were summoned to an apartment fire because a 1-year-old infant was trapped inside. Officers attempted to crawl into the unit but were repelled back because of severe thick smoke and heat. Firefighters subsequently extinguished the flames and found the charred body of an infant lying face down in the bed. Her cranium had ruptured from the extreme heat. Autopsy findings confirmed death from thermal burns and smoke inhalation. Arson investigation revealed the infant's 5-year-old cousin had been playing with matches the day before. She had been reprimanded, but on the day of the fire she had located matches in her grandmother's purse and was "practicing" in anticipation of lighting candles on a birthday cake. The cousin admitted throwing a match on the bed on which the infant had been sleeping. The family had a prior referral to the Department of Children and Family Services for the mother's leaving the children unattended. No charges were filed in the case.

CASE 2

A couple who were baby-sitting their grandchildren were seated in the living room of a two-story house when they smelled smoke. When they went to check, they discovered that a second floor bedroom closest to the staircase, along with the area adjacent to the top of the staircase, was engulfed in flames. The intensity of the fire prevented their entering the bedroom where their 17-month-old granddaughter had been napping. Firefighters subsequently arrived, but the infant could not be resuscitated. An autopsy revealed that the infant had died of smoke inhalation. A 6-year-old cousin had started the fire. The child had learned to light matches the day before during a Fourth of July celebration. The house was not equipped with smoke detectors. When the case was discussed, community representatives revealed that the grandparent's house was in a poor community and that few of the families had smoke detectors in their own homes.

Childhood deaths from burns and fire have decreased, mainly as a result of environmental changes including the development of flame-retardant clothing, temperature–limiting devices on hot water heaters, and the installation of smoke detectors.[41,44] Children in poor urban areas continue to be at risk for fire-related deaths, although in 1999, in Los Angeles County, fires were 10th on the list of accidental child deaths below drowning, falls, and auto-pedestrian collisions.[45] In 1990, the Division of Injury Control reported burn and fire injuries as second only to drowning as a cause of accidental childhood fatalities (2.3 annual fatalities per 100,000).[46] In 1997, the Centers for Disease Control and Prevention (CDC) reported that approximately 15% of unintentional injuries and adverse events in children between 1 and 9 years of age were caused by fires and burns.[34] When children die in fires, parental neglect, poor supervision, or an unsafe environment are key contributing factors. In the 2 cases described above, young children were responsible for igniting fatal household fires.

A 10-year retrospective study of home fires in Scotland reported that household fires were the fifth leading cause of death in children aged 1 to 15 years.[47] In 30% of the cases, the individual responsible for the fire was an inadequately supervised child, and children younger than 5 years were at particular risk from fires started by other young children. Supervision by adults was often suboptimal because the adults were frequently legally intoxicated. For instance, when fires started as a result of cooking mishaps, 84% of the adults killed were intoxicated. In 7% of the cases, no adults were present, and the child had been left at home alone for several hours.

Death was a result of smoke inhalation in 75% of the children.[47] Such deaths are potentially preventable through the appropriate installation and maintenance of smoke detectors. Smoke detectors do not prevent fires, but lessen the risk of injury and death as a result of the fire. Carbon monoxide is one of the most lethal inhalants associated with a fire, producing rapid deterioration of physical and mental competency in an exposed individual. Because young children cannot escape a fire unassisted, they are dependent on a competent adult to assist them. In our second case, the absence of a smoke detector resulted in the death of a young infant. In most areas, landlords are required to install smoke detectors in rented dwellings. Such is not the case in privately owned residences. Additionally, poverty and lack of knowledge place some children at additional risk because their caregivers do not install or maintain smoke detectors. Some communities have provided smoke detectors free to all residents.[48] Having a smoke detector does not ensure its correct operation. Most require a change of batteries every 6 months, although newer units may be equipped with 10-year batteries. Other barriers, such as metal bars on windows to reduce the risk of burglaries, may also compromise a child's ability to escape a fire. Easy access to smoke detectors and the creation of escapable household units are community and societal challenges to reduce the risk of death from household fires. As with drowning, lessening the risk of injury and death from fires requires a combined effort.[49]

CHILD FATALITIES WHEN LEFT UNATTENDED IN CARS

CASE 1

A 5-month-old infant was found dead in a parked car. The story offered by the mother was that she had visited her boyfriend and had left the infant in the car with the windows rolled up. She could not say how long she had been gone, although she thought it was only about 30 minutes. Paramedics reported the infant's temperature to be 108°F (maximum number on the thermometer). The infant was in cardiopulmonary arrest and could not be resuscitated.

CASE 2

A 4-year-old boy was left momentarily in a car parked in the driveway while his mother ran back into the house to get some checks for deposit that she had forgotten. He moved the gearshift into reverse, the car rolled backwards, and ran over his 2-year-old cousin who had wandered out of the house through the open door. The 2-year-old received severe crush injuries to the head and chest and died en route to the hospital.

Children left unattended in parked cars are at risk for death from a number of factors.[50-52] Most commonly death occurs from hyperthermia. On a summer day, the interior of a car can heat up by 30°C (eg, go from 36°C to 66°C) within 15 minutes if the windows in the car are rolled up. The rapidity and degree of temperature rise vary with the type and color of the car. King et al[52] in a study carried out in Brisbane, Australia, reported that light-colored sedans and station wagons reached slightly lower temperatures. They estimated that in so hot an environment, an infant would become 8% dehydrated within 4 hours and develop heat stroke. Gibbs et al[51] found that in Louisiana, the temperature within dark-colored cars with the windows closed and light-colored cars with the windows partially open reached 125°F in 20 minutes and 140°F in 40 minutes. A life-threatening crisis would intervene even after a brief period in such high temperatures.

Most states legislate against leaving children (and pets) unattended in parked vehicles, and parents who do so are cited. If a child then dies as a result of such an action, that action is deemed to be neglectful and a parent can be held criminally responsible. In some areas, signs are visibly posted in parking lots alerting parents to the harmful effects of leaving children within closed vehicles.

Children who are left unsupervised in motor vehicles are also at risk to cause trauma to themselves or others in their vicinity. Agran et al[50] reviewed a series of instances where unsupervised children had set motor vehicles in motion. They uncovered 9 cases during a 24-month period by using a multihospital and coroner's office monitoring system. Three children died. In each case the child had released the brake or placed the car into gear. Sometimes the child jumped or fell from the rolling vehicle; other times the child was in an adjacent area. The authors suggest the following series of measures to safeguard against such mishaps: (1) never leave a child alone in a vehicle; (2) keep vehicles locked to prevent access by a child; and (3) never allow children to play in the vicinity of a parked car.

DEATH FROM FIREARMS

CASE

A 6-year-old boy was showing his 2½-year-old male cousin his father's handgun, which his father kept under his bed. The gun discharged, striking the 2½-year-old boy in the head. The toddler died at the scene. His uncle was prosecuted under California Criminal Storage of Firearms Section 12035.

Unfortunately, the above case scenario is not that uncommon.[53] Although most firearm-related deaths are intentional (homicide and suicide), approximately one third may be unintentional.[11] Absence of a firearm in the home reduces the risk of injury and death most significantly. If firearms are kept, then safe storage measures, including keeping firearms unloaded, locked, and with the ammunition stored separately, are important to endorse. Trigger locks also increase the safety of firearms. The safe storage of firearms may also reduce the risk of death from suicide.[53-55]

DETERMINING THE ROLE OF NEGLECT IN CHILD DEATHS

Different issues need to be examined when assessing the role that neglect may have played in the death of a child. Physicians may be individually asked to render an opinion about whether a parent's actions should be deemed criminally neglectful. Alternatively, they may be asked whether the medical community was negligent. From an advocacy perspective, physicians may be expected to propose legislative or community actions to reduce the risk of death among children. In rendering any of these decisions, the physician should consider all the factors that may have contributed to a neglectful situation (Box 2).

CHILD CHARACTERISTICS

Some children are at increased risk for neglect.[22] Premature infants are at increased risk for all types of child maltreatment.

BOX 2.
Factors Contributing to Child Neglect

Child
- Prematurity
- Low birth weight
- Developmental disability

Parental
- Substance abuse
- Developmental disability
- Mental illness

Family
- Social isolation
- Homelessness
- Unemployment
- Incarceration

Community
- Poor child care
- Limited public transportation
- Limited educational resources

Societal
- Poverty
- Violence

Normal mother-infant bonding may become interrupted by early prolonged separation. The complications of a premature birth may have left the infant with residual medical problems that place undue strains on the family's emotional and financial resources. Neurodevelopmentally disabled infants are particularly challenging because they are often slow feeders and fail to thrive. Sometimes there is a mismatch between children and their biologic parents. Overall, children with disabilities have been identified as having an increased risk of death from unexplained causes. The Oregon Child Fatality Review Team noted this increase to have been 5-fold for 1998.[11]

PARENTAL FACTORS

Limited parenting skills place children at increased risk for neglect.[22] Psychiatric or emotional problems in the primary caregivers may render them emotionally inaccessible. Maternal depression, in particular, is associated with neglect and failure to thrive.[4] Parental substance abuse is a very important risk factor.

Parents who are intoxicated or under the influence of drugs cannot appropriately supervise their youngsters.[56] We have noted the high incidence of caregiver intoxication in cases of home fires. A famous case in Los Angeles several years ago involved a mother who fell asleep on the couch during the day, allegedly under the influence of a cold remedy. While she was asleep, her 1½-year-old and 3-year-old daughters wandered out of the front door and were killed by a train. It was subsequently learned that the mother had a prior history of substance abuse.

Caregivers with developmental disabilities may not be adequately prepared for the challenges of parenting. They may lack independent decision-making skills needed to provide flexible care to their infant.[7,23]

Parental literacy is an important safeguard against neglect.[57] Much medical information is disseminated through brochures, prescription labels, and instructional sheets. A parent who cannot read has a difficult time being compliant. Neglectful mothers are less able to network or access community resources, perhaps in part a reflection of their limited reading skills.[58]

FAMILY CHARACTERISTICS

Families where there has been a death from neglect tend to be larger and have more children than families in which a child has died from physical abuse.[39] Many of the factors affecting parenting skills also affect the ability of the entire family to safeguard the well-being of a child. Our society fosters independence, but this may lead to social isolation. The absence of an extended family places children at risk for neglect. This risk is especially high in single-parent families.[5,39]

Families may struggle with multiple stressors such as homelessness, unemployment, mental illness, substance abuse, and prison. These drain the family resources so that the needs of the child are relegated to the bottom of the family's list of priorities.[22]

COMMUNITY/NEIGHBORHOOD RESOURCES

Factors in the community may place the child at risk.[22] For instance, there may be inadequate access to child care and transportation. Single parents who have no affordable child care may leave children alone, unsupervised, and unattended when they run errands, such as going to the welfare office or when they go to work.

The absence of public transportation in the neighborhood may affect a child's health care. If a parent must take 3 buses to get to a medical appointment, health care may be viewed more as a luxury and inconvenience, and well-child visits seen as less urgent and unimportant.

The absence of educational resources in communities also contributes to neglect.

SOCIETAL FACTORS

Poverty and violence are additional factors that limit the resources and alter the view of one's quality of life.[22]

CHILD FATALITY REVIEW BOARDS

Child fatality review boards assess the factors behind the death of children. The first multidisciplinary child fatality review team began in 1978 in Los Angeles.[12] The team included physicians, mental health workers, law enforcement personnel, district attorneys, dependency attorneys, social workers, and the coroner. Over time additional persons have joined the group including school personnel, public health nurses, epidemiologists, and injury prevention experts. The initial focus of the team was on deaths that could have been attributed to child abuse or neglect. Defining physical abuse is usually less problematic than making a determination of neglect. All contributing factors, including parental skills and family and community resources, should be taken into account when rendering an opinion.[13] Home scene investigations provide invaluable information and may help verify or refute the circumstances alleged by the parents. For instance, a child may be brought to the emergency department in cardiopulmonary arrest, after having supposedly drowned accidentally in a bathtub. But an evaluation of the home may reveal a shower stall, and no bathtub present. The presence of a chaotic, filthy home environment supports the diagnosis of neglect.

Other factors are also worth considering when making an assessment about parental culpability related to neglect.

One consideration is whether any law regulates the circumstances surrounding the child's death.[59] For instance, if a child dies as a result of being left unattended in an enclosed car, is there a regulation prohibiting such an action? Likewise if a child is shot by another child who was playing with an improperly stored loaded gun, is there a law that makes the gun owner both civilly and criminally liable for that action? The existence of such a law helps with decision making, especially in terms of criminal prosecution.

We have already discussed the notion of reasonable and prudent behavior on the part of the parent. Related to this is the issue of the advice that professionals give regarding the situations surrounding the child's death. Is such advice included by all practitioners in their routine anticipatory guidance? In the absence of such advice, is it common knowledge? What does the average person do? For instance, would the average person leave a 3-year-old child alone at home when they went to work? Is it common knowledge that young children require supervision? Besharov[7] states that children younger than 6 years do not have a "sufficient awareness of personal safety." Does an 8-year-old child have such knowledge? At what age is it permissible to allow a child to be without adult supervision? This age would probably vary depending on who was responding to the query. Sometimes this age is legally defined. For instance, Oregon law (ORS 163.545) defines as a misdemeanor leaving a child younger than 10 years unattended for any period that would likely endanger the health or welfare of the child. This law is used by the child fatality review board in defining the role of lack of supervision in the neglect of a child.

The child fatality review team is not only important in assessing the circumstances surrounding the death of an individual child, but also in identifying trends or patterns particularly around unintentional or preventable deaths. Many child fatality review teams develop year-end reports that include recommendations aimed at reducing the risk of death for children.[11,45]

INTERVENTION/PREVENTION

The issue of prevention can be addressed from 3 different perspectives: prevention of the death from neglect of an individual child; prevention of the deaths of children through changes in the environment and through legislative acts; and prevention of such deaths by addressing societal issues such as violence and poverty, noble but more challenging concerns.

Identifying neglectful mothers ahead of time is difficult. Brayden et al[60] reported that neglectful mothers were less likely to have completed high school, had more children younger than 6 years, and answered parenting skills questions more aberrantly. Their infants had lower birth weight and predictably were rated temperamentally more difficult. Polansky et al,[61] through the use of a 99-item inventory, the Childhood Level of Living Scale, identified 3 items that appeared to be associated with the risk of fatal child neglect. One item that was correlated with fatal neglect was the condition of the mattresses within the home. This unusual item may have simply served as a marker for general neglect or poverty. Maternal supervision was an important factor that is more obvious. Did the mother ever leave her child at home alone? What was her level of judgment when she left the child? Did she ever leave the child with insufficiently older children? Third, how vigilant was the mother in storage of medicine? Other areas to consider in assessing the safety of the home also relate to supervision. Are guns accessible? Are lighters and matches within easy reach of a child? Is the mother knowledgeable about bathtub safety? Has she kept her child's medical appointments?

Each child deserves an interventional plan that considers the strengths as well as the weaknesses of the family.[24,62] For any individual child, the health care providers should define the necessary interventions that might reduce risks to the child. Such interventions could include a home assessment by public health nurses who could review with the mother basic issues of child safety, such as coverage of electrical outlets, safe storage of household products and medications, and bathing safety. Health care practitioners can also utilize the excellent program sponsored by the American Academy of Pediatrics, the TIPP (The Injury Prevention Program) program, aimed at age-specific injury prevention.

Likewise, communities need to respond to situational and environmental hazards through the enactment of legislation and public awareness measures. We have already mentioned passenger safety and programs that distribute smoke detectors. A recent series of deaths in Tennessee highlights the needs for constant vigilance on the part of communities. The situation evolved after federal measures aimed at welfare reform removed mothers from the welfare rolls and got them to work. This move resulted in the need for child-care facilities. In June 1997, a 4-month-old infant, being transported to her day-care facility, died of hyperthermia after having been left in a van for 5½ hours. The temperature in the van had risen to 112°F, and the infant died of heat stroke. In July 1999, 2 other children died under similar circumstances. A 22-month-old toddler was "forgotten" in the van transporting her to child care. She was discovered 7 hours later, dead, with a core temperature of 108°F. On the same day, a 2-year-old child was left inside a day-care van for 5 hours. He too died of hyperthermia. The state of Tennessee investigated these deaths and enacted reforms that addressed the core issues behind these deaths, including undertrained day-care workers.[63]

Our society has seen an economic boom over the past decade. Yet not all members of our society have reaped the benefits of this boom. As mentioned above, the Personal Responsibility and Work Opportunity Reconciliation Act of 1996 (PRWORA) has had some unforeseeable consequences. In our effort to achieve economic stability, some families may be experiencing more difficulties with food and housing insecurity. Children, like canaries in the proverbial coal mine, signal the emergence of hunger, homelessness, and poverty, societal issues that increase the risk of neglect and death of children. Health care workers are in an ideal position to recognize and monitor the ill effects of societal conditions and to advocate on behalf of all children.

REFERENCES

1. Anderson R, Ambrosino R, Valentine D, et al: Child deaths attributed to abuse and neglect: An empirical study. *Children and Youth Services Review* 5:75-89, 1983.
2. McCurdy K, Daro D: *Current Trends in Child Abuse Reporting and Fatalities. The National Center on Child Abuse Prevention and Research, Working Paper No 808.* Chicago, National Committee to Prevent Child Abuse, 1994.
3. Munkel WI: Neglect and abandonment, in Monteleone JA, Brodeur AE (eds): *Child Maltreatment: A Clinical Guide and Reference.* St Louis, GW Medical Publishing, 1994, pp 241-257.
4. Black MM: The roots of child neglect, in Reece RM (ed): *Treatment of Child Abuse: Common Ground for Mental Health, Medical and Legal Practitioners.* Baltimore, Johns Hopkins University Press, 2000, pp 157-164.
5. Chronic child neglect. *Virginia Child Protection Newsletter* 54:1-16, 1998.
6. Kessler DB, Dawson P: *Failure to Thrive and Pediatric Undernutrition: A Transdisciplinary Approach.* Baltimore, Paul H. Brookes, 1999.
7. Besharov DJ: *Recognizing Child Abuse: A Guide for the Concerned.* New York, The Free Press, 1990, pp 99-133.
8. US Department of Health and Human Services National Center on Child Abuse and Neglect: *The Third National Incidence Study of Child Abuse and Neglect (NIS-3).* Washington, DC, US Government Printing Office, September 1996.
9. US Department of Health and Human Services, National Center on Child Abuse and Neglect, National Child Abuse and Neglect Data System Child Maltreatment 1995: *Reports from the States to the National Center on Child Abuse and Neglect.* Washington, DC, US Government Printing Office, 1997.
10. Alexander RC: Introduction, special issue on child fatalities. *APSAC Advisor* 7:1-3, 1994.
11. *Child Death in Oregon, 1998: Oregon Child Fatality Review Team Annual Report.* Oregon Department of Human Services, Portland, 1999.
12. Durfee M: History and status of child death review teams: Not mending walls. *APSAC Advisor* 7:4-5, 1994.

13. Thigpen SM, Bonner BL: Child death review teams in action. *APSAC Advisor* 7:5-8, 1994.
14. Committee on Child Abuse and Neglect and Committee on Community Health Services, American Academy of Pediatrics: Investigation and review of unexpected infant and child deaths. *Pediatrics* 104:1158-1160, 1999.
15. Kouno A, Johnson CF: Child abuse and neglect in Japan: Coin-operated locker babies. *Child Abuse Negl* 19:25-31, 1994.
16. Whitaker B: Deaths of unwanted babies bring plea to help parents. *New York Times*, March 6, 2000, pp A1, A19.
17. Rainey RH, Greer DC: Prosecuting child fatality cases. *APSAC Advisor* 7:28-30, 1994.
18. Adelson L: Homicide by starvation: The nutritional variant of the "battered child." *JAMA* 186:458-460, 1965.
19. Rosenberg D: Fatal neglect. *APSAC Advisor* 7:38-40, 1994.
20. Trube-Becker E: The death of children following negligence: Social aspects. *Forensic Sci* 9:111-115, 1977.
21. Meade JL, Brissie RM: Infanticide by starvation: Calculation of caloric deficit to determine degree of deprivation. *J Forensic Sci* 30:1263-1268, 1985.
22. Dubowitz H, Black M: Child neglect, in Reece RM (ed): *Child Abuse: Medical Diagnosis and Management.* Philadelphia, Lea & Febiger, 1994, pp 279-297.
23. Accardo PJ, Whitman BY: Children of mentally retarded parents. *Am J Dis Child* 14:69-70, 1990.
24. Black MM: Long-term psychological management of neglect, in Reece RM (ed): *Treatment of Child Abuse: Common Ground for Mental Health, Medical and Legal Practitioners.* Baltimore, Johns Hopkins University Press, 2000, pp 192-200.
25. Asser S, Swan R: Child fatalities from religion motivated medical neglect. *Pediatrics* 101:625-629, 1998.
26. Dubowitz, H, Giardino A, Gustavon E: Child neglect: Guidance for pediatricians. *Pediatr Rev* 21:111-116, 2000.
27. Silvestri JM, Hufford DR, Durham J, et al: Assessment of compliance with home cardiorespiratory monitoring in infants at risk of sudden infant death syndrome. *J Pediatr* 127:384-388, 1995.
28. Willinger M, Ko CW, Hoffman HJ, et al: Factors associated with caregivers' choice of infant sleep position, 1994-1998. *JAMA* 283:2135-2142, 2000.
29. Swan R: Discrimination de jure: Religious exemptions for medical neglect. *APSAC Advisor* 7:35-37, 1994.
30. Swan R: Children, medicine, religion, and the law, in Barness LA, DeVivo DC, Kaback MM, et al (eds): *Advances in Pediatrics,* vol 44. St Louis, Mosby, 1997, pp 491-543.
31. Bays J: Conditions mistaken for child abuse, in Reece RM (ed): *Child Abuse: Medical Diagnosis and Management.* Philadelphia, Lea & Febiger, 1994, pp 358-385.

32. Risser AL, Mazur LJ: Use of folk remedies in a Hispanic population. *Arch Pediatr Adolesc Med* 149:978-981, 1995.
33. Autotte P: Folk medicine. *Arch Pediatr Adolesc Med* 149:949-950, 1995.
34. Center for Disease Control and Prevention: 10 leading causes of death, United States 1997, all races, both sexes, http://www.cdc.gov/ncipc/wisqars/.
35. Wintemute GJ: Drowning in early childhood. *Pediatr Ann* 21:417-421, 1992.
36. Griest KJ, Zumwalt RE: Child abuse by drowning. *Pediatrics* 83:41-46, 1989.
37. Feldman KW, Monastersky C, Feldman GK: When is childhood drowning neglect? *Child Abuse Negl* 17:329-336, 1993.
38. Nixon J, Peam J: Non-accidental immersion in bathwater: Another aspect of child abuse. *BMJ* 1:271-272, 1977.
39. Margolin L: Fatal child neglect. *Child Welfare* 69:309-319, 1990.
40. Schmidt P, Madea B: Death in the bathtub involving children. *Forensic Sci Int* 72:147-155, 1995.
41. Feldman KW: Accidental injuries. *APSAC Advisor* 7:14-16, 1994.
42. Peterson L: Swimming pool, child drowning link sought. *Daily Breeze*, Torrance, Calif, May 1, 2000, pp Al, A7.
43. Rivara FP: Injury control: Issues and methods for the 1990's. *Pediatr Ann* 21:411-413, 1992.
44. Hall JR: U.S. experience with smoke detectors. Quincy, Mass, National Fire Protection Association, 1988.
45. *ICAN Child Death Review Team Report for 1999. Report Compiled from 1998 Data.* Los Angeles County, 1999.
46. Division of Injury Control, Center for Environmental Health and Injury Control, CDC: *Am J Dis Child* 144:627-646, 1990.
47. Squires T, Busuttil A: Child fatalities in Scottish house fires 1980-1990: A case of child neglect? *Child Abuse Negl* 19:865-873, 1995.
48. Gorman RL, Chamey E, Holtzman NA, et al: A successful city-wide smoke detection giveaway program. *Pediatrics* 75:14-18, 1985.
49. McLoughlin E, Brigham PA: Stop carelessness? No, reduce burn risk. *Pediatr Ann* 21:423-428, 1992.
50. Agran P, Winn D, Castillo D: Unsupervised children in vehicles: A risk for pediatric trauma. *Pediatrics* 87:70-73, 1991.
51. Gibbs LI, Lawrence DW, Kohn M: Heat exposure in an enclosed vehicle. *J La State Med Soc* 147:545-546, 1995.
52. King K, Negus K, Vance JC: Heat stress in motor vehicles: A problem in infancy. *Pediatrics* 68:579-582, 1981.
53. Wintemute GJ, Teret SP, Kraus JF, et al: When children shoot children: 88 unintentional deaths in California. *JAMA* 257:3107-3109, 1987.
54. Christoffel K: Pediatric firearm injuries: Time to target a growing population. *Pediatr Ann* 21:430-436, 1992.
55. Powell EC, Christoffel KK: Firearms: A culture of violence. *APSAC Advisor* 7:8-11, 1994.
56. Cantwell HB: The neglect of child neglect, in Helfer ME, Kempe RS,

Krugman RD (eds): *The Battered Child,* ed 5. Chicago, University of Chicago Press, 1990, pp 347-373.

57. Christian CW, Seidl T, Cervone FP: Initial treatment of child neglect: Medical, psychosocial, and legal considerations, in Reece RM (ed): *Treatment of Child Abuse: Common Ground for Mental Health, Medical and Legal Practitioners.* Baltimore, Johns Hopkins University Press, 2000, pp 165-182.
58. Coohey C: Neglectful mothers, their mothers, and partners: The significance of mutual aid. *Child Abuse Negl* 19:885-895, 1995.
59. Helfer RE: The neglect of our children. *Pediatr Clin North Am* 37:923-942, 1990.
60. Brayden RM, Altemeier WA, Tucker DD, et al: Antecedents of child neglect in the first two years of life. *J Pediatr* 120:426-429, 1992.
61. Polansky NA, Halley C, Polansky NF: *Profile of Neglect: A Survey of the State of Knowledge.* Washington, DC, US Department of Health, Education, and Welfare, 1977.
62. Dubowitz H: Prevention and ongoing medical management of child neglect, in Reece RM (ed): *Treatment of Child Abuse: Common Ground for Mental Health, Medical and Legal Practitioners.* Baltimore, Johns Hopkins University Press, 2000, pp 183-191.
63. Goldstein A: It took three dead babies. *Time*, July 20, 2000, pp 80-81.

CHAPTER 12

Thrombophilia in the Infant and Child

Marilyn J. Manco-Johnson, MD
Professor of Pediatrics, University of Colorado Health Sciences Center, Director, Mountain States Regional Hemophilia and Thrombosis Center, Aurora, Colo

Rachelle Nuss, MD
Associate Professor of Pediatrics, University of Colorado Health Sciences Center, Associate Director, Mountain States Regional Hemophilia and Thrombosis Center, Aurora, Colo

Thrombophilia is a term indicating a genetic predisposition to form excessive blood clots or thrombi. Many genetic traits associated with thrombophilia have been described during the past several years, and new ones are being discovered at a rapid rate (Table 1).[1,2] In addition to thrombophilia, a number of acquired traits predispose to thrombosis (Box 1). Vascular occlusions including cerebral, coronary, and venous thrombi often occur as part of the aging process. Adults with thrombophilia manifest these signs of vascular disease prematurely (defined as before 40-50 years of age). Recently, there has been recognition that thrombophilia may also predispose to vascular disease in infants and children.[3-6] This chapter reviews the presentation, etiology, diagnosis, and management of thrombophilia in the pediatric population.

PRESENTATION OF THROMBOPHILIA IN INFANTS AND CHILDREN

Thromboses occur more frequently during the perinatal period than during any other phase of childhood. Subsequently, the incidence of thrombosis is lower during infancy and childhood, increases with puberty, and rises steadily thereafter. By young adulthood, the rate of venous thrombosis is 23 cases per 100,000 and increases 15-fold over the next 3 decades.[2] Cumulatively, the rate of thrombosis is approximately 5% to 10% over a lifetime. Thrombosis in children is charac-

TABLE 1.
Genetic Etiologies of Thrombophilia in Children

Trait	Frequency
Excessive Primary Hemostasis	
These disorders result in platelet clumping and clearance but usually manifest with bleeding rather than thrombosis.	
Congenital hemolytic uremic syndrome/ thrombotic thrombocytopenia purpura	
-caused by deficient vWF-cleaving metallo-proteinase	Rare
-caused by vascular endothelial cyclo-oxygenase deficiency	Rare
Platelet GP Ib mutations resulting in increased platelet/vWF interactions (platelet or pseudo von Willebrand disease)	Rare
Excessive Thrombin Generation	
Elevated factor VIII	11% of whites
Factor V G1691A mutation	3% to 8% of whites
Prothrombin G20210A mutation	1% to 2% of whites
Deficient Thrombin Regulation	
Antithrombin deficiency	1/5000
Protein C deficiency	1/500
Protein S deficiency	Unknown
Deficient Fibrinolysis	
Dysfibrinogenemia	Rare
Plasminogen deficiency	Rare
Multiple Effects	
Cystathionine β-Synthase Deficiency	Rare
Sickle cell anemia	1/400 African Americans
β Thalessemia	Population dependent

Abbreviation: vWF, von Willebrand factor.

terized by a predilection for large vessels and an increased incidence of arterial lesions. Infants and children with thrombophilia present with thrombi similar in site and extent to thrombi that develop from other causes. Thrombophilic children typically develop thrombi in a setting complicated by other predisposing medical conditions and provoking factors (Box 2). Indwelling catheters frequently precipitate thrombi. The presence of predisposing and provoking factors does not diminish the odds of detecting thrombophilia and, in general, should not dissuade pursuing laboratory evaluation. In addition, detection of a single thrombophilic trait in a child should not limit the complete evaluation. Recent studies suggest that thrombosis in the young is multifactorial, and the coexistence of multiple thrombophilic genes in symptomatic children is common.[6-8] Occasionally, thrombophilia may be suggested by the occurrence of thrombi in unusual locations or without other apparent provocation.

The incidence of thrombosis in the newborn infant has been estimated at 5.1 cases per 100,000.[9] In the term newborn infant, thromboses may occur prenatally and usually present clinically within the first 48 hours of life. The cerebral arteries and veins, renal veins, aorta, and vena cava are most commonly affected.[10] Renal vein thrombosis presents with a flank mass that may be palpable in the delivery room or in the nursery before discharge. Hematuria, thrombocytopenia, and hypertension form a classic clinical triad

BOX 1.
Acquired Abnormalities Predisposing to Thrombosis in Children

Excessive Primary Hemostasis
- Polycythemia/hyperviscosity
- Essential thrombocythemia
- Hemolytic uremic syndrome/thrombotic thrombocytopenia purpura
- Heparin-associated thrombocytopenia and thrombosis syndrome (HITS)
- Postsplenectomy (eg, sideroblastic anemia)

Excessive Thrombin Generation
- Lupus anticoagulant ± anticardiolipin antibody
- Increased tissue factor expression with infection, inflammation, malignancy

Deficient Thrombin Regulation
- Acquired antithrombin deficiency with nephrotic syndrome
- Decreased synthesis of hepatic proteins (eg, chemotherapy with L-asparaginase)
- Disseminated intravascular coagulation
- Acquired antibodies to coagulation regulatory proteins

Mixed Effects
- Hyperhomocysteinemia
  - Dietary deficiencies of folate, vitamin B_6, or vitamin B_{12}
  - Inactivity
  - Smoking
  - Coffee
- Primary antiphospholipid antibody syndrome

BOX 2.
Underlying Predisposing Medical Conditions and Provoking Factors Associated With Thrombosis in Children

Indwelling vascular catheter
Vascular damage
Trauma
Surgery
Infection, inflammation
Vascular malformation or damage
Malignancy/chemotherapy
Cardiac disease
Prosthetic cardiac valves
Systemic lupus erythematosus
Rheumatoid arthritis
Crohn disease
Ulcerative colitis
Sickle cell anemia and other hemoglobinopathies
Renal disease
Diabetes mellitus
Inflammation, appendicitis
Oral contraceptive agents

in neonatal renal vein thrombosis. Neonatal stroke generally manifests with seizures within the first 24 hours of life. The level of consciousness may be normal or depressed. Massive aortic thromboses present with absent pulses in the lower extremities, upper extremity hypertension, and cardiovascular collapse. Occasionally, an infant is delivered with an obviously ischemic, pale, pulseless extremity or a frankly necrotic limb.

A rare syndrome of neonatal purpura fulminans with disseminated intravascular coagulopathy is caused by homozygous or compound heterozygous deficiencies of protein C or protein S.[11-14] Affected infants often manifest blindness and retinal hemorrhage in addition to cerebral infarcts and renal vein thrombosis.[15] Neonates who have extensive, multiple, or unusual thrombi are likely to carry 2 or more thrombophilia traits or acquired coagulopathies resulting from transplacentally acquired antiphospholipid antibodies.[16-20]

In preterm infants, thrombi most commonly develop in association with indwelling umbilical arterial and venous catheters.

Vascular obstruction by a catheter nearly as large as the vessel, longer duration of use, and endothelial irritation by materials infused (eg, antibiotics, high-concentration glucose, and amino acids) contribute to catheter thrombogenicity.

The rate of arterial and venous stroke in infants and children beyond the neonatal period is 2 cases per 100,000. One third of children with stroke test positive for anticardiolipin antibodies.[21,22] Many genetic thrombophilic traits have been associated with stroke in children.[23]

The prevalence of venous thrombosis in pediatric patients beyond the neonatal period has been estimated at 0.7 cases per 100,000.[24] Thrombophilia is often found in conjunction with an acquired predisposing condition. Arterial thrombosis not associated with an indwelling catheter is rare in children and has been associated with genetic and acquired thrombophilia.

ETIOLOGY OF THROMBOPHILIA

Balanced coagulation is dependent on primary hemostasis (platelet-vessel interaction), thrombin generation, fibrin clot formation, thrombin regulation, and fibrinolysis or clot dissolution. Thrombophilia can be caused by genetic mutations affecting any of these processes, as shown in Figure 1. The list of genetic mutations that have been associated with thrombophilia is long and continues to grow.

Genetic disorders causing enhanced primary hemostasis are rare. They generally present in infancy with recurrent thrombocytopenia and features of hemolytic uremic syndrome or thrombotic thrombocytopenia purpura.

Genetic mutations resulting in increased thrombin generation are receiving heightened attention currently. Elevated levels of circulating factor VIII (greater than 150% of normal) are transmitted in an autosomal dominant inheritance pattern and are found in 11% of the population. An increased incidence of venous thrombosis is associated with such elevations in factor VIII activity.[25,26] Elevated factor VIII activity may prove to be the most frequent thrombophilic trait identified to date. The genetic mutation causing the elevated factor VIII activity has not yet been identified.

The G1691A mutation of factor V (also known as factor V Leiden) affects 5% to 8% of the white population.[2] Although this mutation is not found in Africa or Asia, because of genetic mixing it is present in all US populations, although to a lesser extent than that found in the white population. The mutation causing factor V

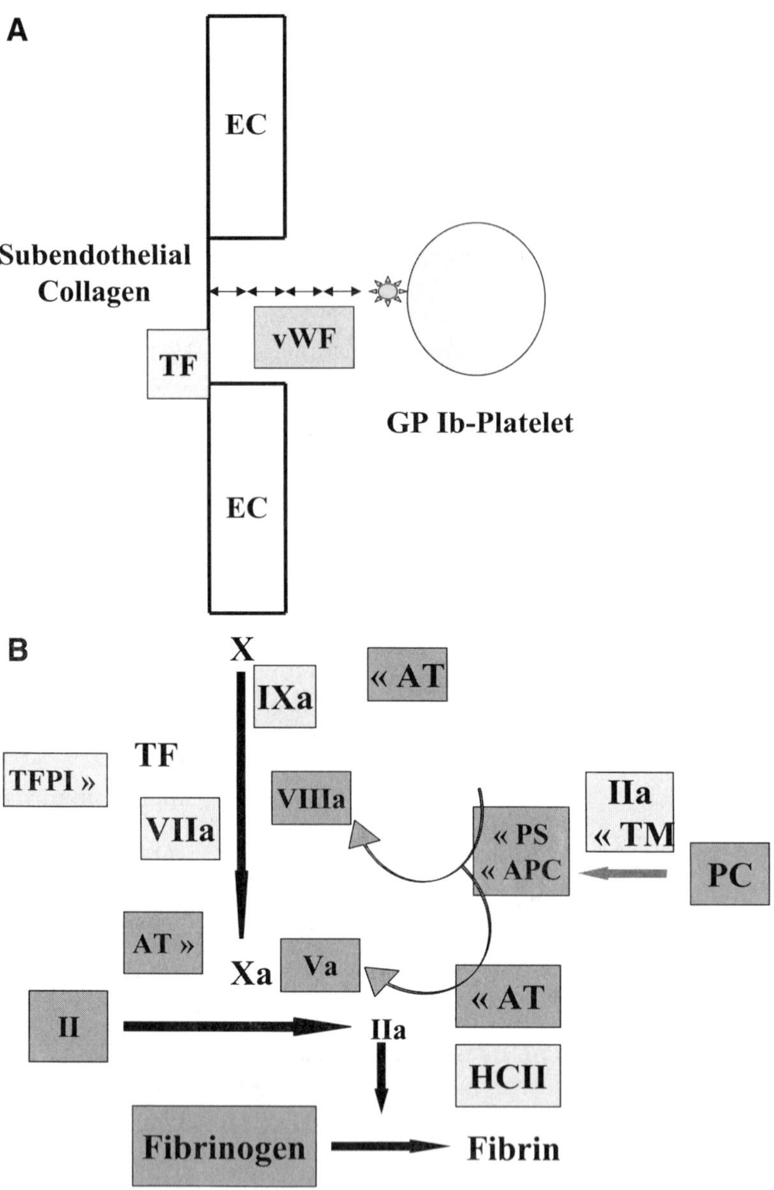

FIGURE 1.

Thrombophilic traits in clot formation and dissolution. **A,** The first or primary phase of hemostasis. Platelets interact with subendothelial collagen and tissue factor that are exposed in areas of vascular damage. **B,** The coagulation cascade. Thrombin is generated, resulting in fibrin formation.

(continued)

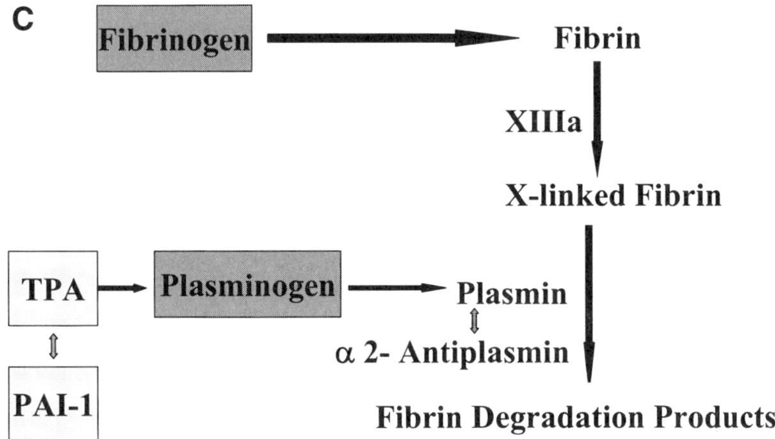

FIGURE 1. (continued)
C, Fibrinolysis or clot dissolution. *Darker gray tinting* indicates proteins whose abnormal levels or functions have been proven to be associated with thrombophilia. *Lighter gray tinting* indicates proteins in which gene mutations could cause thrombophilia, although no such mutations have yet been proven. *Abbreviations: EC,* Endothelial cell; *TF,* tissue factor; *vWF,* von Willebrand factor; *TFPI,* tissue factor pathway inhibitor; *AT,* antithrombin; *PS,* protein S; *PC,* protein C; *APC,* activated protein C; *TM,* thrombomodulin; *HCII,* heparin cofactor II; *II,* prothrombin; *IIa,* thrombin; *Va,* activated factor V; *VIIa,* activated factor VII; *VIIIa,* activated factor VIII; *IXa,* activated factor IX; *Xa,* activated factor X; *XIIIa,* activated factor XIII; *TPA,* tissue plasminogen activator; *PAI-1,* plasminogen activator inhibitor, type 1.

Leiden appears to have occurred as a single, conserved event exhibiting what is known as a "founder effect." Factor V G1691A contains a single amino acid substitution, resulting in a replacement of glutamine for arginine in the active site of factor V where activated protein C cleaves activated factor V (Va) in the process of inactivation. Consequently, children with the factor V mutation have a factor V that, after activation by thrombin, is resistant to inactivation.[27] Heterozygous factor V G1691A increases the risk of venous thrombosis by 6-fold; homozygous mutations increase the rate of venous thrombosis by 80-fold.[28] Arterial thrombi are not common but have been reported in infants and children with this mutation. Spontaneous and provoked thrombi have been reported in children with factor V G1691A from the neonatal period through adolescence.[29-36] Factor V G1691A shows some hormonal interaction and increases the risk of thrombosis, especially stroke, in adolescents in association with oral contraceptive agents or pregnancy, and during the perinatal period.[8,23,37] There is some suggestion that maternal factor V G1691A may cause thrombus formation in the maternal circulation, fetal-placental circulation, or both.[38] The contribution of fetal factor V G1691A has not yet been determined. Factor V G1691A is usually present with other genetic or acquired prothrombotic risks in children who develop thrombosis. The combination of the factor V mutation with a mutation in protein C or its cofactor protein S is synergistic in its thrombogenic potential. Factor V G1961A has been reported in a neonate with purpura fulminans and bilateral renal vein thrombosis.[36] Because the trait is so common and disastrous outcomes are uncommon in heterozygous children, severe clinical disorders should be considered multifactorial, and contributing causes for thrombosis should be sought. Other less common mutations in the factor V gene have been described that result in a similar thrombotic tendency.

A mutation in prothrombin, prothrombin G20210A, found in 1% to 2% of the white population, is the next most common cause of thrombophilia.[39] Prothrombin G20210A is caused by a single, conserved point mutation in the untranslated 3´ region of the prothrombin gene and results in a modest increase in circulating levels of prothrombin, the zymogen precursor of thrombin.[40] Prothrombin G20210A has been associated with venous and arterial thrombosis in infants, children, and adolescents, including those with thrombotic lesions of the central nervous system.[31,32] The prothrombin mutation behaves clinically very similar to the factor V mutation, but does not appear to be hormonally regulated.

Elevated levels of factors XI,[41] IX,[42]and VII[43] have also been associated with an increased incidence of thrombotic disease in adults. An association between factor XII deficiency and thrombosis has been suspected but not proven.[44] At this time, there are no data regarding these factors as thrombophilic traits in infants or children.

Abnormalities of any one of the regulatory proteins, antithrombin (AT), protein C, or protein S, are associated with thrombosis. AT is a physiologic inhibitor of activated serine proteases, including factors XIIa, XIa, IXa, Xa, and IIa (and to a lesser extent VIIa and the tissue factor complex). Familial AT deficiency was the first thrombophilic trait described in 1965.[45] Antithrombin deficiency results from more than 100 different gene mutations.[46] Type I AT deficiency connotes a decrease in the plasma concentration of a structurally normal protein. Type II AT deficiency signifies a dysfunctional molecule, which may be present in normal or reduced concentrations. Antithrombin deficiency is relatively rare, affecting approximately 1 in 4000 persons. However, the clinical severity of the disease is far greater than those traits previously discussed. Essentially all affected heterozygotes develop symptomatic thromboses if they live long enough, and most affected women develop pregnancy-related thromboses unless they are given prophylactic anticoagulation during pregnancy and the postpartum period. Homozygous or compound heterozygous mutations cause very low AT levels, resulting in severe thrombophilia. True absence of AT has never been described and is probably incompatible with life.

The protein C system is critical in downregulation of the potent augmentors of the coagulation cascade (Fig 1, B). The protein C system includes protein C whose activated form, APC, inactivates activated factors V (Va) and VIII (VIIIa). In addition, the system includes the protein C cofactor, protein S, the endothelial cell surface receptor for protein C activation, thrombomodulin, the endothelial cell protein C cofactor, and protein Z.[47] Types I and II deficiencies of protein C result from quantitative and qualitative defects similar to those seen with AT deficiency. Heterozygous protein C deficiency occurs in 1 in 500 individuals; most persons are asymptomatic. However, some heterozygous defects are associated with a moderately severe clinical syndrome. Levels of protein C develop slowly in utero and postnatally. The mean protein C level at 24 weeks' gestation is 0.20 U/mL and at term, 0.40 U/mL. Levels plateau at 6 months of age until puberty when they increase to the full adult potential. Therefore, it is often difficult to interpret borderline plasma activity levels in children before adolescence.

Protein S has a unique biochemistry. Sixty-percent of protein S circulates in the plasma bound to the C4b-binding protein.[48] The C4b-bound compartment of protein S functions to localize C4b to cell surfaces and has no anticoagulant function. The remaining 40% of protein S circulates in the "free" form and participates as a cofactor for the APC-mediated inactivation of factors Va and VIIIa. The anticoagulant portion of protein S is estrogen responsive and decreases during pregnancy and with oral contraceptive agents. Protein S deficiency exists as 3 types of genetic mutations. Type I is characterized by a concordant decrease in protein antigen (absolute amount) and activity. Type II has normal total and free protein S compartments with a decrease in protein S clotting activity. Type III protein S deficiency has a normal total protein S with a decrease in both free protein S as well as protein S clotting activity. Decreased levels of free protein S correlate best with thrombotic risk.[49] Clinically, protein S deficiency manifests similar to protein C deficiency in severity. The newborn infant has a mean plasma level of total protein S antigen of only 0.20 U/mL. However, because the level of C4b-binding protein is extremely low in the normal infant at birth (approximately 0.1 U/mL), almost all neonatal protein S is functional.[50]

Abnormalities of a number of coagulation factors should theoretically result in thrombophilia, but convincing evidence for their associations with thrombosis in a large number of families has not been obtained. This is true for deficiency of the inhibitor heparin cofactor II.[51] Proteins such as thrombomodulin and tissue factor pathway inhibitor that are normally associated with cell surfaces or other compartments may be genetically altered but are difficult to study. Gene sequencing has been applied to detect abnormalities of these proteins, but gene mutations are not always synonymous with protein deficiencies.[52,53]

Other rare genetic coagulation defects have been associated with thrombophilia. Decreases in the amount or activity of plasminogen[54] as well as some dysfibrinogenemias[55] have been associated with deficiencies in fibrinolysis. Whether tissue plasminogen activator (TPA) deficiency or elevated plasminogen activator inhibitor type 1 (PAI-1) predisposes to familial thrombosis is being studied.

The metabolic disease homocystinuria, caused by decreased activity of the enzyme cystathionine β-synthase, is associated with a 50% incidence of early-onset arterial and venous thrombosis as well as premature atherosclerotic vascular disease.[56] Other enzyme deficiencies in the metabolism of homocysteine also result in increased vascular disease. There appear to be multiple mechanisms of hyperhomocysteinemia in the pathogenesis of endothelial damage.[56] Mild to moderate hyperhomocysteinemia, diagnosed by elevated levels of homocysteine either fasting or after a methionine load, has been identified as a risk factor for venous thrombosis.[57] The most common genetic defect of homocysteine metabolism is caused by a thermolabile variant of the methyltetrahyrofolate reductase gene (MTHFRC677T), which is found in a homozygous (MTHFR 677TT) form in 10% of the population. MTHFR polymorphisms (677 CC, CT, or TT) have been correlated with levels of homocysteine in children as well as in adults.[58,59] However, not all affected individuals have hyperhomocysteinemia. The presence of the MTHFR 677TT in the absence of elevated homocysteine levels does not appear to be an independent risk factor for thrombosis.[60]

Elevations of the genetically regulated lipoprotein, Lp(a), have been statistically linked with a predisposition to coronary heart disease.[61] This association appears to have a mild effect. Levels of Lp(a) more than 2 standard deviations above the mean (generally greater than 30 mg/dL) have been reported by German colleagues in association with thromboses, both arterial and venous, in newborns and children.[62,63] The data for this association, while convincing, have not yet been confirmed in other populations.

ACQUIRED TRAITS PREDISPOSING TO THROMBOSIS

The most common acquired disorders predisposing to thrombosis in children and adolescents are caused by antiphospholipid antibodies, both the lupus anticoagulant and anticardiolipin antibodies.[3,4,64,65] Criteria for diagnosis of the lupus anticoagulant include prolongation of a functional clotting assay (usually either the activated partial thromboplastin time [APTT] or the dilute Russell viper venom time [dRVVT]) and failure to correct the clotting prolongation with addition of normal plasma, but correction with addition of excess phospholipid.[66] The anticardiolipin antibody is detected by using an enzyme-linked immunosorbent assay (ELISA).[67] Both of these autoantibodies can be of IgG, IgM, or IgA specificity, although IgG antibodies are most reliably correlated with clinical pathology.

The lupus anticoagulant is an antibody directed against complexes of coagulation proteins with negatively charged phospholipid surfaces. Lupus anticoagulants probably result from the association of coagulation proteins with altered (damaged) endothelial cell or platelet membranes. In children, transient lupus anticoagulants may follow acute infections with organisms that infect endothelial cells, including streptococcus, adenovirus, herpesviruses, and varicella-zoster viruses.[68] The thrombotic tendency related to postinfectious antiphospholipid antibody is transient and generally persists for days to months after the onset of the inciting infection. Lupus anticoagulants occur as true autoantibodies in approximately 40% of children with systemic lupus erythematosus, and occasionally in children with juvenile rheumatoid arthritis, ulcerative colitis, Crohn disease, and other collagen vascular diseases.

The antiphospholipid antibody syndrome often presents in adolescents. This clinical syndrome is characterized by the lupus anticoagulant or anticardiolipin antibody along with other autoantibodies, most often directed against blood elements including platelets, red blood cells, and white blood cells. Antithyroid antibodies are also common.

The lupus anticoagulant is associated with a high rate of venous thrombosis and primary pulmonary thrombi or pulmonary emboli. Thrombosis associated with the lupus anticoagulant had a 67% rate of recurrence within 6 weeks of discontinuing therapeutic anticoagulation.[64] Anticardiolipin antibodies are found in one third of children with stroke.[21] In adult women, anticardiolipin antibodies are most commonly found in a clinical constellation including thrombocytopenia, migraine headache, stroke, and recurrent fetal wastage. A few case reports have included familial variants of the antiphospholipid antibody syndrome with lupus anticoagulants.

Autoantibodies causing acquired deficiencies of protein S, protein C, or antithrombin with or without evidence of a concomitant lupus anticoagulant occasionally are present in children.[68-72]

Protein S levels are affected by hormonal status. Adolescent girls treated with high-dose estrogen may have acquired deficiencies.[73] Therapy with OCAs may provoke thrombosis in an adolescent with an underlying factor V G1691A mutation or deficiency of protein S or antithrombin.

Acquired deficiencies of coagulation regulatory proteins and thrombosis occur in disseminated intravascular coagulation as well as disorders affecting hepatic protein synthesis, such as chemotherapy with L-asparaginase for acute leukemia. Nephrosis is associated with urinary losses of antithrombin along with other proteins. An acquired increase in homocysteine secondary to deficiencies of folic acid or vitamins B_6 or B_{12} is a more common etiology of hyperhomocysteinemia than are genetic mutations. Smoking and coffee consumption are other risk factors for hyperhomocysteinemia.

Heparin-associated antibodies form against complexes of heparin with platelet factor 4 on the surface of the platelet and result in platelet clumping, thrombocytopenia, and paradoxic thrombosis during heparin administration. Heparin-associated antibodies have been described in children and probably occur more commonly in pediatric patients than is currently recognized.[74-76] Evidence for heparin-associated antibodies should be sought in children with thrombocytopenia and progressive thrombosis while receiving heparin therapy.

Normal newborn infants manifest a unique hemostatic balance that would appear to predispose to thrombosis, as shown in Box 3. These traits are physiologic and are not considered causes of thrombophilia.

BOX 3.
Physiologic Characteristics of Neonatal Coagulation That Predispose to Thrombosis

Increased Primary Hemostasis
- Increased concentration and size of vWF multimers
- Increased hematocrit and viscosity

Increased Thrombin Generation
- Increased concentration of factor VIII
- Increased tissue factor expression on monocytes and endothelial cells

Decreased Thrombin Regulation
- Decreased levels of coagulation inhibitors AT, protein C, and protein S

Decreased Fibrinolysis
- Decreased concentration of plasminogen
- Fetal plasminogen with reduced and delayed activation
- Decreased TPA
- Increased α_2-antiplasmin and PAI-1

Abbreviations: vWF, von Willebrand factor; *AT,* antithrombin; *TPA,* tissue plasminogen activator; *PAI-1,* plasminogen activator inhibitor, type 1.

TESTING FOR THROMBOPHILIA IN CHILDREN

WHO TO TEST FOR THROMBOPHILIA

All children who have arterial or venous thrombosis should be evaluated for thrombophilia, regardless of the presence of underlying predisposing or provoking medical conditions. All term neonates who have clinical signs of thrombosis should be evaluated similarly. There is still controversy regarding whether it is medically indicated or whether the cost-benefit ratio favors evaluating the preterm infant with catheter-related thrombosis.

The first measure to decrease the cost of screening is to apply a very extensive and complete personal and family history for thrombosis. One such screening history is shown in Table 2. However, sometimes one or more thrombophilic traits are inherited from an asymptomatic parent, and the child who develops a predisposing condition or is exposed to a provoking factor is the family proband.

For the purpose of genetics counseling to determine the potential for thrombotic disease in offspring, when an adult has thrombosis and is found to carry one or more thrombophilic traits, it is useful to evaluate the spouse. Genetic or functional prenatal test-

TABLE 2.
Suggested Personal and Family History for Thrombophilia

	DVT	PE	MI	Stroke	Arterial	Age at 1st onset	Predisposing/ Provoking Factors	Recur	Long-term anticoag
Pro band									
Mother									
Father									
Sibling 1									
Sibling 2									
Sibling 3									
Mat GM									
Mat GF									
Pat GM									
Pat GF									
Aunt									
Uncle									
Cousin									
Other									

Abbreviations: DVT, Deep vein thrombosis; *PE,* pulmonary embolism; *MI,* myocardial infarct; Recur, recurrent thrombosis; *Long-term anticoag,* long-term anticoagulant therapy.

ing can be performed using chorionic villus sampling, periumbilical blood sampling, or amniocentesis.

The decision whether to test clinically asymptomatic siblings of a symptomatic family member is difficult. There may be problems with acquiring health insurance if abnormalities are identified, even if the person is asymptomatic. There are psychological consequences to knowing that there is an increased risk for thrombosis that may occur many years in the future or never at all. On the other hand, an asymptomatic child who carries thrombophilic traits can be treated prophylactically with short courses of anticoagulant therapy for high-risk events including surgery, immobilization, inflammation, or serious infection. Prophylactic therapy is particularly important for children with multiple risk factors for thrombosis.

WHAT TESTS TO PERFORM TO EXCLUDE THROMBOPHILIA

Unfortunately, there are no global screening tests for hypercoagulability similar to the APTT or prothrombin time that are used to screen for bleeding disorders. In addition, a minority of individuals with a single thrombophilic trait develop thrombosis. Most children develop clinical thrombosis in association with 2 or more thrombophilic traits, in addition to acquired medical conditions. Therefore, each thrombophilic trait must be individually determined by functional assay or genetic testing. The complete battery of tests should be performed together.

HOW TO TEST FOR THROMBOPHILIA

Table 3 displays the progressive levels of laboratory testing to diagnose thrombophilia. Once a decision is made to test a child for thrombophilia, a complete level I basic evaluation should be obtained. If all of these test results are normal in a child who had a life-threatening, recurrent, or unusual thrombosis, or in a child with a very positive family history for thrombosis, then a level II evaluation should be performed. Factors listed on level III are currently under investigation but have not yet been definitively linked to thrombophilia.

In general, functional clotting or chromogenic assays are preferred over immunologic assays because both types I and II deficiencies are detected in functional assays. Vitamin K–dependent protein C and protein S should not be measured while a patient is receiving oral anticoagulation with warfarin. In addition, the clotting assay for protein S is altered by hormones, heparin, and other influences. An immunologic assay for the free (unbound) protein S is a more reliable assay and will detect types I and III deficiencies, which account for the vast majority of genetic protein S defects.

WHEN TO TEST CHILDREN FOR THROMBOPHILIA

Recommendations for evaluation of thrombophilia in adults call for delaying the thrombophilia evaluation until the adult is in a stable state and not receiving oral anticoagulation. There are compelling reasons to perform a thrombophilia evaluation in a child at the time of presentation with acute thrombosis. A child with thrombosis is more likely, as compared with the adult, to have multiple thrombophilic genes. Successful management of the acute thrombosis may require replacement of a severely deficient protein, such as protein C or AT, regardless of whether the cause of the deficiency is familial or acquired. In the common case of AT deficiency during L-asparaginase therapy for acute leukemia, knowledge of the acute deficiency may be critical to planning future replacement therapy or altering subsequent chemotherapy. Tests that yield

TABLE 3.
Recommendations for Laboratory Testing of Thrombophilia in Children

Level I: Basic evaluation for all children with thrombosis
Complete blood count with hematocrit, white blood cell count, differential, and platelet count
Antithrombin activity
Protein C activity
Protein S, free or activity
Factor VIII activity
Factor V A1691G gene test and/or functional activated protein C resistance assay
Prothrombin G20210A gene test
Homocysteine level
Lupus anticoagulant test
Anticardiolipin antibody test
Sickle Cell/thalassemia: screen or hemoglobin electrophoresis
Level II: Extended evaluation for children with normal level I values and recurrent thrombosis, a positive family history for thrombosis or severe thrombosis
Euglobulin clot lysis time (ELT)
Plasminogen activity
Dysfibrinogenemia evaluation: fibrinogen activity, antigen, thrombin time, reptilase time, fibrin degradation products, consider crossed immunoelectrophoresis
Paroxysmal nocturnal hemoglobinuria (PNH; sucrose hemolysis)
If not previously performed:
Functional activated protein C resistance (modified assay)
Hemoglobin electrophoresis
Erythrocyte sedimentation rate (ESR), C-reactive protein (CRP)
Level III: (Currently under investigation)
Lp(a)
Factor XII deficiency
Elevated factor XI
Elevated factor IX
Elevated factor VII
Elevated von Willebrand factor level; larger molecular weight multimers
Spontaneous platelet aggregation
Platelet receptor polymorphisms
Heparin cofactor II activity deficiency
Elevated plasminogen activator inhibitor (PAI)
Tissue plasminogen activator (TPA) deficiency
Tissue factor pathway inhibitor (TFPI) deficiency
Thrombomodulin deficiency
MTHFR gene test

abnormal results may be repeated 3 to 6 months later, with the patient off anticoagulant and other therapies, to confirm or exclude the genetic nature of the deficiency.

CLINICAL MANAGEMENT OF CHILDREN WITH THROMBOPHILIA

All children with acute thrombosis require initial therapy with thrombolysis or anticoagulation, followed by at least 3 months of anticoagulant therapy with heparin or warfarin. Children in whom only an acute, transient risk factor is found (eg, cardiac catheterization, infection, or trauma) have a low risk of thrombus recurrence after 3 months of therapy. Children with genetic or acquired thrombophilia must be treated for at least 6 to 12 months. If the child has a homozygous or compound heterozygous deficiency of a single protein or two or more combined thrombophilic traits, then indefinite anticoagulation is probably needed. Children with a single thrombophilic trait can probably be treated 6 to 12 months and then watched expectantly. Decisions regarding the duration of long-term anticoagulant therapy should be directed by the severity of the initial clinical presentation and the family history of severity. In general, children with severe deficiencies of protein C, protein S, or AT, the lupus anticoagulant, or multiple combined defects have a high rate of recurrence, whereas children with single defects, including the factor V or prothrombin mutation, may not experience recurrence until after puberty or not at all. Children for whom continuous indefinite anticoagulation is not prescribed may benefit from short-term anticoagulation targeted to high-risk events, including episodes of surgery, immobilization, casting, or inflammatory conditions and infections. These children may be treated with short courses of prophylactic unfractionated or low-molecular weight heparin around high-risk events.

REFERENCES

1. Rosendaal FR: Risk factors for venous thrombosis. *Thromb Haemost* 82:610-619, 1999.
2. Rosendaal FR: Thrombosis in the young: Epidemiology and risk factors. A focus on venous thrombosis. *Thromb Haemost* 78:1-6, 1997.
3. Manco-Johnson MJ: Disorders of hemostasis in childhood: Risk factors for venous thromboembolism. *Thromb Haemost* 78:710-714, 1997.
4. Nuss R, Manco-Johnson M: Childhood thrombosis. *Pediatrics* 96:291-294, 1995.
5. DeVeber F, Monagle P, Chan A, et al: Prothrombotic disorders in infants and children with cerebral thromboembolism. *Arch Neurol* 55:1539-1543, 1998.

6. Zimbelman J, Lefkowitz J, Schaeffer C, et al: Unusual complications of warfarin therapy: Skin necrosis and priapism. *J Pediatr* 137:266-268, 2000.
7. Kosch A, Junker R, Kurnik K, et al: Prothrombotic risk factors in children with spontaneous venous thrombosis and their asymptomatic parents. *Thromb Res* 99:531-537, 2000.
8. Ehrenforth S, for the Childhood Thrombophilia Study Group: Multicentre evaluation of combined prothrombotic defects associated with thrombophilia in childhood. *Eur J Pediatr* 158:97S-104S, 1999.
9. Nowak-Göttl U, vonKries R, Goebel U: Neonatal symptomatic thromboembolism in Germany: Two year survey. *Arch Dis Child Fetal Neonatal Ed* 76:F163, 1997.
10. Schmidt B, Andrew M: Neonatal thrombosis: Report of a prospective Canadian and international registry. *Pediatrics* 96:939-943, 1995.
11. Hartman KR, Manco-Johnson M, Rawlings JS, et al: Homozygous PC deficiency: Early treatment with warfarin. *Am J Pediatr Hematol Oncol* 11:395-401, 1989.
12. Kemahli S, Alhenc-Gelas M, Gandrille M, et al: Homozygous protein C deficiency with a double variant His 202 to Tyr and Ale 346 to Thr. *Coagulation and Fibrinolysis* 9:351-354, 1998.
13. Long GL, Tomczak JA, Rainville IR, et al: Homozygous type I protein C deficiency in two unrelated families exhibiting thrombophilia related to Ala136—> Pro or Arg 286—> His mutations. *Thromb Haemost* 72:526-533, 1994.
14. Pung-amritt P, Poort SR, Vos HL, et al: Compound heterozygosity for one novel and one recurrent mutation in a Thai patient with severe protein S deficiency. *Thromb Haemost* 81:189-192, 1999.
15. Hattenbach LO, Beeg R, Kreuz W, et al: Ophthalmic manifestations of congenital protein C deficiency. *J AAPOS* 3:188- 190, 1999.
16. Brenner B, Zivelin A, Lanir N, et al: Venous thromboembolism associated with double heterozygosity for R506Q mutation of factor V and for T298M mutation of protein C in a large family of a previously described homozygous protein C-deficient newborn with massive thrombosis. *Blood* 88:877-880, 1996.
17. Formstone CJ, Hallam PJ, Tuddenham EG, et al: Severe perinatal thrombosis in double and triple heterozygous offspring of a family segregating two independent protein S mutations and a protein C mutation. *Blood* 87:3731-3737, 1996.
18. Schild RL, Lobb MO, Voke JM: Hereditary thrombophilia in a family with three independent protein S and protein C mutations. A cause of adverse perinatal outcome. *Eur J Obstet Gynecol Reprod Biol* 80:283-285, 1998.
19. De Klerk OL, de Vries TW, Sinnige LGF: An unusual cause of neonatal seizures in a newborn infant. *Pediatrics* 100:E8, 1997.
20. Deally C, Hancock BJ, Giddins N, et al: Primary antiphospholipid syndrome: A cause of catastrophic shunt thrombosis in the newborn. *J Cardiovasc Surg (Torino)* 40:261-264, 1999.

21. Baca V, Garcia-Ramirez R, Ramirez-Lacayo M, et al: Cerebral infarction and antiphospholipid syndrome in children. *J Rheumatol* 23:1428-1431, 1996.
22. DeVeber G, Monagle P, Chan A, et al: Prothrombotic disorders in infants and children with cerebral thromboembolism. *Arch Neurol* 55:1539-1543, 1998.
23. Nowak-Göttl U, Sträter R, Heinecke A, et al: Lipoprotein (a) and genetic polymorphisms of clotting factor V, prothrombin, and methylenetratrahydrofolate reductase are risk factors of spontaneous ischemic stroke in childhood. *Blood* 94:3678-3682, 1999.
24. Andrew M, David M, Adams M, et al: Venous thromboembolic complications (VTE) in children: First analyses of the Canadian Registry of VTE. *Blood* 83:1251-1257, 1994.
25. Kraaijenhagen RA, Anker PS, Koopman MMW, et al: High plasma concentration of factor VIIIc is a major risk factor for venous thromboembolism. *Thromb Haemost* 83:5-9, 2000.
26. Kyrle PA, Minar E, Hirschl M, et al: High plasma levels of factor VIII and the risk of recurrent venous thromboembolism. *N Engl J Med* 343:457-462, 2000.
27. Dahlbäck B, Carlsson M, Svensson PJ: Familial thrombophilia due to a previously unrecognized mechanism characterized by poor anticoagulant response to activated protein C: Prediction of a cofactor to activated protein C: *Proc Natl Acad Sci U S A* 90:1004-1008, 1993.
28. Rosendaal FR, Koster T, Vandenbroucke JP, et al: High risk of thrombosis in patients homozygous for factor V Leiden (activated protein C resistance). *Blood* 85:1504-1508, 1995.
29. Sifontes M, Nuss R, Jacobson L, et al: Thrombosis in otherwise well children with the factor V Leiden mutation. *J Pediatr* 128:324-328, 1996.
30. Sifontes MT, Nuss R, Hunger SP, et al: Activated protein C resistance and the factor V Leiden mutation in children with thrombosis. *Am J Hematol* 57:29-32, 1998.
31. Zenz W, Bodó Z, Plotho J, et al: Factor V Leiden and prothrombin gene G 20210 A variant in children with ischemic stroke. *Thromb Haemost* 80:763-766, 1998.
32. Harum KH, Hon AH Jr, Kato GJ, et al: Homozygous factor-V mutation as a genetic cause of perinatal thrombosis and cerebral palsy. *Dev Med Child Neurol* 41:777-780, 1999.
33. Gorbe E, Nagy B, Varadi V, et al: Mutation in the factor V gene associated with inferior vena cava thrombosis in newborns. *Clin Genet* 55:65-66, 1999.
34. Newman RS, Spear GS, Kirschbaum N: Postmortem DNA diagnosis of factor V Leiden in a neonate with systemic thrombosis and probable antithrombin deficiency. *Obstet Gynecol* 92:702-705, 1998.
35. Kodish E, Potter C, Kirschbaum NE, et al: Activated protein C resistance in a neonate with venous thrombosis. *J Pediatr* 127:645-648, 1995.

36. Pohl M, Zimmerhackl LB, Heinen F, et al: Bilateral retinal vein thrombosis and venous sinus thrombosis in a neonate with factor V mutation (FV Leiden). *J Pediatr* 132:159-161, 1998.
37. Schobess R, Junker R, Auberger K, et al: Factor V G1691 A and prothrombin G20210A in childhood spontaneous venous thrombosis: Evidence of an age-dependent thrombotic onset in carriers of factor V G1691A and prothrombin G20210A mutation. *Eur J Pediatr* 158:105S-108S, 1999.
38. Kraus FT, Acheen VI: Fetal thrombotic vasculopathy in the placenta: Cerebral thrombi and infarcts, coagulopathies, and cerebral palsy. *Hum Pathol* 30:759-769, 1999.
39. Poort SR, Rosendaal FR, Reitsma PH, et al: A common genetic variation in the 3' untranslated region of the prothrombin gene is associated with elevated prothrombin levels and an increase in venous thrombosis. *Blood* 88:3698-3703, 1996.
40. Zivelin A, Rosenberg N, Faier S, et al: A single genetic origin for the common prothrombotic G20210A polymorphism in the prothrombin gene. *Blood* 92:1119-1124, 1998.
41. Meijers JC, Tekelenburg WL, Bouma BN, et al: High levels of coagulation factor XI as a risk factor for venous thrombosis. *N Engl J Med* 342:696-701, 2000.
42. Van Hylckama VA, van der Linden IK, Bertina RM, et al: High levels of factor IX increase the risk of venous thrombosis. *Blood* 95:3678-3682, 2000.
43. Girelli D, Russo C, Ferraresi P, et al: Polymorphisms in the factor VII gene and the risk of myocardial infarction in patients with coronary artery disease. *N Engl J Med* 343:774-780, 2000.
44. Zeerleder S, Schloesser M, Redondo M, et al: Reevaluation of the incidence of thromboembolic complications in congenital factor XII deficiency. *Thromb Haemost* 82:1240-1246, 1999.
45. Egeberg O: Inherited antithrombin deficiency causing thrombophilia. *Thromb Diath Haemorrh* 13:516-530, 1965.
46. Lane DA, Bayston R, Olds RJ, et al: Antithrombin mutation database: 2nd (1997) update. *Thromb Haemost* 77:197-211, 1997.
47. Esmon CT, Ding W, Yasuhiro K, et al: The protein C pathway: New insights. *Thromb Haemost* 78:70-74, 1997.
48. Dahlbäck B: Purification of human C4b-binding protein and formation of its complex with vitamin K–dependent protein S. *Biochem J* 209:847, 1983.
49. Makris M, Leach M, Beauchamp NJ, et al: Genetic analysis, phenotype diagnosis and risk of venous thrombosis in families with inherited deficiencies of protein S. *Blood* 15:1935-1941, 2000.
50. Schwarz HP, Muntean W, Watzke H, et al: Low total protein S antigen but high protein S activity due to decreased C4b-binding protein in neonates. *Blood* 71:562-565, 1988.
51. Frenkel EP, Bick RL: Prothrombin G20210A gene mutation, heparin cofactor II defects, primary (essential) thrombocythemia, and throm-

bohemorrhagic manifestations. *Semin Thromb Hemost* 25:375-386, 1999.
52. Kleesiek K, Schmidt M, Götting C, et al: The 536C→T Transition in the human tissue factor pathway inhibitor (TFPI) gene is statistically associated with a higher risk for venous thrombosis.
53. Öhlin A-K, Norlund L, Marlar MR: Thrombomodulin gene variations and thromboembolic disease. *Thromb Haemost* 78:396-400, 1997.
54. Hong JJ, Kwaan HC: Hereditary defects in fibrinolysis associated with thrombosis. *Semin Thromb Hemost* 25:321-331, 1999.
55. Matsuda M, Sugo R, Yoshida N, et al: Structure and function of fibrinogen: Insights from dysfibrinogenemias. *Thromb Haemost* 82:283-290, 1999.
56. Wilcken DEL, Dudman NPB: Mechanisms of thrombogenesis and accelerated atherogenesis in homocysteinaemia. *Haemostasis* 19:14S-23S, 1989.
57. Heijer MD, Koster R, Blom HJ, et al: Hyperhomocysteinemia as a risk factor for deep-vein thrombosis. *N Engl J Med* 334:759-762, 1996.
58. Balasa VV, Gruppo RA, Glueck CJ, et al: The relationship of mutations in the MTHFR, prothrombin, and PAI-1 genes to plasma levels of homocysteine, prothrombin and PAI-1 in children and adults. *Thromb Haemost* 81:739-744, 1999.
59. Gaustadnes M, Rüdiger N, Rasmussen K, et al: Intermediate and severe hyperhomocysteinemia with thrombosis: A study of genetic determinants. *Thromb Haemost* 83:554-558, 2000.
60. Kluijtmans LAJ, den Heijer M, Reitsma PH, et al: Thermolabile methylenetetrahydrofolate reductase and factor V Leiden in the risk of deep-vein thrombosis. *Thromb Haemost* 79:254-258, 1998.
61. Danesh J, Collins R, Peto R: Lipoprotein(a) and coronary heart disease: Meta-analysis of prospective studies. *Circulation* 102:1082-1085, 2000.
62. Nowak-Göttl U, Junker R, Hartmeier M, et al: Increased lipoprotein (a) is an important risk factor for venous thromboembolism in childhood. *Circulation* 100:743-748, 1999.
63. Nowak-Göttl U, Sträter R, Heinecke A, et al: Lipoprotein(a) and genetic polymorphisms of clotting factors V, prothrombin, and methylenetetrahydrofolate reductase are risk factors of spontaneous ischemic stroke in childhood. *Blood* 94:3678-3682, 1999.
64. Manco-Johnson MJ, Nuss R: Lupus anticoagulant in children with thrombosis. *Am J Hematol* 48:240-243, 1995.
65. Nuss, R, Hays T, Chudgar U, et al: Antiphospholipid antibodies and coagulation regulatory protein abnormalities in children with pulmonary emboli. *J Pediatr Hematol Oncol* 19:202-207, 1997.
66. Brandt J, Triplett D, Alving B, et al: Criteria for the diagnosis of lupus anticoagulants: An update. *Thromb Haemost* 74:1185-1190, 1995.
67. Hughes GRV, Harris EN, Gharavi AE: The anticardiolipin syndrome. *J Rheumatol* 133:486-489, 1986.
68. Manco-Johnson MJ, Nuss R, Key N, et al: Lupus anticoagulant and

protein S deficiency in children with postvaricella purpura fulminans or thrombosis. *J Pediatr* 128:319- 323, 1996.

69. Ruiz-Arguelles GJ, Ruiz-Arguelles A, Deleze M, et al: Acquired protein C deficiency in a patient with primary antiphospholipid syndrome. Relationship to reactivity of anticardiolipin antibody with thrombomodulin. *J Rheumatol* 16:381- 383, 1989.
70. Garbrecht F, Gardner S, Johnson V, et al: Deep vein thrombosis in a child with nephrotic syndrome associated with a circulating anticoagulant and acquired protein S deficiency. *Am J Pediatr Hematol Oncol* 13:330-333, 1991.
71. Korte W, Otremba H, Lutz S, et al: Childhood stroke at three years of age with transient protein C deficiency, familial antiphospholipid antibodies and F XII deficiency: A family study. *Neuropediatrics* 25:290-294, 1994.
72. Prince HM, Thurlow PJ, Buchanan RC, et al: Acquired protein S deficiency in a patient with systemic lupus erythematosus causing central retinal vein thrombosis. *J Clin Pathol* 48:387-389, 1995.
73. Van Ommen CH, Fijnvandraat K, Vulsma R, et al: Acquired protein S deficiency caused by estrogen treatment of tall stature. *J Pediatr* 135:477-481, 1999.
74. Ranze O, Ranze P, Magnani HN, et al: Heparin-induced thrombocytopenia in paediatric patients: A review of the literature and a new case treated with danaparoid sodium. *Eur J Pediatr* 158:130S-133S, 1999.
75. Spadone D, Clark F, James E, et al: Heparin-induced thrombocytopenia in the newborn. *J Vasc Surg* 15:306-312, 1992.
76. Butler TJ, Sodoma LJ, Doski JJ, et al: Heparin-associated thrombocytopenia and thrombosis as the cause of a fatal thrombus on extracorporeal membrane oxygenation. *J Pediatr Surg* 32:768-771, 1997.

CHAPTER 13

Iron Deficiency Anemia

Alexander K. C. Leung, MBBS, FRCPC, FRCP(UK & Ire), FRCPCH
Clinical Associate Professor of Pediatrics, The University of Calgary; Pediatric Consultant, Alberta Children's Hospital, Alberta, Canada

Ka Wah Chan, MBBS, FRCPC
Professor of Pediatrics, The University of Texas M.D. Anderson Cancer Center, Houston

ABSTRACT

Iron deficiency anemia is the most common cause of anemia worldwide and results from inadequate iron supply for erythropoiesis. Iron deficiency is most prevalent during periods of rapid body growth: in infancy and again at puberty. Insufficient intake accounts for most cases. The clinical manifestations of iron deficiency anemia can be subtle, but irreversible delayed psychomotor development may occur if the anemia is severe and prolonged. The optimal approach is prevention and early treatment.

Iron deficiency is the most common nutritional deficiency and the leading cause of anemia in children.[1] When present in early childhood, especially if severe and prolonged, iron deficiency can adversely affect behavior and psychomotor development.[2] These effects may not always be fully reversible even with complete correction of the iron deficiency.[3,4] In recent years, its prevalence has declined and the methods of laboratory diagnosis have become more precise. This article reviews the epidemiology, etiology, clinical manifestations, diagnosis, and management of iron deficiency anemia, as well as strategies for its prevention.

DEFINITION

Iron deficiency denotes a deficit in total-body iron, resulting from iron requirements that exceed iron supply. Three successive stages of iron deficiency may be distinguished. Storage iron deficiency

TABLE 1.
Estimated Normal Mean Values and Lower Limits of Normal (95% Range) for Hemoglobin, Hematocrit, Mean Corpuscular Volume *(MCV)*, and Mean Corpuscular Hemoglobin *(MCH)*

	Hemoglobin (g/L)		Hct (%)		MCV (fL)		MCH (pg)	
Age (y)	**Mean**	**Lower Limit**	**Mean**	**Lower Limit**	**Mean**	**Lower Limit**	**Mean**	**Lower Limit**
0.5-4	125	110	36	32	80	72	28	24
5-10	130	115	38	33	83	75	29	25
11-14F	135	120	39	34	85	77	29	26
11-14M	140	120	41	35	85	77	29	26
15-19F	135	120	40	34	88	79	30	27
15-19M	150	130	43	37	88	79	30	27
20-44F	135	120	40	35	90	80	31	27
20-44M	155	135	45	39	90	80	31	27

(Adapted from Dallman PR, Shannon K: Developmental changes in red blood cell production and function, in Rudolph AM, Hoffman JF, Rudolph CD (eds): *Rudolph's Pediatrics*. Stamford, Conn, Appleton & Lange, 1996, pp 1170.)

develops first and is recognized by a decreased serum ferritin concentration in the absence of other biochemical evidence of iron deficiency. Next, erythropoiesis becomes affected, although the values of hemoglobin (Hb) remain within the normal range. The stage is characterized by a low serum ferritin concentration, low serum iron concentration, and low serum transferrin saturation. Finally, anemia occurs when the supply of iron to the bone marrow is sufficiently impaired to cause a clear decrease in Hb concentration to below the 5th percentile of the reference range for age and sex. The limits of normal at various ages for Hb, hematocrit (Hct), mean corpuscular volume (MCV), and mean corpuscular Hb (MCH) are shown in Table 1.

IRON METABOLISM

Iron is essential for the adequate functioning of all cells. Iron compounds that serve known metabolic functions account for about 70% to 90% of the total iron in the body.[5] The remaining 10% to 30% is stored primarily in the reticuloendothelial cells of the bone marrow, liver, and spleen as ferritin, a labile and readily accessible source of iron. Some is stored in an insoluble form as hemosiderin. Storage iron exists primarily in ferric salt–protein complexes.

Term infants have approximately 75 mg of elemental iron per kilogram of body weight, two thirds of it as Hb.[6] Total-body iron changes very little during the first 4 months of life. Although blood volume increases, Hb concentration decreases during this time. Thereafter, approximately 1 mg of iron must be absorbed each day during childhood to maintain a positive iron balance for growth and to replace basal losses.[7] Because absorption of dietary iron is approximately 10%, a diet containing at least 10 mg of iron daily is necessary for optimal nutrition.

Iron is absorbed mainly in the duodenum and upper jejunum.[8] It is transported in blood by transferrin to erythroid precursor cells in the bone marrow.[9] The amount that is absorbed by the small intestine is tightly regulated.

Iron absorption increases when the body's iron stores are low. On the other hand, when iron stores are high, much of the iron that is taken up by the mucosal cells is returned into the intestinal lumen by desquamation. An increased rate of erythrocyte production also enhances the intestinal uptake of iron.[10] Iron absorption is also higher during pregnancy. Heme and nonheme iron are the 2 major sources of iron in the diet. Heme iron found in meat, poultry, and fish is highly bioavailable.[11] It is 2 to 3 times more absorbable than nonheme iron.[11] Within the intestinal mucosal cell, an enzyme splits heme and releases ionic iron to the circulation. Iron is then shuttled to cells active in the synthesis of iron-containing proteins by transferrin. Nonheme iron is found in plant-based foods, eggs, and iron-fortified foods,[12] primarily in the form of ferric complexes. In the process of digestion, the iron is reduced from the ferric to the ferrous form, which is more readily absorbed. The absorption of nonheme iron is enhanced by ascorbic acid, and hydrochloric acid in the gastric juice, and inhibited by phytates (in bran), polyphenols (in certain vegetables and legumes), tannins (in tea), calcium, and phosphate (in high concentration in unmodified cow's milk).[10,11,13]

The percentage of iron absorbed from a cow's milk formula decreases as the concentration increases, so that 6% of iron is absorbed from a formula containing 6 mg of iron per liter, compared with only 4% from a formula containing 12 mg of iron per liter.[13]

EPIDEMIOLOGY

The prevalence of iron deficiency anemia varies widely depending on a variety of factors such as the age, ethnic composition, socioeconomic status, dietary habits, and the criteria used to establish the diagnosis. In general, iron deficiency anemia is most common among children aged 6 months to 3 years.[14,15] The prevalence drops among school-age children but increases again during adolescence. Iron deficiency anemia is more common among children living in poverty, in blacks, and in areas with endemic parasitic infestation. In the United States, its prevalence has declined in the past 3 decades. In the early 1970s, iron deficiency anemia affected as many as 30% to 76% of children 1 to 2 years of age who attended public health clinics.[16,17] Between 1975 and 1985, the prevalence of iron deficiency anemia in children younger than 2 years decreased from 8% to 14%, to 3%.[18,19] The third National Health and Nutrition Examination Survey, conducted during 1988-1994, showed that 3% or less of children younger than 2 years and less than 1% of children aged 3 to 5 years had iron deficiency anemia.[20] These trends most likely reflect the widespread use of iron-fortified infant formulas and cereals and the increasing popularity of breast-feeding.

ETIOLOGY

The various causes of iron deficiency anemia are listed in Table 2.

INCREASED PHYSIOLOGIC DEMANDS

Rapid Growth

Growth is particularly rapid during the first 2 years of life and again during adolescence. Iron deficiency anemia may result

TABLE 2.
Causes of Iron Deficiency Anemia

A. Increased physiologic demands
   1. Rapid growth
   2. Menstruation
   3. Pregnancy
B. Inadequate iron intake
C. Malabsorption
D. Blood loss
   1. Gastrointestinal
   2. Genitourinary
   3. Pulmonary
   4. Iatrogenic
   5. Perinatal hemorrhage
E. Defective plasma iron transport

unless there is a corresponding increase in iron uptake. In a term infant, the body weight triples and the blood volume doubles in the first year of life.[21] Because of the abundance of iron stores at birth, iron deficiency anemia is uncommon before 6 months of age. Preterm infants and twins have lower iron stores at birth. Because of a more rapid growth rate and more rapid expansion of the blood volume, their iron stores may be depleted by 2 to 3 months of age.

A second growth spurt occurs during adolescence, with rapid expansion of blood volume and body mass. The iron requirement is increased to maintain positive balance.

Menstruation

Menstruation is a common cause of iron deficiency anemia in adolescent girls. The average menstrual blood loss is about 40 mL (20 mg iron) per period. However, in 10% of females, menstrual blood loss exceeds 80 mL per period.[22] The use of an intrauterine device further increases menstrual blood loss.[23]

Pregnancy

During pregnancy, an additional 680 mg of iron is required for the expansion of maternal blood volume and diversion of iron to the fetus for erythropoiesis.[21] Most of this need occurs in the third trimester. Blood loss at delivery may result in another 150 to 200 mg of iron loss.[24] Although menstruation ceases and iron absorption increases, most pregnant women who do not take iron supplements become anemic. This problem is especially exaggerated with teen pregnancy.

INADEQUATE IRON INTAKE

A diet poor in iron is a major contributing factor to the development of iron deficiency anemia. Both breast milk and cow's milk are notoriously poor in iron, containing less than 0.3 to 1 mg/L. Iron in breast milk is highly bioavailable, possibly because of the lower calcium content and the presence of lactoferrin.[13] Approximately 50% of the iron in the breast milk is absorbed, in contrast to about 10% of that in cow's milk.[4] Nevertheless, prolonged exclusive breast-feeding without iron supplementation may also lead to iron deficiency anemia in 30% of these infants at 12 months of age.[25] The usual dietary pattern of infants with iron deficiency anemia is consumption of large amounts of milk not supplemented with iron.[7] In adolescence, lack of nutrition knowledge, concern about body image, and food fads lead to inadequate iron intake and the development of anemia.

MALABSORPTION

Malabsorption of iron is an uncommon cause of iron deficiency anemia, except after gastrointestinal surgery and in malabsorption syndromes such as tropical and nontropical sprue.[26] Rarely, impaired iron absorption and utilization may be inherited as an autosomal recessive trait.[27,28]

BLOOD LOSS

Gastrointestinal

Iron deficiency anemia may develop in children with cow's milk allergy secondary to gastrointestinal blood loss.[29] Blood loss may be caused by milk-induced enterocolitis, milk-induced colitis, allergic eosinophilic gastroenteritis, and Heiner syndrome. Ziegler et al[30] randomly assigned 52 infants at 168 days of age to receive either cow's milk or a milk-based formula. With the feeding of cow's milk, the proportion of guaiac-positive stools increased from 3% at baseline to 30% during the first 28 days of the trial ($P < .01$), whereas the proportion of guaiac-positive stools remained low (5%) with the feeding of formula. Fomon et al[31] found that 15 (40%) of 38 children aged 4 to 7 months fed pasteurized cow's milk compared with 4 (9%) of 43 children fed nutritional supplement (Enfamil) or heat-treated cow's milk had occult blood in the stool ($P < .001$). It has been suggested that a heat-labile protein in the milk such as lactalbumin is responsible for the intestinal bleeding.[32]

Iron deficiency anemia may also result from Meckel diverticulum, peptic ulcer, intestinal polyp, intestinal hemangioma, hereditary hemorrhagic telangiectasia, and inflammatory bowel disease. Hookworm infestation is an important cause of intestinal blood loss in some geographic areas.[33,34]

Conversely, severe iron deficiency may lead to histologic changes in the mucosal lining of the intestinal tract with resultant occult bleeding. Iron deficiency may also induce an enteropathy, or leaky gut syndrome, further aggravating the anemia.[35]

Genitourinary

Menorrhagia may lead to iron deficiency anemia. Occasionally, urinary loss of Hb may be secondary to intravascular hemolysis in paroxysmal nocturnal hemoglobinuria and in prosthetic heart valve replacement.[24] Rarely, iron deficiency anemia may result from hematuria.

Pulmonary

Iron deficiency anemia resulting from hemoptysis is uncommon. It can be seen in idiopathic pulmonary hemosiderosis or Goodpasture syndrome.[5] The pulmonary macrophages ingest and degrade the red blood cells and store the iron derived from the heme as hemosiderin.[21,36] As pulmonary macrophages are isolated from the circulation, iron trapped within these cells is effectively lost to the body metabolism.[36]

Iatrogenic

Iron deficiency anemia may result from frequent phlebotomies or excessive blood donations. Patients undergoing hemodialysis are particularly at risk because of blood loss into the dialysis machine and tubing, regular blood sampling, and occult bleeding from the gastrointestinal tract.[37]

Perinatal Hemorrhage

Iron deficiency anemia may be secondary to perinatal hemorrhage such as fetal-maternal transfusion, fetal-to-fetal transfusion, and bleeding from the placenta. Early clamping of the umbilical cord reduces the newborn's iron content by 15% to 30%.[38,39]

DEFECTIVE PLASMA IRON TRANSPORT

Very rarely, iron deficiency anemia may result from congenital atransferrinemia or defective transferrins.[36,40] In congenital atransferrinemia, the iron that is absorbed is either free in the circulation or loosely bound to other plasma proteins. The condition is inherited as an autosomal recessive disorder.[21] Much of the iron is taken up by the liver because such uptake is not mediated by transferrin.[36] However, the uptake of iron by normoblasts is insufficient because such a process is mediated by transferrin. Defective transferrin molecules are extremely rare. However, when they do occur, the defective transferrins disrupt the delivery of iron to the bone marrow with resultant iron deficiency anemia.[36]

CLINICAL MANIFESTATIONS

The symptoms and signs of iron deficiency anemia are varied and often nonspecific. The prominence of the symptoms and signs depends on both the degree and the rate of development of the anemia. Pallor is the most frequent presenting feature. In mild to moderate iron deficiency anemia, weakness, easy fatigability, dizziness, irritability, and anorexia may be seen. In severe iron deficiency anemia, diaphoresis, dyspnea, tachycardia, soft ejection systolic flow murmurs, and cardiomegaly may occur.[41] Because the anemia is often of insidious onset and prolonged duration, adaptive circulatory and respiratory responses may minimize these manifestations.[9] Children can often tolerate Hb concentrations of 30 to 40 g/L with remarkably few symptoms, unless an intercurrent infection triggers tachycardia and cardiac decompensation. The spleen is palpable in 10% to 15% of patients.[7] Retinal hemorrhages and exudates may be seen in patients with severe iron deficiency anemia.[24] In long-standing cases, widening of the diploë of the skull may occur because of an expansion of the medullary space by the bone marrow.[7]

CONDITIONS ASSOCIATED WITH IRON DEFICIENCY

Iron deficiency may also produce clinical manifestations independent of anemia. Headache, paresthesia, angular stomatitis, glossitis, postcricoid eosphageal web or stricture, and gastric atrophy are caused presumably by iron deficiency within tissue cells.[21,36] A rare complication of iron deficiency is the Plummer-Vinson or Patterson-Kelly syndrome, which is characterized by postcricoid esophageal web, glossitis, and dysphagia.[36,42] In chronic severe iron deficiency, atrophy of the skin and koilonychia (spoon-shaped nails) may result.[9] The blue sclerae seen in children with iron deficiency is caused by impairment of collagen synthesis with resultant thinning of the sclerae.

Numerous studies have shown that iron deficiency anemia in children, especially during the first 2 years of life, is associated with delayed psychomotor development.[43-45] It has been postulated that either iron deficiency causes low brain iron and reduced neurotransmitter levels, or the systemic effects of hypoxia directly affect cognition.[46] Usually, no impairment in cognitive functions is detected in iron deficiency of lesser severity not manifest as overt anemia.[47] The severity and duration of anemia correlate with poorer performance. Delays in mental development may not always be fully reversible with iron therapy.[3,44] Walter et al[44] followed up 196 healthy full-term Chilean infants who were randomly assigned in an iron supplementation study. At 1 year of age, 39 infants were found to be anemic, 127 nonanemic but iron deficient, and 30 healthy (controls). Anemic infants had significantly lower developmental scores than did control infants or nonanemic iron-deficient infants. Control infants and nonanemic iron-deficient infants performed comparably. Correction of anemia or even complete reversal of iron status to normal values with iron therapy for 3 months did not yield improvement of cognitive abilities in the anemic group. Lozoff et al[43] conducted a study on 191 Costa Rican infants, 12 to 23 months of age, with various degrees of iron deficiency. Infants with moderate iron deficiency anemia (Hb, ≤ 100 g/L) had lower mental and motor test scores than did appropriate controls. Infants with mild anemia (Hb, 101-105 g/L) had lower motor but not mental scores. Infants with lesser degrees of iron deficiency did not have impairments in developmental test performance. After 3 months of iron therapy, lower mental and motor test scores were no longer observed among iron-deficient anemic infants whose anemia and iron deficiency were both corrected (36%). However, significantly lower mental and motor test scores persisted among most initially anemic infants (64%) who had more severe or chronic iron deficiency. Of the 196 children, 163 (85%) were re-evaluated at 5 years of age.[3] All the children had excellent hematologic status and growth. However, children who had moderately severe iron deficiency anemia as infants (Hb, ≤ 100 g/L) had lower scores on tests of mental and motor functioning than the rest of the children. Idjradinata and Pollitt[45] conducted a randomized, double-blind study with infants 12 to 18 months of age (50 iron deficient and anemic, 29 nonanemic but iron deficient, and 47 iron sufficient) in Indonesia. Within each group, infants were randomly assigned to receive dietary ferrous sulfate or placebo for 4 months. Before intervention, the mean mental and motor scores of the iron-deficient anemic infants were significantly lower than those of the nonanemic iron-deficient and iron-sufficient classes. After intervention, developmental delays were reversed among iron-deficient anemic infants who had received iron, but they remained unchanged among placebo-treated iron-deficient anemic infants. Neither ferrous sulfate nor placebo had significant effects on the scores of the other two iron status classes. Further studies are necessary to determine the effects of the severity, chronicity, and the time of onset of the anemia, as well as the duration of treatment, on the reversibility of cognitive function later in life.

It is generally believed that severely iron-deficient children are irritable, apathetic, and have a short-attention span.[21] Oski et al[48] observed that iron-deficient nonanemic infants were less irritable, more perseverant, easier to engage in play, and less solemn after treatment with parenteral iron. Lozoff et al[49] compared the behavior of 52 Costa Rican children, aged 12 to 23 months, who had iron deficiency anemia with that of 139 children without iron deficiency anemia. These investigators found that children with iron deficiency anemia maintained closer contact with caregivers;

showed less pleasure and delight; were more wary, hesitant, and easily tired; made fewer attempts at test items; were less attentive to instructions and demonstrations; and were less playful. Such behaviors could make it more difficult for children with iron deficiency anemia to learn from their environments. Ballin et al[50] treated 29 girls, aged 16 and 17 years, with a syrup that contained 105 mg of elementary ferrous iron and 30 girls with a placebo liquid daily for 2 months. By the end of the study, a statistically significant improvement in lassitude, the ability to concentrate in school, and mood was reported by the girls who ingested iron compared with the controls. Seventy-five percent, 100%, and 65% of the girls, respectively, who reported improvement in the above-mentioned characteristics, were hypoferremic initially and became normoferremic by the end of the study.

Chronic severe iron deficiency is often associated with reduced growth rate, especially among preschool children.[51] Although both conditions may be secondary to an overall nutritional deficiency, several studies have shown that iron supplementation improves physical growth in anemic children independent of their nutritional status.[52-54] Chwang et al[52] investigated the effect of oral iron supplementation on physical growth in 119 rural Indonesian schoolchildren in a double-blind study. The children were classified into anemic (n = 78) and normal (n = 41) groups according to their initial Hb and transferrin saturation levels and were randomly assigned to either iron or placebo treatment. Before treatment, anemic children were smaller than nonanemic children. Treatment with ferrous sulfate, 10 mg/kg per day for 12 weeks, resulted in a significant improvement in anemic children's hematologic status and growth velocity. The direct action of iron on oxidative processes and alleviation of the irritability and anorexia associated with iron deficiency may be responsible for the stimulated growth rate.[51,53]

Iron deficiency anemia impairs exercise capacity in adults and possibly in children as well. The impairment is roughly proportional to the degree of anemia. Gardner et al[55] studied 75 women who worked on a tea estate in Sri Lanka. These women performed a standard, multistage treadmill test in which the speed and grade were gradually increased for a maximum period of 18 minutes. Eleven women with an Hb concentration of 130 g/L or greater all completed the exercise task. In contrast, 5 women with an Hb concentration between 60 and 70 g/L were all unable to reach the peak workload. The work time of those women with an Hb concentration between 110 and 119 g/L was 20% less than that of women with an

Hb concentration of 130 g/L or greater. Edgerton et al[56] studied the quantity of tea picked per day by 199 tea estate workers in Sri Lanka before and after iron supplementation or treatment with a placebo. These investigators found a significant increase in productivity among those workers whose initial Hb concentration was between 60 and 90 g/L and who were treated with iron. Likewise, Viteri and Torún[57] showed decreased performance among anemic agriculture laborers in Guatemala. Within 1 month, performance was substantially improved in the iron-treated group compared with the placebo-treated group. Rowland et al[58] studied 14 non-anemic iron-deficient female adolescent runners. Treadmill endurance times improved significantly in the iron-treated runners compared with the controls. Bhatia and Seshadri[59] described poorer work capacity in a group of 8- to 12-year-old anemic Indian boys ($n = 52$) compared with nonanemic controls ($n = 52$). The anemic children made significantly fewer jumps than did the nonanemic controls (71 vs 96, $P < .001$). The number of anemic children who could persist in the task started declining at the sixth minute, and there was a significant reduction in the number continuing to jump at the ninth minute in the anemic group, whereas for the nonanemic group, there was no appreciable reduction at this time.

The association of pica with iron deficiency is well documented. Geophagia or compulsive eating of dirt is more common in children with iron deficiency, whereas pagophagia or compulsive eating of ice is more common in adults with iron deficiency.[21] It can be argued that pica may induce iron deficiency by replacing dietary iron sources or inhibiting the absorption of iron. Clays bind iron in the gastrointestinal tract, resulting in its poor absorption.[36] However, considerable evidence suggests that iron deficiency is usually the cause and pica the consequence.[60] Iron therapy is characteristically followed by an abrupt loss of interest in dirt eating.[61] Iron deficiency anemia may contribute to lead poisoning in children by increasing the intestinal absorption of lead.[62]

In chronic severe iron deficiency, the intestinal function may be impaired with decreased absorption of fat and xylose.[5] Conversely, iron deficiency may result from a malabsorptive disease.

Existing research has yielded conflicting data regarding the role of iron in host response to infection.[63,64] On the one hand, iron deficiency is known to adversely affect immune functions by causing decreased myeloperoxidase activity, reduced bactericidal capacity, a quantitative decrease in the number of circulating T cells, impaired mitogenic response, and poor natural killer activity.[21,65] On the other hand, unsaturated transferrin has been shown to inhibit the growth of bacteria in vitro.[21] Clinical studies have also yielded controversial results, except for very specific infections such as malaria and brucellosis, for which iron deficiency may have a protective effect.[64,66] Further studies are necessary before this important issue can be elucidated. Conversely, recurrent infections may impair iron absorption and predispose to iron deficiency.[67] The relation is further confounded by environmental and socioeconomic variables that may predispose to both anemia and infection.[51]

A causal relationship between iron deficiency anemia and breath-holding spells has been recognized.[68-70] Bhatia et al[68] found that children with breath-holding spells (n = 50) in an outpatient immunization clinic had significantly lower Hb and serum iron levels than did a control group (n = 50) ($P < .001$). These investigators further demonstrated that all anemic children with breath-holding spells had a decrease in severity and frequency of breath-holding spells with oral iron therapy, paralleling an increase in Hb levels to 110 g/L or greater in 82% of cases. Yilmaz and Kukner[70] found iron deficiency anemia in 51 of 86 patients aged 6 to 24 months who were admitted to a pediatric neurology department with breath-holding spells. The Hb levels were between 63 and 110 g/L. All the patients with anemia were given oral iron therapy at a dosage of 6 mg/kg per day. After 3 months, complete resolution of breath-holding spells was detected in 11 patients (21.5%). Thirty-seven patients (72.5%) showed a significant decrease in severity and frequency of the spells. Mocan et al[69] prospectively evaluated 91 children (56 boys, 35 girls) with breath-holding spells. In 49 of the children, the frequency of breath-holding spells was less than 10 each month, in 22 children it was 10 to 30 each month, and in 20 children it was more than 30 each month. Sixty-three children were found to have iron deficiency anemia and were treated with iron, 6 mg/kg per day for 3 months. Other patients were not given any treatment. After 3 months, 84% of the patients treated with iron showed complete or partial remission, whereas only 21% of the patients in the nontreated group improved. It is known that children with iron deficiency are more irritable and tend to have more instances of crying. These behavioral characteristics, coupled with decreased cerebral oxygen tension, may account for the increased prevalence of breath-holding spells in children with iron deficiency anemia. The role of iron in catecholamine metabolism and the functioning of enzymes and neurotransmitters in the central nervous system cannot be ignored.[69]

Iron deficiency anemia may predispose to febrile convulsions. Pisacane et al[71] compared the hematologic status of 156 children aged 6 to 24 months admitted to a hospital in Naples, Italy, with the diagnosis of febrile convulsions with that of 2 control groups. The latter consisted of a random sample of children admitted to the same ward with the diagnosis of respiratory and gastrointestinal infection during the same period, and a group of healthy children randomly selected from the provincial birth register for an iron deficiency survey in Greater Naples during 1994. They found that iron deficiency anemia was significantly more common in children with febrile convulsions (30%) than in hospital (14%) and population (12%) controls. On the other hand, Kobrinsky et al[72] prospectively evaluated 51 children who presented to a pediatric emergency department with a febrile illness with (n = 26) or without (n = 25) an associated febrile convulsion. Iron deficiency was less frequently observed in the group of children with febrile convulsions (8.7%) than in the control group (40%).

Rarely, iron deficiency anemia may lead to stroke in both the adult and pediatric populations. Hartfield et al[73] reported a series of 6 children, 6 to 18 months of age, who presented with ischemic stroke or venous thrombosis in whom iron deficiency was the only consistent positive laboratory finding after complete investigations. It has been postulated that stroke may be caused by thrombosis secondary to thrombocytosis, a hypercoagulable state, and anemic hypoxia. Rigidity of the red blood cells caused by iron deficiency anemia may also be a contributing factor.[7]

The relationship between iron deficiency anemia and an increased risk of preterm delivery has been supported by several[74,75] but not all studies.[76] In the study by Scholl et al,[75] the odds of preterm delivery were more than doubled with iron deficiency anemia, but not increased with anemia from other causes. When vaginal bleeding at or before entry to care accompanied anemia, the odds of a preterm delivery were increased 5-fold for iron deficiency anemia and doubled for other anemias.

DIAGNOSIS

Anemia caused by iron deficiency should be suspected if there is a history of poor dietary intake of iron, a history of excessive blood loss, and pallor on physical examination. If iron deficiency appears likely on clinical grounds, a therapeutic trial of iron therapy may be indicated without confirmatory tests. A therapeutic trial consists of the oral administration of 3 mg/kg per day of elemental iron as ferrous sulfate for a month.[4,14] An increase of 10 g/L or more in the Hb concentration is generally considered diagnostic of iron deficiency anemia.[4,11] However, if a child is recovering from a recent infection, the Hb level may increase spontaneously, making it difficult, if not impossible, to determine whether iron deficiency truly existed in the first place.[4] Laboratory confirmatory studies are necessary in patients who are not at high risk for nutritional deficiency, such as children between the ages of 3 and 10 years; in patients who have severe iron deficiency anemia; or in patients who fail to respond after 1 month of iron therapy.

LABORATORY FEATURES

Although a low Hb level is necessary for the diagnosis of iron deficiency anemia, anisocytosis is the earliest recognizable hematologic manifestation of iron deficiency.[4] The red blood cell distribution width (RDW), a measure of the variation in the size of erythrocytes, can be used to detect increased anisocytosis. It is calculated by dividing the standard deviation of the MCV by the MCV and multiplying by 100.[11,47] RDW values greater than 14% are consistent with iron deficiency anemia.[11] As iron deficiency progresses, the erythrocytes become smaller than normal (microcytosis), with decreased Hb content (hypochromia), and have abnormal shapes (poikilocytosis). The plasma membranes of iron-deficient erythrocytes are abnormally stiff, which may contribute to the poikilocytic changes.[36] The Hb, Hct, MCV, MCH, and mean corpuscular Hb concentration (MCHC) are lower than normal for age.

The relative number of reticulocytes is usually normal or slightly elevated. The absolute reticulocyte count, however, is often low and indicates an insufficient response to anemia.[7] Recently, reticulocyte Hb content has been shown to be very sensitive in detecting iron-deficient erythropoiesis.[1,77] When incorporated into an automated hematology analyzer, the measurement of reticulocyte Hb content is an inexpensive and rapidly available alternative to biochemical studies for the detection of iron deficiency before the onset of anemia.[78]

The white blood cell count is usually normal. The platelet count varies from thrombocytosis to thrombocytopenia. In general, thrombocytosis is more common in those patients with associated bleeding, whereas thrombocytopenia is often seen with more severe anemia.[35]

Trace amounts of ferritin are found in the serum, and its level parallels the iron stores in the body. It is a sensitive indicator of early iron deficiency and is not affected by diurnal variation. A serum ferritin level in the range of 10 to 20 μg/L indicates depletion of iron stores; a level less than 10 μg/L is diagnostic of iron deficiency. The serum ferritin level may be elevated in infectious, inflammatory, malignant, or hepatic disease.[9,21] However, a level greater than 50 μg/L argues against the diagnosis of iron deficiency, even in the presence of other conditions that may cause an elevation of the serum ferritin level.[79] The serum ferritin level increases rapidly to normal when iron therapy is started, long before iron stores are fully restored.

Serum iron levels have a low diagnostic value. There is normally a diurnal variation in the serum iron concentration, with higher values in the morning and lower values at night.[24,80] The serum iron concentration also decreases in the presence of menstruation, inflammation, or malignancy.[24] The total iron-binding capacity (TIBC) reflects the total amount of transferrin available in the blood, normally ranging from 200 to 400 μg/dL.[79] A TIBC greater than 400 μg/dL suggests iron deficiency, whereas a value less than 200 μg/dL is characteristic of an inflammatory disease. Transferrin saturation, calculated by dividing the concentration of serum iron by the TIBC and multiplying by 100 to express the result as a percentage, is generally considered the most relevant index of iron supply to the bone marrow.[21] In adults, a transferrin saturation level less than 16% is consistent with iron deficiency.[47,79] However, the lower limits of transferrin saturation in normal children are at 7% to 10%.

The serum transferrin receptor reflects the amount of specific membrane receptors that are required for iron uptake by cells. The level is elevated with increased erythropoiesis and depressed with decreased erythropoiesis with the notable exception of iron deficiency, in which it is also elevated.[5,8] The test, however, is not generally available in most laboratories.

Protoporphyrin combines with iron to form heme. As such, free erythrocyte protoporphyrin (FEP) reflects the adequacy of iron delivery to the erythroid precursors in the bone marrow. Its level is increased in disorders of heme synthesis, such as iron deficiency, lead poisoning, and sideroblastic anemia.[24] Values greater than 3 μg/g of Hb are considered abnormal.[14]

Although no single test can reliably document iron deficiency in all clinical situations, low values of Hb, MCV, and MCH, and high values of RDW and FEP provide strong supportive evidence. A serum ferritin level of less than 10 μg/L or a transferrin saturation of less than 7% provides confirmation of the diagnosis in most cases.

DIFFERENTIAL DIAGNOSIS

The differential diagnosis of a hypochromic microcytic anemia includes thalassemias and lead poisoning. The thalassemias represent a diverse group of inherited anemias of varying degrees of severity. The underlying genetic defects include total or partial deletions of globin chain genes and nucleotide substitutions, deletions, or insertions. The gene frequency of thalassemia is greatest among persons of African, Middle Eastern, and Asian descent. Thalassemia major is characterized by severe hemolysis and anemia, and the clinical presentation is easily distinguishable from iron deficiency anemia. Mild or no anemia characterizes thalassemia minor, but red blood cell morphology shows prominent hypochromia, microcytosis, and anisocytosis, out of proportion to the degree of anemia. Target cells and basophilic stippling, rarely seen in iron deficiency anemia, can be found easily in thalassemia. The serum ferritin level, the transferrin saturation, and the FEP level are normal.[1]

Confirmatory tests include Hb electrophoresis and DNA studies. The HbA_2 level is elevated in β-thalassemia minor, but the value is falsely low if iron deficiency coexists. If clinical suspicion is strong, repeated testing is necessary after iron replacement therapy. In lead poisoning, there is coarse basophilic stippling, an elevated blood lead level, and marked elevation of FEP (>18 μg/g of Hb).

The anemia of chronic disease is the result of a decreased erythropoietic response to anemia, decreased red blood cell survival, diminished reutilization of iron, impaired iron mobilization from macrophages by transferrin, and decreased intestinal absorption of iron.[21] The anemia is usually normochromic and normocytic, but hypochromic microcytic anemia occurs in 20% to 30% of cases.[24] Mild anemia, an elevated FEP level, and a low serum iron concentration can be found in both iron deficiency anemia and anemia of chronic disease. Unlike iron deficiency anemia, chronic disorders are associated with a decreased TIBC, a normal RDW, an increased serum ferritin level, and a normal serum transferrin receptor level. An elevated serum transferrin receptor level is characteristic of iron deficiency anemia irrespective of whether the patient has coexisting anemia of chronic disease.[81] The serum transferrin receptor to ferritin ratio can be used to distinguish combined anemia from that purely of inflammation. In the study by Pettersson et al,[82] the ratio was less than 50 in all patients with anemia of inflammation, but more than 50 in 11 of 13 patients with combined anemia.

MANAGEMENT

The goals of treatment of iron deficiency should be 2-fold: replenishment of body iron stores and correction of underlying disorders. Iron replacement therapy should consist of oral administration of one of the ferrous salts. Ferric salts are less well absorbed. Ferrous sulfate is usually preferred because of its low cost and high bioavailability. Ferrous sulfate is 20% elemental iron by weight. Optimal response is achieved with a dosage of elemental iron of 6 mg/kg per day in 2 to 3 divided doses. For best absorption, iron should be given between meals and not with milk. Transient staining of teeth may occur with liquid iron preparations and can be minimized by placing the medication with a dropper toward the back of the tongue.[32] Gastrointestinal side effects consist mainly of nausea, constipation, diarrhea, and abdominal pain.[79] They are uncommon and are dose related.[79] Reducing the dosage of the medication or by giving it with food minimizes these side effects. Once the Hb level is within the normal range, iron replacement should continue for 3 months to replenish iron stores.[8]

Failure to respond to oral iron therapy may be caused by poor compliance, an inadequate iron dose, an ineffective iron preparation, ongoing blood loss, coexistent disease that interferes with absorption or utilization of iron, or an incorrect diagnosis.[7,8,17]

Use of parenteral (intramuscular or intravenous) iron therapy will not increase the rate of response. Indications for its use include genuine intolerance of oral iron, compromise of gastrointestinal iron absorption, and iron losses exceeding maximal oral replacement.[8,79] Parenteral iron therapy may also be considered in patients who are noncompliant with oral administration of iron and in patients with chronic renal failure undergoing hemodialysis who are treated with erythropoietin.[8,17] The dosage of iron (mg) may be calculated by using the following formula: deficient Hb (g/L) $\times$ body weight (kg) $\times$ 0.22.[79] The most feared complication is anaphylaxis. Tolerance to parenteral iron should therefore be checked by administering a test dose of iron dextran, 0.5 mg. Other side effects of intravenous infusion of iron include nausea, vomiting, abdominal pain, flushing, fever, headache, malaise, shivering, myalgia, arthralgia, urticaria, lymphadenopathy, pleural effusion, hypotension, and shock.[79] Intramuscular injection of iron is painful and may be associated with permanent staining of the skin, muscle necrosis, and sterile abscesses.

Red blood cell transfusion should be reserved for patients with very severe anemia. Packed red blood cell transfusion should be administered slowly in an amount sufficient to raise the Hb to a safe level (about 70 g/L), at which the response to iron therapy can be awaited.[7] Children with impending cardiac decompensation (usually precipitated by fever of an intercurrent infection) may be best managed by a partial exchange transfusion with fresh erythrocytes.[17]

PREVENTION

Because growth and diet are almost always contributing factors for iron deficiency anemia in childhood, education about feeding practices in high-risk groups should prove beneficial. Primary prevention can be achieved by giving supplementary iron or by the fortification of foods. Human milk has iron that is highly bioavailable and is the preferred feeding for all infants. Nevertheless, if not given supplement, exclusively breast-fed infants remain at risk for reduced iron.[25,83] Pisacane et al[25] investigated the iron status of 30 infants who had been breast-fed until their first birthday and who had never received cow's milk, medicinal iron, or iron-enriched formula and cereals; 30% of these infants were anemic at 12 months of age. The Committee on Nutrition of the American Academy of Pediatrics recommends that iron supplementation for breast-fed infants should start at 4 to 6 months of age for full-term infants and no later than 2 months of age in preterm infants.[14] The dosage of iron should be 1 mg/kg per day for term infants. The iron requirements for preterm infants range from 2 mg/kg per day for infants with birth weights between 1500 and 2500 g, to 4 mg/kg per day for infants less than 1500 g at birth. Iron-fortified cereal and iron drops are good sources of iron. Infants who are not breast-fed or are partially breast-fed should receive an iron-fortified formula (containing 4-12 mg/L of iron) from birth to 12 months.[14] Whole cow's milk should be avoided in infants younger than 12 months of age. In addition to being a poor source of iron, cow's milk may induce occult gastrointestinal blood loss that may contribute to the development of iron deficiency anemia.[84,85] Tunnessen et al[85] followed up 2 groups of infants, one fed whole cow's milk commencing at 6 months of age (n = 69), and the other continuing to receive iron-fortified infant formula (n = 98). At 12 months of age, infants fed cow's milk had significantly lower serum ferritin levels and MCV, higher FEP values, and a greater incidence of Hb levels less than 110 g/L than did formula-fed infants. Children aged 1 to 5 years should consume no more than 24 oz of cow's milk per day.[11]

Secondary prevention involves screening for, diagnosing, and treating iron deficiency.[11] A brief, 3-component dietary history is a useful screening tool.[86] A diet of less than 5 servings each of meat, grains, vegetables, and fruit per week; more than 16 oz of milk per day; or daily intake of fatty snacks, sweets, or more than 16 oz of soft drink is considered deficient. This brief dietary history can correctly identify children 15 to 60 months of age at low risk for iron deficiency anemia 97% of the time.[86] Measurement of Hb and MCV values by electronic cell counter is the preferred laboratory test for screening.[14] In general, screening should not be done if the child has a recent or current infection during the preceding 2 to 3 weeks because this may affect the result of the screening.[87] The decision as to whom to screen should be based on the prevalence of iron deficiency in that population.[11] For children in the community at high risk for iron deficiency anemia, screening should be performed between 9 and 12 months of age, 6 months later, and annually from 2 to 5 years of age.[11] On the other hand, in populations not at high risk, only those children with known risk factors need to be screened.[11] Prematurity, low birth weight, early consumption of cow's milk, fast growth rate, a low-iron diet, limited access to food because of poverty or neglect, or special health care needs are considered the main risk factors.[11] Screening for anemia should be considered before 6 months of age for preterm and low birth weight infants who are not fed an iron-fortified infant formula.

CONCLUSION

Iron fortification of formulas and cereals has reduced the prevalence of iron deficiency anemia. This may render the patient population less well defined and its diagnosis more difficult. Worldwide iron deficiency is still the most common cause of anemia, and physicians should be cognizant of its presence in children who have come from outside the United States.

REFERENCES

1. Brugnara C, Zurakowski D, DiCanzio J, et al: Reticulocyte hemoglobin content to diagnose iron deficiency in children. *JAMA* 281:2225-2230, 1999.
2. de Andraca I, Castillo M, Walter T: Psychomotor development and behavior in iron-deficient anemic infants. *Nutr Rev* 55:125-132, 1997.
3. Lozoff B, Jimenez E, Wolf AW: Long-term developmental outcome of infants with iron deficiency. *N Engl J Med* 325:687-694, 1991.
4. Oski FA: Iron deficiency in infancy and childhood. *N Engl J Med* 329:190-193, 1993.
5. Dallman PR, Shannon K: Developmental changes in red blood cell production and function, in Rudolph AM, Hoffman JF, Rudolph CD (eds): *Rudolph's Pediatrics*. Stamford, Conn, Appleton & Lange, 1996, pp 1167-1172.
6. Committee on Nutrition, American Academy of Pediatrics: Iron fortification of infant formulas. *Pediatrics* 104:119-123, 1999.

7. Schwartz E: Iron deficiency anemia, in Behrman RE, Kliegman RM, Jenson HB (eds): *Nelson Textbook of Pediatrics.* Philadelphia, WB Saunders, 2000, pp 1469-1471.
8. Provan D: Mechanisms and management of iron deficiency anaemia. *Br J Haematol* 105:19S-26S, 1999.
9. Frewin R, Henson A, Provan D: Iron deficiency anemia. *BMJ* 314:360-363, 1997.
10. Bothwell TH: Overview and mechanisms of iron regulation. *Nutr Rev* 53:237-245, 1995.
11. CDC: Recommendations to prevent and control iron deficiency in the United States. *MMWR* 47(RR-3):1-29, 1998.
12. Hallberg L: Bioavailability of dietary iron in men. *Annu Rev Nutr* 1:123-147, 1981.
13. Booth IW, Aukett MA: Iron deficiency anaemia in infancy and early childhood. *Arch Dis Child* 76:549-554, 1997.
14. Committee on Nutrition, American Academy of Pediatrics: Iron deficiency, in Barness LA (ed): *Pediatric Nutrition Handbook.* Elk Grove Village, Ill, American Academy of Pediatrics, 1993, pp 227-236.
15. Kwiatkowski JL, West TB, Heidary N, et al: Severe iron deficiency anemia in young children. *J Pediatr* 135:514-516, 1999.
16. Andelman MB, Sered BR: Utilization of dietary iron by term infants: A study of 1,048 infants from a low socioeconomic population. *Am J Dis Child* 111:45-55, 1966.
17. Lanzkowsky P: Iron deficiency anemia. *Pediatr Ann* 3:6-33, 1974.
18. Miller V, Swaney S, Deinard A: Impact of the WIC program on the iron status of infants. *Pediatrics* 75:100-105, 1985.
19. Yip R, Walsh KM, Goldfarb MG, et al: Declining prevalence of anemia in childhood in a middle-class setting: A pediatric success story? *Pediatrics* 80:330-334, 1987.
20. Looker AC, Dallman PR, Carroll MD, et al: Prevalence of iron deficiency in the United States. *JAMA* 277:973-976, 1997.
21. Lukens JN: Iron metabolism and iron deficiency, in Miller DR, Baehner RL (eds): *Blood Diseases of Infancy and Childhood.* St Louis, Mosby, 1995, pp 193-219.
22. Cole SK, Billewicz WZ, Thomas AM: Sources of variation in menstrual blood loss. *Br J Obstet Gynaecol* 78:933-939, 1971.
23. Kivijarvi A, Timonen H, Rajamaki A, et al: Iron deficiency in women using modern copper intrauterine devices. *Obstet Gynecol* 67:95-98, 1986.
24. Fairbanks VF, Beutler E: Iron deficiency, in Beutler E, Lichtman MA, Coller BS, et al (eds): *Williams Hematology.* New York, McGraw-Hill, 1995, pp 490-511.
25. Pisacane A, deVizia B, Valiante A, et al: Iron status in breast-fed infants. *J Pediatr* 127:429-431, 1995.
26. Anand BS, Callender ST, Warner GT: Absorption of inorganic and haemoglobin iron in coeliac disease. *Br J Haematol* 37:409-414, 1977.

27. Buchanan GR, Sheehan RG: Malabsorption and defective utilization of iron in three siblings. *J Pediatr* 98:723-728, 1991.
28. Hartman KP, Barker JA: Microcytic anemia with iron malabsorption: An inherited disorder of iron metabolism. *Am J Hematol* 51:269-275, 1996.
29. Leung AK: Food allergy: A clinical approach. *Adv Pediatr* 45:145-177, 1998.
30. Ziegler EE, Fomon SJ, Nelson SE, et al: Cow milk feeding in infancy: Further observations on blood loss from the gastrointestinal tract. *J Pediatr* 116:11-18, 1990.
31. Fomon SJ, Ziegler EE, Nelson SE, et al: Cow milk feeding in infancy: Gastrointestinal blood loss and iron nutritional status. *J Pediatr* 98:540-545, 1981.
32. Dallman PR: Iron deficiency, in Rudolph AM, Hoffman JI, Rudolph CD (eds): *Rudolph's Pediatrics*. Stamford, Conn, Appleton & Lange, 1996, pp 1176-1180.
33. Olsen A, Magnussen P, Ouma JH, et al: The contribution of hookworm and other parasitic infections to haemoglobin and iron status among children and adults in western Kenya. *Trans R Soc Trop Med Hyg* 92:643-649, 1998.
34. Stoltzfus RJ, Chwaya HM, Tielsch JM, et al: Epidemiology of iron deficiency anemia in Zanzibari schoolchildren: The importance of hookworms. *Am J Clin Nutr* 65:153-159, 1997.
35. Lanzkowsky P: Iron deficiency anemia, in Lanzkowsky P (ed): *Manual of Pediatric Hematology and Oncology*. New York, Churchill Livingstone, 1995, pp 35-50.
36. Andrews NC, Bridges KR: Iron deficiency, in Nathan DG, Orkin SH (eds): *Nathan and Oski's Hematology of Infancy and Childhood*. Philadelphia, WB Saunders, 1998, pp 437-461.
37. Nissenson AR, Strobos J: Iron deficiency in patients with renal failure. *Kidney Int* 55:18S-21S, 1999.
38. Geethanath RM, Ramji S, Thirupuram S, et al: Effect of timing of cord clamping on the iron status of infants at 3 months. *Indian Pediatr* 34:103-106, 1997.
39. Grajeda R, Pérez-Escamilla R, Dewey KG: Delayed clamping of the umbilical cord improves hematologic status of Guatemalan infants at 2 mo of age. *Am J Clin Nutr* 65:425-431, 1997.
40. Goya N, Miyazaki S, Kodate S, et al: A family of congenital atransferrinemia. *Blood* 40:239-245, 1972.
41. Hetzel TM, Losek JD: Unrecognized severe anemia in children presenting with respiratory distress. *Am J Emerg Med* 16:386-389, 1998.
42. Anthony R, Sood S, Strachan DR, et al: A case of Plummer-Vinson syndrome in childhood. *J Pediatr Surg* 34:1570-1572, 1999.
43. Lozoff B, Brittenham GM, Wolf AW, et al: Iron deficiency anemia and iron therapy effects on infant developmental test performance. *Pediatrics* 79:981-995, 1987.
44. Walter T, de Andraca I, Chadud P, et al: Iron deficiency anemia:

Adverse effects on infant psychomotor development. *Pediatrics* 84:7-17, 1989.
45. Idjradinata P, Pollitt E: Reversal of developmental delays in iron-deficient anaemic infants treated with iron. *Lancet* 341:3-4, 1993.
46. Youdim MB, Ben-Shachar D, Yehuda S: Putative biological mechanisms of the effect of iron deficiency on brain biochemistry and behavior. *Am J Clin Nutr* 50:607S-615S, 1989.
47. Graham EA: The changing face of anemia in infancy. *Pediatr Rev* 15:175-183, 1994.
48. Oski FA, Honig AS, Helu B, et al: Effect of iron therapy on behavior performance in nonanemic, iron-deficient infants. *Pediatrics* 71:877-880, 1983.
49. Lozoff B, Klein NK, Nelson EC, et al: Behavior of infants with iron-deficiency anemia. *Child Dev* 69:24-36, 1998.
50. Ballin A, Berar M, Rubinstein U, et al: Iron state in female adolescents. *Am J Dis Child* 146:803-805, 1992.
51. Moy RJ, Early AR: Iron deficiency in childhood. *J R Soc Med* 92:234-236, 1999.
52. Chwang L, Soemantri AG, Pollitt E: Iron supplementation and physical growth of rural Indonesian children. *Am J Clin Nutr* 47:496-501, 1988.
53. Angeles IT, Schultink WJ, Matulessi P, et al: Decreased rate of stunting among anemic Indonesian preschool children through iron supplementation. *Am J Clin Nutr* 58:339-342, 1993.
54. Aukett MA, Parks YA, Scott PH, et al: Treatment with iron increases weight gain and psychomotor development. *Arch Dis Child* 61:849-857, 1986.
55. Gardner GW, Edgerton VR, Senewiratne B, et al: Physical work capacity and metabolic stress in subjects with iron deficiency anemia. *Am J Clin Nutr* 30:910-917, 1977.
56. Edgerton VR, Gardner GW, Ohira Y, et al: Iron-deficiency anaemia and its effect on worker productivity and activity patterns. *BMJ* 2:1546-1549, 1979.
57. Viteri FE, Torún B: Anaemia and physical work capacity. *Clin Haematol* 3:609-626, 1974.
58. Rowland TW, Deisroth MB, Green GM, et al: The effect of iron therapy on the exercise capacity of nonanemic iron-deficient adolescent runners. *Am J Dis Child* 142:165-169, 1988.
59. Bhatia D, Seshadri S: Anemia, undernutrition and physical work capacity of young boys. *Indian J Pediatr* 24:133-139, 1987.
60. Moore DF, Sears DA: Pica, iron deficiency, and the medical history. *Am J Med* 97:390-393, 1994.
61. McDonald R, Marshall SR: The value of iron therapy in pica. *Pediatrics* 34:558-562, 1964.
62. Goyer RA: Nutrition and metal toxicity. *Am J Clin Nutr* 61:646S-650S, 1995.
63. Walter T, Olivares M, Pizarro F, et al: Iron, anemia, and infection. *Nutr Rev* 55:111-124, 1997.

64. Oppenheimer SJ: Iron and infection in the tropics: Paediatric clinical correlates. *Ann Trop Med* 18:81S-87S, 1998.
65. Macdougall LG, Anderson R, McNab GM, et al: The immune response in iron-deficient children: Impaired cellular defense mechanisms with altered humoral components. *J Pediatr* 86:833-843, 1975.
66. Murray MJ, Murray AB, Murray MB, et al: The adverse effect of iron repletion on the course of certain infections. *BMJ* 2:1113-1115, 1978.
67. Reeves JD, Yip R, Kiley VA, et al: Iron deficiency in infants: The influence of mild antecedent infection. *J Pediatr* 105:874-879, 1984.
68. Bhatia MS, Singhal PK, Dhar NK, et al: Breath holding spells: An analysis of 50 cases. *Indian Pediatr* 27:1073-1079, 1990.
69. Mocan H, Yildiran A, Orhan F, et al: Breath holding spells in 91 children and response to treatment with iron. *Arch Dis Child* 81:261-262, 1999.
70. Yilmaz S, Kukner S: Anemia in children with breath-holding spells. *J Pediatr* 128:440-441, 1996.
71. Pisacane A, Sansone R, Impagliazzo N, et al: Iron deficiency anemia and febrile convulsions: Case-control study in children under 2 years. *BMJ* 313:343, 1996.
72. Kobrinsky NL, Yager JY, Cheang MS, et al: Does iron deficiency raise the seizure throhold? *J Child Neurol* 10:105-109, 1995.
73. Hartfield DS, Lowry NJ, Keene DL, et al: Iron deficiency: A cause of stroke in infants and children. *Pediatr Neurol* 16:50-53, 1997.
74. Murphy JF, Newcombe RG, O'Riordan J, et al: Relation of haemoglobin levels in first and second trimesters to outcome of pregnancy. *Lancet* 1:992-994, 1986.
75. Scholl TO, Hediger ML, Fisher RL, et al: Anemia vs iron deficiency: Increased risk of preterm delivery in a prospective study. *Am J Clin Nutr* 55:985-988, 1992.
76. Lu ZM, Goldenberg R, Cliver S, et al: The relationship between maternal hematocrit and pregnancy outcome. *Obstet Gynecol* 77:190-194, 1991.
77. Schaefer RM, Schaefer L: Hypochromic red blood cells and reticulocytes. *Kidney Int* 55:44S-48S, 1999.
78. Cohen AR: Choosing the best strategy to prevent childhood iron deficiency. *JAMA* 281:2247-2248, 1999.
79. Massey AC: Microcytic anemia: Differential diagnosis and management of iron deficiency anemia. *Med Clin North Am* 76:549-566, 1992.
80. Statland BE, Winkel P: Relationship of day-to-day variation of serum iron concentrations to iron-binding capacity in healthy young women. *Am J Clin Pathol* 67:84-90, 1977.
81. Punnonen K, Irajala K, Rajamaki A: Serum transferrin receptor and its ratio to serum ferritin in the diagnosis of iron deficiency. *Blood* 89:1052-1057, 1997.
82. Pettersson T, Kivivuori SM, Siimes MA: Is serum transferrin receptor useful for detecting iron-deficiency in anaemic patients with chronic inflammatory diseases? *Br J Rheumatol* 33:740-744, 1994.

83. Duncan B, Schifman RB, Corrigan JJ Jr, et al: Iron and the exclusively breast-fed infant from birth to six months. *J Pediatr Gastroenterol Nutr* 4:421-425, 1985.
84. Gill DG, Vincent S, Segal DS: Follow-on formula in the prevention of iron deficiency: A multicentre study. *Acta Paediatr* 86:683-689, 1997.
85. Tunnessen WW Jr, Oski FA: Consequences of starting whole cow milk at 6 months of age. *J Pediatr* 111:813-816, 1987.
86. Boutry M, Needlman R: Use of dietary history in the screening of iron deficiency. *Pediatrics* 98:1138-1142, 1996.
87. US Public Health Service: Anemia in children. *Am Fam Physician* 51:1121-1123, 1995.

CHAPTER 14

Enuresis

Wm. Lane M. Robson, MD, FRCP(C), FRCP(Glasg), FAAP
Chief of Pediatrics, Memorial Hospital of Rhode Island; Professor of Pediatrics, Brown University, Providence

Significant recent advances in our understanding of the factors involved with enuresis have improved the outcome for children treated for this problem.[1] The high level of international scientific interest in continence suggests an even brighter future for the estimated 5 million American children who have enuresis. This article reviews the causes, genetics, management, investigation, definitions, historical aspects, epidemiology, psychological and social impact, normal achievement of continence, pathophysiologic factors, and prognosis of enuresis.

DEFINITIONS

The word "enuresis" is derived from the Greek word *εvoup εiv* (*enour ein),* and according to Liddell and Scott's Greek-English Lexicon, means *to make water.*[2] The International Children's Continence Society (ICCS) suggests that enuresis should refer only to nocturnal enuresis and should not refer to other forms of urinary incontinence.[3] The ICCS separates enuresis into primary and secondary forms based on whether a child experiences a minimum 6-month period of continence before onset of the enuresis.[3]

HISTORICAL ASPECTS

Papyrus records from 1550 BC are the first written record of enuresis.[4-6] The recorded treatment of the day in Ebers was a mixture of cypress, juniper berries, and beer.[4] The first known description of an enuretic patient was by Lucretius in the first century BC.[7] Later healers included Dioscorides, who in 50 AD recommended the *cerebrum of the hare, ground and imbibed.*[4] Perhaps this ancient healer considered an abnormality in the CNS as the most probable cause of enuresis. If so, and considering our current understand-

TABLE 1.
Treatment of Enuresis in the 19th Century[4,5]

Silver nitrate cautery of the urethral meatus
Collodion poured into the prepuce
Blisters to the penis
Penile bandages
Electric shock to the urethral meatus

ing, Dioscorides might therefore be considered the father of modern enuresis.

Many affected families are reluctant to discuss enuresis, and similarly some physicians are reluctant to treat the condition; the reasons for this reluctance might derive from the still-remembered anachronistic attitudes and treatments in the 19th and early-to-mid 20th century (Table 1).[4,5] Some 19th century physicians attributed enuresis to "madness," and this legacy, together with Freud's reference to enuresis as a "pollution," imparted a negative psychiatric implication to the problem, which sadly persists today.[8]

Nocturnal polyuria was considered a possible cause by Chambers,[9] who in 1846 recommended limiting fluid intake for 3 hours before bedtime and emptying the bladder at bedtime. An arousal-related cause was considered by Ruddock,[10] who in 1878 recommended awakening the child during the second hour of sleep to avoid deep sleep.

A German physician who supervised a home for handicapped children discovered alarm therapy at the turn of the century.[11] Many of the children wet at night, and Dr Pfaundler[11] arranged an alarm system to identify those children who required changing. He noted that some of the children became dry with the alarm. Notwithstanding this early success, alarm treatment was uncommon until about 50 years ago when Professors Mowrer and Mowrer[8] developed and reported a practical alarm system. Some variations on the alarm system set back the use of this therapy. Alarms were developed that administered an electric shock as the arousal method, sometimes to the genitalia. These barbaric systems continued in use until at least the 1970s.

Modern pharmacologic treatment approaches have only several decades of historical precedence. Soon after investigators realized that the pituitary gland was identified as a source of an antidiuretic chemical, clinicians recognized a potential treatment for enuresis. In 1956, Holt[12] reported dryness in 8 (13%) of 60 patients treated with posterior-pituitary snuff (Di-sipidin), a product derived from desiccated animal pituitaries. 1-Deamino-8-D-arginine vasopressin (DDAVP) was synthesized in 1967[13] and first reported as a treatment for enuresis in 1977.[14]

EPIDEMIOLOGY

The prevalence of enuresis varies by age, sex, and perhaps geography. Enuresis is more common in boys. Byrd et al[15] studied 10,960 American children aged 5 to 17 years who wet at least once every 24 days. The prevalence of enuresis in boys at ages 7 and 10 years was 9% and 7%, respectively, compared with 6% and 3%, respectively, in girls.[15] The prevalence of enuresis gradually decreases throughout childhood. At 5 years of age, 23% of children still have enuresis at least once every 3 weeks.[16] During the elementary school years, the condition continues to be common, with 20% of 7-year-old and 4% of 10-year-old children still bothered by enuresis.[16] At 18 years of age, and through adulthood, at least 2% of individuals still wet the bed.[16] This figure is likely an underestimate because many adults prefer not to discuss this condition. Table 2 lists the prevalence by geography.[15,17-21]

GENETICS

The familial nature of enuresis was likely evident thousands of years ago, but the first reported study emerged just over a century ago.[22] Numerous studies report a varying but high prevalence of enuresis in other family members.[23-27] The highest reported, but still possibly underestimated familial prevalence, suggests that 56% of fathers, 36% of mothers, and 40% of siblings experience

TABLE 2.
Prevalence (Percent) of Enuresis by Geography

Country		Prevalence
Scotland[17]	> several times/wk	3.6
Sweden[18]	> once/wk	3.8
Netherlands[19]*	> once/wk (7-9 y)	3.8
Australia[20]	> twice/wk (5-12 y)	5.1
Italy[21]*		8.1
United States[15]		9.0

Data include only reports of enuresis at least once per month and are for 7-year-old boys unless otherwise noted.[15,17-21]
*Boys and girls reported in study.

enuresis.[25] Viewed forward on the genetic path, enuresis is reported in 43% and 44% of the children of enuretic fathers and mothers, respectively, and 77% of children when both the mother and father had enuresis.[26]

Chromosome 22 was identified as the site of an enuresis locus in a Danish family reported in 1995.[28] The heterogeneous nature of enuresis is evident at the chromosome level. Subsequent reports link enuresis to chromosomes 8, 12, and 16.[29-31]

Future research might clarify the physiologic factors controlled by these loci.

PSYCHOLOGICAL AND SOCIAL IMPACT

Psychological problems are almost always the result of the enuresis and only rarely the cause.[32,33] The emotional impact of enuresis on a child and family can be enormous.[32,34-37] Children with enuresis are commonly punished[38] and are at significant risk for emotional and physical abuse.[39] Numerous studies report feelings of embarrassment and anxiety, loss of self-esteem, and effects on self-perception, interpersonal relationships, quality of life, and school performance.[36,37,40] A significant negative impact on self-esteem is reported in children with enuretic episodes as infrequent as once per month.

NORMAL ACHIEVEMENT OF CONTINENCE

Dryness at night usually follows achievement of continence by day.[41] Table 3 shows the percentage of American children who achieve daytime and nighttime continence at varying ages.[41] At approximately 4 years of age, a child is able to initiate a micturition even in the absence of the desire to void, by voluntary relaxation of the external urethral sphincter.[42]

PATHOPHYSIOLOGIC FACTORS AND CAUSES

Enuresis is a symptom and not a disease. It is convenient to consider the pathophysiologic factors that might be operative in chil-

TABLE 3.
Percent of Children Dry by Day and Night at Various Preschool Ages[41]

Age (y)	Dry by Day (%)	Dry by Night (%)
2.0	25	10
2.5	85	48
3.0	98	78

TABLE 4.
Pathophysiologic Factors in Children With Enuresis as an Isolated Symptom

Disorder of sleep arousal
Nocturnal polyuria
Small nocturnal bladder capacity

dren with this isolated symptom separate from the causes of enuresis in children who also experience daytime symptoms. Although "developmental delay" has enjoyed historical popularity as a cause of enuresis, the use of this term is nonspecific and in our view should not be included in the lexicon of this problem.[43] Research does not support developmental delay of a specific causal factor. The pathophysiologic factors that might be operative when a meticulous history does not reveal any daytime symptoms are shown in Table 4.

DISORDER OF SLEEP AROUSAL

Notwithstanding the observation by parents that their children with enuresis sleep "deeper" than nonenuretic siblings, the association of depth of sleep with enuresis was not generally accepted until the last decade. Earlier studies that examined the relationship of the stage of sleep with enuresis failed to reveal a consistent or significant association.[44] However, recent studies show that children with enuresis do not wake up normally in response to an auditory signal and confirm a defect in arousal.[45-47]

Arousal to the sensation of a full or contracting bladder involves interconnected anatomical areas that include the cerebral cortex, reticular activating system, locus ceruleus, pontine micturition center, hypothalamus, spinal cord, and bladder. The reticular activating system controls for depth of sleep, the locus ceruleus for arousal, and the pontine micturition center initiates the command for a detrusor contraction.[1,48,49] A variety of neurotransmitters are involved including noradrenaline, serotonin, and antidiuretic hormone (ADH). ADH is theorized to prevent enuresis by minimizing nocturnal production of urine. It is possible that another and perhaps more important role of ADH is to facilitate arousal.[1,49]

Until recently, the conventional wisdom suggested that infants did not arouse with voiding and that in normal children this relationship "evolves" during the second or third years of life. Yeung et al[50] showed cortical arousal in newborn and older infants immediately before voiding. Further studies are necessary to determine whether cortical arousal is abnormal from birth in children with enuresis or whether arousal becomes abnormal later in childhood.

Professors Mowrer and Mowrer[8] noted the absence of enuresis and early achievement of daytime continence in some less developed cultures. They theorized that because the infant and mother in these cultures slept together, whenever the infant voided at night, the mother would immediately wake to the wetness and change the infant, and this process might lead to conditioned dryness.[8] Professors Mowrer and Mowrer did not have the benefit of the knowledge that cortical arousal precedes voiding in infants.[50] It is also possible that the mother might wake to the preceding arousal, and facilitate voiding without wetting the common bed, a process that might also lead to conditioned dryness.

Obstructive sleep apnea (OSA) is a disorder associated with an abnormality in both arousal and enuresis.[51-53] Simmons et al[54] described an 8-year-old boy and a 15-year-old girl with enuresis that resolved subsequent to surgical treatment of airway obstruction with adenotonsillectomy and tracheostomy, respectively. Subsequent studies confirmed this association.[55,56] Most children with airway obstruction sufficient to cause OSA develop the problem over time, which might account for the more common improvement noted after adenotonsillectomy in children with secondary enuresis.[56] The dramatic resolution of enuresis after surgical treatment of airway obstruction suggests that OSA influences a critical pathophysiologic factor.[56] A disorder of sleep arousal is suggested as the most likely. Nocturnal polyuria is reported in OSA and is another possible causative factor.[56] The decrease in nocturnal secretion of ADH and increase in atrial natriuretic peptide (ANP) reported in individuals with OSA are possible explanations for nocturnal polyuria.[56] The most common cause of OSA in childhood is adenotonsillar hypertrophy, which has a peak incidence at 2 to 5 years of age.[56]

NOCTURNAL POLYURIA

Nocturnal polyuria was long suspected as a pathophysiologic factor.[9] Studies reveal nocturnal polyuria in some but not all children with enuresis.[57-61] Although nocturnal polyuria is important in the pathophysiology of enuresis, overproduction of urine cannot be the sole causal factor. Nocturnal polyuria does not explain why children with enuresis do not wake to the sensation of a full or contracting bladder, or why incontinence occurs during daytime naps.

TABLE 5.
Factors That Might Cause Nocturnal Polyuria in Children With Enuresis[62,63]

Fluid ingestion in the evening before bedtime
Eating in the evening before bedtime
Low nocturnal secretion of ADH
Increased nocturnal solute excretion

Abbreviation: ADH, Antidiuretic hormone.

Factors that might cause nocturnal polyuria in children with enuresis are shown in Table 5.[62,63] Ingestion of fluids in the evening before bedtime is a common cause. Solid food ingestion is also a cause because excretion of solute by the kidney is accompanied by an obligate amount of water. Production of urine is controlled by several factors that include ADH,[64] which directly controls water absorption, and ANP and aldosterone, which control solute and therefore indirectly affect water excretion. Nørgaard et al[62,63] reported an absence of the expected nocturnal increase in ADH secretion in children with enuresis. Subsequent reports suggest that a low nocturnal secretion of ADH is present in some but not all children with enuresis.[65,66] This finding supports the heterogeneous nature of enuresis.

Urine sodium and potassium excretion are increased in some children with enuresis, but the reasons for these observations are not clear.[67,68] Rittig et al[67] reported that the secretion of ANP in children with enuresis shows a normal circadian rhythm, and the renin-angiotensin-aldosterone system is intact. Further studies are necessary to corroborate these observations.

Bladder distension might have an influence on nocturnal secretion of ADH. Some studies report that ADH secretion is increased in response to bladder distension and reduced with bladder emptying.[1,69-71] If ADH secretion does decrease with bladder emptying, the observed low nocturnal blood levels of ADH might be a consequence rather than a cause of enuresis.

Any disease that affects the ability of the kidney to concentrate urine might be expected to have a higher prevalence of enuresis. In support of this concept, enuresis is more common in children with a sickle cell hemoglobinopathy.[72-74] The prevalence at the age of 8 years is reported to be at least twice that found in nonaffected children. Although nocturnal polyuria caused by an impaired ability to concentrate the urine is the most common suggested reason to account for the enuresis, Readett et al[73] report that bed-wetting in these patients does not correlate with disease severity and that other pathophysiologic factors might be operative. Studies that correlate nocturnal urine output and osmolality, arousal, and nocturnal bladder capacity are necessary to clarify the cause of enuresis in patients with a sickle cell hemoglobinopathy.

LOW NOCTURNAL BLADDER CAPACITY

Small bladder capacity is a long suspected pathophysiologic factor. This theory has engendered much controversy and until recently was considered a less likely explanation for enuresis in children without daytime symptoms. Reports include normal and reduced bladder capacity, but few studies report on carefully selected patients with only bed-wetting.[75-77] Results of daytime urodynamic studies in carefully selected children with enuresis without daytime symptoms are reported to be normal.[77] Urodynamic studies during sleep reveal that some of these children have a low nocturnal bladder capacity.[78] The reasons for the diurnal-nocturnal difference are not clear. The rate of bladder filling might be a factor. Spontaneous detrusor contractions are reported to be more common with active compared with passive filling.[79] Although a study by Kirk et al[80] did not support a relationship between the rate of bladder-filling and enuresis, these authors did show that enuresis-like episodes could be provoked in normal children by administering large volumes of fluid at bedtime.

Mattsson and Lindström[81] reported that functional bladder capacity (FBC) was positively correlated with nighttime urine output. Children with enuresis might maintain a smaller nocturnal bladder volume, and this might "condition" the detrusor to contract at a lower volume. According to this theory, the low nocturnal bladder capacity might be a consequence rather than a cause of enuresis.

Bloom et al[82,83] suggest a problem with the external urethral sphincter as a possible cause of a low nocturnal bladder capacity. Heretofore, most theories have focused on a detrusor contraction as the cause of the enuresis. Bloom et al suggest that the control of voiding rests at the external urethral sphincter where constant activity is present as a "guarding reflex" to preserve continence. The activity of the external urethral sphincter might fall below a critical level during sleep and thereby trigger a detrusor contraction. Schacter[84] offered a similar explanation in 1932 with the suggestion that enuresis was "a deficiency of inhibitory control over an essentially autonomic function."

Prostaglandins affect detrusor tone and might be involved in the pathogenesis of enuresis.[75,85] Şener et al[85] reported elevation of blood and urine prostaglandin E_2 levels in children with enuresis.

CAUSES OF ENURESIS WHEN DAYTIME SYMPTOMS ARE ALSO PRESENT

Daytime symptoms can be present from birth. In this situation the causes include neurogenic bladder secondary to conditions such as cerebral palsy, myelomeningocele, and sacral agenesis; congenital urethral obstruction; ectopic ureter; and congenital diabetes insipidus. Daytime symptoms can also develop after birth or after the age when dryness might otherwise be expected. The causes include urge syndrome and dysfunctional voiding, urinary tract infection (UTI), daytime frequency syndrome, constipation, acquired neurogenic bladder, acquired urethral obstruction, emotional stress, diabetes mellitus, and acquired diabetes insipidus (Table 6).[86]

URGE SYNDROME AND DYSFUNCTIONAL VOIDING

Urge syndrome and dysfunctional voiding are more frequent in girls of preschool and elementary school age[86-88] and in children with attention-deficit/hyperactivity disorder (ADHD).[89] Vesicoureteral reflux is common, and UTI and constipation are frequent complicating problems. Squatting behavior, a common and distinct symptom of urge syndrome and dysfunctional voiding, is a learned response to suppress an unexpected and unwelcome detrusor contraction. To avoid embarrassment, older children might choose not

TABLE 6.
Causes of Enuresis When Daytime Symptoms Are Also Present[86]

Urge syndrome and dysfunctional voiding
Urinary tract infection
Daytime frequency syndrome
Constipation
Neurogenic bladder
Urethral obstruction
Significant emotional stress
Ectopic ureter
Diabetes mellitus
Diabetes insipidus

to squat, but rather pretend that something has dropped to the floor or that a shoelace is untied, and a sitting child might shift to the hard edge of the chair. The detrusor contraction can last for more than a minute. Urodynamic studies reveal unstable detrusor contractions early in the filling phase,[88] but are not necessary for a clinical diagnosis. In some children, a period of normal voiding occurs before the onset of the problem. The symptoms tend to improve or resolve with time, and are less common after puberty.

UTI

UTI is a common cause of secondary enuresis and an aggravating factor associated with other causes. UTI associated with enuresis can present at any age. Cystitis causes uninhibited detrusor contractions,[90] which can lead to episodes of daytime and nighttime wetting. When UTI is the only cause of enuresis, other symptoms of infection are usually present, and the wetting resolves with appropriate treatment. UTI is more common in children with urge syndrome and dysfunctional voiding, neurogenic bladder, urethral obstruction, ectopic ureter, and diabetes mellitus. In these conditions, daytime symptoms do not completely resolve with antibiotic treatment.

DAYTIME FREQUENCY SYNDROME

Daytime frequency syndrome occurs in children of preschool and elementary school age (mean age, 5 years), is more common in boys, and presents with the sudden onset of frequent voiding, often every 5 to 10 minutes.[91] Although frequency is the predominant symptom, secondary enuresis is present in about 20% of the children.[91] Daytime wetting occurs in about 25%, typically the younger children who are unable to reach the bathroom on time. Suggested etiologies include a viral or chemical cystourethritis and emotional stress.[91]

CONSTIPATION

Constipation per se can cause secondary enuresis[92-94] and is a common aggravating factor that should be considered when other causes are present. Although the mechanism is not clear, it is possible that the pressure effect of stool in the descending or sigmoid colon can trigger an uninhibited detrusor contraction. Constipation is usually present in children with neurogenic bladder and is more common in those with urge syndrome and dysfunctional voiding.

NEUROGENIC BLADDER

Neurogenic bladder can develop as a result of a lesion at any level in the nervous system, including the cerebral cortex, the spinal cord, or the peripheral nerves.[95,96] As many as 37% of children with cerebral palsy have enuresis.[97] Specific dysfunction in the external urethral sphincter can develop after pelvic extirpative surgery, radiation therapy for pelvic malignancy, pelvic fracture, and incontinence surgery.[98] Sacral agenesis can be associated with a neurogenic bladder.[99] Up to 5% of patients with imperforate anus have a neurogenic bladder and most also have a lumbosacral anomaly.[100]

URETHRAL OBSTRUCTION

Urethral obstruction can be congenital, such as with posterior urethral valves, congenital stricture, or urethral diverticuli, or acquired as a result of traumatic or infectious stricture. Meatal stenosis is a common cause of distal urethral obstruction in circumcised males.

EMOTIONAL STRESS

Enuresis might present as an intermittent or short-term problem associated with specific and limited duration stresses, such as change of residence, school difficulties, or temporary parental discord, or as a persistent problem if the stress is prolonged, such as severe emotional distress associated with ongoing child abuse.

ECTOPIC URETER

Ectopic ureter is a rare congenital abnormality that is caused by the insertion of the ureter in a location other than the lateral angle of the bladder trigone. Incontinence results when the insertion is distal to the external urethral sphincter. Girls with ectopic ureter are always wet. Boys are usually continent because the ureter inserts proximal to the external urethral sphincter.

DIABETES MELLITUS AND DIABETES INSIPIDUS

Enuresis caused by diabetes mellitus and diabetes insipidus is usually attributed to nocturnal polyuria. Diabetes mellitus is associated with abnormalities in the afferent sensory pathways to the bladder, which might contribute to the enuresis.[101]

EVALUATION

The best time to investigate enuresis is when the parent first raises the issue in the office. A common and less appropriate recommendation is to consider enuresis a problem only if the wetting persists after the age of 6 years.

HISTORY

The most important aspect of the investigation is a meticulous history, which not only establishes the diagnosis, but also can lead to more precise treatment recommendations, and minimizes the need for invasive and costly investigations. A careful voiding history is necessary in every patient. The frequency and exact schedule of voiding is necessary to determine whether daytime symptoms are present. Most school-age children void 4 to 6 times a day and do not get up at night to void.[102]

Questions about the urinary stream should include whether the child needs to wait or push to initiate voiding, if the stream is strong and continuous, and in boys, whether the stream is straight. Precise questions are required. An inquiry about whether a child wets by day might result in a negative response from a parent, whereas a question about the presence of dampness might lead to a positive response. Dampness is so common that many parents apparently consider this important symptom "normal" or unworthy of comment. Many parents are unable to answer questions about the voiding pattern in their child. These parents should be instructed to maintain a precise voiding diary for several weeks before a follow-up visit.

A sleep history should include the times when a child goes to bed, falls asleep, and awakens in the morning. When possible, the timing and number of wetting episodes should be determined. Whether the child has experienced prolonged periods of dryness should be determined and the circumstances of these episodes. Parents should be asked to comment on the depth of sleep and to offer examples why they consider their child to sleep deep or not. The presence of restless sleep, snoring, and the type and frequency of nocturnal arousals such as nightmares, sleep terrors, and sleepwalking should be determined.

The family history should include questions about enuresis in parents, grandparents, and siblings.

A diet history should include the timing, quantity, and type of fluid and solid food intake from the end of school to bedtime.

An assessment of the emotional impact on the child is important. Information should be solicited from the parents and the child. Whether the child has been teased by family or friends, or has self-restricted participation in sleepovers, or school or other trips are basic and revealing questions.

For children with enuresis and daytime symptoms, the history should also focus on specific symptoms of the conditions that may be causing the enuresis. Children with urge syndrome and dysfunctional voiding present with frequency, urgency, and squatting behavior. In children with UTI, there are usually associated symptoms of dysuria, frequency, urgency, and cloudy, foul-smelling urine. Daytime frequency syndrome presents with the sudden onset of voiding as frequently as every 5 to 10 minutes. Children with constipation have hard, infrequent bowel movements. Children with a neurogenic bladder can have symptoms related to the specific neurologic problem. Spinal cord lesions can be associated with constipation, encopresis, or a gait disturbance. Children with urethral obstruction usually need to wait or push to initiate or sustain voiding, and have a weak, interrupted, or narrow-caliber urinary stream. It is helpful to review the symptoms and signs of a urinary stream abnormality with the parents and ask them to observe the stream at home, and report their observations at the next visit. When emotional stress is the cause of regular enuresis, the situation at home is usually significantly dysfunctional. Diabetes mellitus and diabetes insipidus present with thirst and the frequent need to void large volumes of urine. Symptoms suggestive of OSA in childhood include snoring, restless or interrupted sleep, parental observation of episodes of apnea or hypopnea during sleep, and daytime mouth breathing.[51] Excessive daytime sleepiness is not as common a symptom of OSA in children as in adults.[51]

PHYSICAL EXAMINATION

A thorough physical examination is important for every child with enuresis. Abnormal physical findings are usually not present in children with enuresis as the sole symptom, or in children with urge syndrome and dysfunctional voiding, daytime frequency syndrome, or diabetes mellitus or insipidus. Abnormal physical findings can be found in patients with UTI, constipation, neurogenic bladder, urethral obstruction, ectopic ureter, and OSA.

In patients with UTI there can be fever, tenderness of the kidneys or bladder, or inflammation or discharge in the genital area. Constipation is suggested by the presence of hard stool in the left lower quadrant and hard, impacted stool by rectal examination. The examination for neurogenic bladder should specifically assess the motor power, tone, sensation, and spinal and plantar reflexes in the lower extremities. The anal area should be tested for an intact anal wink, and the lumbosacral spine should be checked for abnormalities including tufts of hair, dimples, masses, or abnormal skin coloration. In patients with urethral obstruction, the bladder and kidneys can be enlarged to palpation. It is helpful to observe the urinary stream in children with suspected urethral obstruction. If there is an audible "grunt," the child uses the abdominal muscles to push, or if the stream is weak or interrupted, a urethral obstruction might be present. Meatal stenosis in boys is recognized by inspection of the caliber of the urethral meatus and the urinary stream, which is of narrow caliber and deflected off center. In girls with ectopic ureter, a constant moistness is observed in the introitus, and regular drying with tissue will reveal the persistent leak of urine. Tonsillar size in a child examined in the awake and sitting position may not correlate with OSA symptoms.[56] Examination of the child in the prone position and during sleep may be necessary to visibly document obstruction.[56]

NONINVASIVE INVESTIGATIONS

The urinalysis is the most important screening test in a child with daytime wetting. Children with UTI usually have white blood cells or bacteria in the microscopic urinalysis. If the history or the urinalysis suggests UTI, urine should be sent for culture and sensitivity. Urethral obstruction may be associated with red blood cells in the urine. A random or first-morning specific gravity greater than 1.020 rules out diabetes insipidus, and the presence of glucose suggests diabetes mellitus.

Uroflowmetry is a simple noninvasive measurement of urine flow that is helpful to screen patients for neurogenic bladder and urethral obstruction. Children are instructed to void into a special toilet with a pressure-sensitive rotating disc at the base. A normal uroflow study shows a single bell-shaped curve with a normal peak and average flow rate for age and size.[103] Patients with urethral obstruction, neurogenic bladder, and some patients with urge syndrome and dysfunctional voiding, have a prolonged curve or an interrupted series of curves and a low peak and average urine flow rate. Failure to empty the bladder is a significant risk factor for UTI and is common in patients with urge syndrome and dysfunctional voiding, neurogenic bladder, and urethral obstruction. A portable bladder ultrasound is available to assess residual urine. The residual volume of urine is normally less than 10 mL.[104]

An ultrasound of the kidney and bladder is an excellent noninvasive screening study and should be considered in all patients with enuresis and persistent daytime symptoms. Patients with neurogenic bladder and urethral obstruction have a thick, trabeculated bladder wall and evidence of hydronephrosis or cortical scarring on renal ultrasound.

In patients with significant daytime symptoms who have normal findings on ultrasound of the kidneys and bladder, more invasive investigations should be deferred pending a 3-month period during which the voiding routine and emptying are improved, UTI is treated or prevented, and constipation is treated.[105]

OTHER INVESTIGATIONS

If a neurogenic bladder is suspected, a voiding cystourethrogram (VCUG) should be performed. The lumbosacral spine should be visualized during the VCUG to look for sacral agenesis or spinal dysraphism. A video-urodynamic study measures filling phase parameters such as bladder capacity, presence or absence of unstable detrusor contractions, bladder compliance, and the state of the bladder neck, and voiding phase parameters such as voiding pressures, bladder emptying, and the state of the external urethral sphincter. Patients with evidence of a neurogenic bladder without an obvious cause should have an MRI of the spine to look for a spinal cord abnormality. If urethral obstruction is suspected based on an abnormal urinary stream or ultrasound, a VCUG should be performed. If OSA is possible, a lateral radiograph of the neck or referral to a pediatric otolaryngologist for direct visualization of the nasopharynx should be considered.

MANAGEMENT

One of the most important reasons to treat enuresis is to minimize the embarrassment and anxiety of the child. All children with enuresis benefit from a caring and patient approach by their parents. A positive attitude and motivation to be dry are important components of treatment. Most children with enuresis feel very much alone with their problem. Family members with a past history of enuresis should be encouraged to share their experience and offer moral support to the child. The knowledge that another family member had and outgrew the problem can be very therapeutic.

Children should be instructed not to overeat or drink to excess with dinner, and to minimize fluid and solid food intake after dinner and before bed. Commonsense modifications of fluid intake are necessary to maintain hydration in children who play sports or who are otherwise physically active in the evening after dinner. Fluid or solid food restriction should not be presented in a fashion that might be construed by the child as a punishment for the enuresis.

Children should be instructed to go to bed at an hour calculated to offer the optimal hours of sleep for age (Table 7).[106] Children

TABLE 7.
Recommended Hours of Sleep by Age[106]

Age (y)	Recommended Hours of Sleep
5	11
6	11
7	10.5
8	10
9	10
10	10
11	9.5
12	9
13	9
14	9
15	9
16	8.5
17	8
18	8

should be instructed to void immediately before bedtime. Parents should be asked to take the child to the bathroom to void before their bedtime. Because this therapeutic measure is only designed to minimize the quantity of fluid in the bladder, full wakefulness is neither necessary nor desirable. Because the children do not usually wake fully, careful monitoring by a parent is necessary for the trip from bed to bathroom and back.

An explanation of the probable cause of the enuresis is important for every family. When a child has no daytime symptoms and has experienced prolonged dry spells in the past, the presence of a structural abnormality as a cause of the enuresis is unlikely. This should be explained to the parents to allay any fears about other causes and also to reassure that invasive investigations are not necessary. Parents should be asked to provide specific examples of what they are worried may be the cause so these often irrational fears can be discussed and relieved.

MANAGEMENT OF CHILDREN WITH ENURESIS AS THE SOLE SYMPTOM

Alarm Therapy

Alarm therapy offers the possibility of sustained improvement of enuresis and should be considered in every patient.[8,107,108] The mechanism of therapeutic action of alarm therapy is not known.

Some successfully treated children replace enuresis with nocturia, and others sleep dry without the need to void at night.[109] Some improve within the first 2 weeks of treatment and others only after several months. Alarm therapy is reported to increase nocturnal bladder capacity.[110] For optimal results, alarm therapy requires a motivated child and family, and a significant commitment of effort and time. Analysis of 25 reported studies suggest an average success rate of 68%.[107]

A number of practical considerations limit the usefulness of alarm therapy and should be discussed with the family before selecting this approach. Optimal results occur when the child is well motivated. Older children have increased motivation. Parental motivation is also critical. The parent should believe the approach worthwhile and be prepared to participate every night for at least 3 consecutive months. The impact on other family members should be considered. If the alarm might interrupt the sleep of an infant sibling, sibling in the same bedroom, shift-working parent, or live-in grandparent, alarm therapy may not be suitable.

Numerous alarms are available. The alarm should be attached at bedtime to the underwear or pajamas in a position chosen to promptly sense wetness. Although most children with enuresis will not awaken to the alarm, they will stop emptying the bladder. When the alarm sounds, a parent must assist the child to the bathroom to finish voiding. It is not necessary for the child to be awakened to full consciousness. After changing the sheets and underwear or pajamas, the child should be returned to bed and the alarm reset. Close follow-up is important to sustain motivation, trouble-shoot technical problems, and otherwise monitor the therapy.

In successfully treated children, alarm therapy should be continued for at least 2 weeks after sustained dryness. Relapses are common, occurring in 29% to 66% of children, and may respond to further alarm therapy.[107] If the child is still wet after a minimum of 3 months of consecutive use, alarm therapy can be discontinued and considered unsuccessful.[107] Failure does not preclude future successful treatment in an older more motivated child.

Pharmacologic Therapy

DDAVP is the preferred medication to treat children with enuresis. Numerous studies report total dryness in 38% to 55% of children treated with DDAVP.[111-116] DDAVP is the synthetic analogue of the natural pituitary hormone ADH and was synthesized as a treatment for patients with diabetes insipidus. Removal of the amino group in position 1 and substitution of D-arginine for L-arginine in position 8 preserves the antidiuretic action but minimizes the vasopressor action. Although most authorities suggest the therapeutic benefit of DDAVP results from a reduction in the nocturnal production of urine, it is possible that effects on arousal may be more important.[1,49]

The tablet and nasal spray formulations have similar efficacy.[117] The more recently approved tablet formulation has several advantages over the nasal spray. The precise and time-consuming instructions necessary for optimal administration of the nasal spray are obviated with a tablet. The nasal spray has reduced effectiveness in children with nasal congestion caused by infection or allergy. For sleepovers and other special occasions, the tablet formulation is more discrete. A blood test to check serum electrolytes is recommended in the product monograph for the nasal spray but not for the tablet.

The pharmacokinetic data for the tablet and nasal spray are different (Table 8).[118,119] Pharmacokinetic action is measured with respect to antidiuretic effect. The time to onset and time to maximal effect are less for the nasal spray than for the tablet. The duration of effect, however, is less for the tablet than for the spray.[118,119] A shorter duration of action with less likelihood of next-day antidiuretic effect reduces the risk of water intoxication and favors the tablet formulation.

Numerous studies have attempted to identify those patients most likely to respond to DDAVP. Whether family history of enuresis has predictive value is controversial.[120,121] A family history of enuresis did not predict response to DDAVP in a large Swedish study[121] but did in an American study.[120] Neither study clarifies the issue because both reported on a heterogeneous population. The predictive value of family history requires study of the response to DDAVP within families with specific chromosomal loci that control for enuresis. Older children are reported to be more responsive to

TABLE 8.
Pharmacokinetic Data on DDAVP Tablets and Nasal Spray[118,119]

	Tablets (h)	Nasal Spray (h)
Onset	1	<1
Maximum effect	4-7	1-3
Duration	8-12	8-20

Abbreviation: DDAVP, 1-deamino-8-D-arginine vasopressin.

DDAVP.[122-124] Rushton et al[125] reported that children with a normal FBC are more likely to respond to DDAVP than those with an FBC less than 70% predicted. Nocturnal polyuria is suggested by a history of a significant first-morning volume of urine notwithstanding enuresis the preceding night, and a low first-morning urine osmolality. The results of studies that compare nocturnal urine output or first-morning urine osmolality, with response to DDAVP are contradictory.[112,122,126-130] Low nocturnal levels of ADH do not predict response to DDAVP.[65] However, ADH levels are reported to increase after treatment with DDAVP.[131] Long-term treatment with DDAVP is reported to increase the resolution rate beyond that observed in untreated patients.[113,121,132,133]

Patients with enuresis associated with sickle cell hemoglobinopathy and with myelomeningocele respond to DDAVP.[74,134] Figueroa et al[74] reported that 6 (60%) of 10 patients with sickle cell hemoglobinopathy responded to DDAVP, and Horowitz et al[134] reported that 14 (78%) of 18 patients with myelomeningocele responded to DDAVP.

DDAVP tablets should be administered at bedtime. The recommended starting dose is 0.2 mg, and the drug can be titrated as necessary to a maximum of 0.6 mg. Failure to respond does not preclude future successful treatment with the drug. The immediate onset of action of DDAVP allows the flexibility of intermittent administration for special occasions.

The side effect profile of DDAVP is favorable.[135,136] For the tablet, the incidence of minor side effects is not significantly different than that with placebo.[119] The most frequently reported side effects with the nasal spray are nasal discomfort, epistaxis, abdominal pain, and headache.[135,136] The only serious adverse effect reported in patients with enuresis treated with DDAVP is seizure or other CNS symptoms caused by water intoxication.[137] We reviewed the case reports of water intoxication associated with DDAVP and confirmed excess fluid intake was a feature of at least 6 of 11 cases.[137] This serious adverse effect is preventable with careful patient education not to overdo fluids on any evening that DDAVP is administered. We recommend a maximum of 1 cup (8 ounces) of fluid at dinner, no more than a cup between dinner and bedtime, and nothing to drink in the 2 hours before bedtime.[137] Early symptoms of water intoxication include headache, nausea, and vomiting.[137] If these symptoms develop, the medication should be discontinued and the child promptly assessed by a physician. Children with ADHD are often impulsive, and their fluid intake requires especially close monitoring to avoid water intoxication.

Combination Therapies

The combinations of alarm therapy with DDAVP,[138,139] and oxybutynin chloride (Ditropan) with DDAVP[140] are reported to result in dryness not achievable with either therapy alone. The combination of DDAVP and oxybutynin chloride is particularly efficacious in children with urge syndrome and dysfunctional voiding who respond to anticholinergic therapy with daytime dryness but who continue to wet at night.

Therapies Not Recommended

Punishment has no role in the treatment of enuresis. Punishment can be subtle and unrecognized by an otherwise well-meaning parent. A child easily interprets fluid restriction and requests to wear pull-ups or launder sheets and clothes as punishment. Parents should be very sensitive to the presentation of these requests to minimize any sense of punishment.

We do not recommend use of imipramine or other antidepressant medications in the treatment of children with enuresis. Imipramine has an unfavorable profile of side effects and is associated with a significant risk for adverse effects with overdose, including fatal arrhythmia. Because of the potential for morbid consequences, imipramine is not recommended for the treatment of enuresis by the World Health Organization.

MANAGEMENT OF CHILDREN WITH ENURESIS AND DAYTIME SYMPTOMS

Children who hold the urine to the last minute should be counseled to respond promptly to the need to void. Parents should remind children to void when they wake, about every 1.5 to 2.0 hours during the day, before leaving the house for any reason, after any significant fluid intake, and before bedtime. The child should be advised that it does not matter whether any urine is produced, but it is important to try. When parents note that a child is fidgeting or adopting a posture otherwise suggestive of the need to void, the parents should ask the child to void. There is no role for punishment. Children do not wet to create a problem. Appropriate instruction, patience, and reward encourage resolution of the problem. Preschool children who hold the urine may respond to a reward system of praise or a sticker chart.

Antibiotics are necessary if UTI is the cause of the daytime wetting. If UTI is the only cause, the wetting should resolve with an appropriate antibiotic. If daytime symptoms continue notwithstanding successful treatment of the UTI, another cause of wetting should be suspected. Parents of children with the daytime frequency syndrome should be patient and supportive. For children with constipation, 3 regular meals a day and treatment with a high-fiber diet, mineral oil, a laxative, or an enema program will help evacuate the bowel and normalize the bowel movements.

Urotherapy may be helpful in some patients with enuresis caused by urge syndrome and dysfunctional voiding or neurogenic bladder.[141,142] With voiding, children should relax and take enough time to completely empty the bladder. Optimal posture is important.[142] Children should sit well back on the commode and lean slightly forward with a straight back.[142] Most preschool children need an over-the-toilet seat and a stool to support their feet. Proper breathing is important. Children should relax, take a full breath, and initiate voiding with exhalation. Some children have difficulty relaxing the pelvic floor muscles during voiding. Biofeedback therapy can be helpful for these children.

Anticholinergic medications are helpful in patients with urge syndrome and dysfunctional voiding or neurogenic bladder. These medications reduce uninhibited detrusor contractions, increase the threshold volume at which an uninhibited detrusor contraction occurs, and enlarge the FBC. Oxybutynin chloride and hyoscyamine sulfate (Levsin) are commonly prescribed anticholinergic medications. Oxybutynin chloride also has antispasmodic and analgesic properties.[143] Hyoscyamine sulfate is available in a long-acting preparation with a half-life of 8 hours compared with the relatively shorter half-life of less than 4 hours for oxybutynin chloride. Flavoxate hydrochloride (Urispas), a urinary spasmolytic, is helpful in some patients with unstable bladder, but is only approved for children older than 12 years. Tertolidine (Detrol) is an antimuscarinic medication that is helpful in some patients but is not approved for use in children less than 12 years.

Children with enuresis associated with ADHD should be encouraged to void regularly, not hold the urine to the last minute, and take time to completely empty the bladder. Consistency with daily practice of these measures often improves the daytime wetting but not the enuresis. Specific pharmacologic treatment of the ADHD may improve the enuresis in some children.

Neurosurgical treatment is available for spinal cord tumors and tethered cord. For patients with myelomeningocele, those with neurogenic bladder caused by central lesions, or patients with residual neurogenic damage after surgical intervention, management considerations include regular voiding every 1.5 to 2 hours, manual expression of the bladder, clean intermittent self-catheterization, and an anticholinergic medication.[95] Urinary diversion, bladder augmentation, or an artificial urinary sphincter is appropriate in selected cases. If urethral obstruction or ectopic ureter is identified, the child should be referred to a pediatric urologist for operative repair. Children with OSA should be referred to an otolaryngologist for possible surgical management.

PROGNOSIS

The most important reason to treat children with enuresis is to improve the loss in self-esteem and other secondary emotional problems that develop consequent to enuresis. Hägglöf et al[40] reported improvement in self-esteem to levels comparable to control children after 6 months of treatment. The spontaneous cure rate for children who are not treated is reported to be about 15% per year.[144] This often-reported rate is based on a 1974 study of 1129 children in Belfast, Ireland, and included a heterogeneous group with nighttime and daytime wetting.[144] When enuresis is the sole symptom, treatment with DDAVP results in total dryness in up to 55% of children and improvement in more than 75%.[113,127] When daytime symptoms are also present, the prognosis depends on the underlying cause. The prognosis is excellent when enuresis is caused by UTI, daytime frequency syndrome, ectopic ureter, OSA, diabetes mellitus, and diabetes insipidus. Enuresis caused by UTI should resolve with appropriate antibiotic therapy. Time resolves enuresis in children with daytime frequency syndrome. Ectopic ureter and OSA respond to specific surgical intervention. Diabetes mellitus and diabetes insipidus respond to specific medical intervention.

The prognosis is very good for children with enuresis caused by constipation. Loening-Baucke[92] reported resolution of associated enuresis in 63% of patients successfully treated for chronic constipation. Enuresis caused by urge syndrome and dysfunctional voiding usually resolves, but daytime symptoms continue after puberty and into adulthood in up to 20% of patients.[87,145] The prognosis of enuresis caused by neurogenic bladder depends on the neurologic cause and whether a surgical solution is possible. Continence is possible in up to 24% of children with myelomeningocele.[146]

ACKNOWLEDGMENT

We thank Debbie Mills, BSc, Lois Geuder, and Spike Jones for expert transcription assistance, and the library staff at Greenville Memorial Hospital.

REFERENCES

1. Nørgaard JP, Djurhuus JC, Watanabe H, et al: Experience and current status of research into the pathophysiology of nocturnal enuresis. *Br J Urol* 79:825-835, 1997.
2. Liddell HG, Scott RA: in Jones HS, McKenzie E (eds): *Greek-English Lexicon.* New ed. Oxford, The Clarendon Press, 1953.
3. Nørgaard JP, van Gool JD, Hjälmås K, et al: Standardization and definitions in lower urinary tract dysfunction in children. *Br J Urol* 81:1-16, 1998.
4. Glicklich LB: An historical account of enuresis. *Pediatrics* 8:859-876, 1951.
5. Salmon MA: An historical account of nocturnal enuresis and its treatment. *Proc R Soc Med* 68:443-445, 1975.
6. Gill D: Enuresis through the ages. *Pediatr Nephrol* 9:120-122, 1995.
7. Bloom D: Personal communication, 1999.
8. Mowrer OH, Mowrer WM: Enuresis: A method for its study and treatment. *Am J Orthopsychiatry* 8:436-459, 1938.
9. Chambers R: On incontinence of urine in children. *Prov M & SJ* 10:617, 1846.
10. Ruddock H: *Diseases of Infants and Children and Their Homeopathic and General Treatment.* London, Homeopathic Publishing, 1878, p 190.
11. Pfaundler M: Demonstration eines Apparates zur Selsttätigen Singalisierung Subchabter Bettnässung. *Verhandlungen der Gesellschaft Für Kinderheilkunde* 21:219-220, 1904.
12. Holt KS: Drug treatment of enuresis controlled trials with propantheline, amphetamine, and pituitary snuff. *Lancet* 2:1334-1336, 1956.
13. Zaoral M, Kolo J, Šorm F: Amino acids and peptides: LXXI. Synthesis of 1-deamino-8-D-lysine-vasopressin and 1-deamino-8-D-arginine-vasopressin. *Coll Czech Chem Commun* 32:1250-1257, 1967.
14. Dimson SB: Desmopressin as a treatment for enuresis. *Lancet* 1:1260, 1977.
15. Byrd RS, Weitzman M, Lanphear NE, et al: Bed-wetting in US children: Epidemiology and related behavior problems. *Pediatrics* 98:414-419, 1996.
16. Bloom DA, Seeley WW, Ritchey ML, et al: Toilet habits and continence in children: An opportunity sampling in search of normal parameters. *J Urol* 149:1087-1090, 1993.
17. Blomfield JM, Douglas JWB: Bedwetting prevalence among children aged 4-7 years. *Lancet* 2:850-852, 1956.
18. Hellström AL, Hanson E, Hasson S, et al: Micturition habits and incontinence in 7-year-old Swedish school entrants. *Eur J Pediatr* 149:434-437, 1990.
19. Spee-van der Wekke J, Hirasing RA, Meulmeester JF, et al: Childhood nocturnal enuresis in the Netherlands. *Urology* 51:1022-1026, 1998.
20. Bower WF, Moore KH, Shepherd RB, et al: The epidemiology of childhood enuresis in Australia. *Br J Urol* 78:602-606, 1996.

21. Chiozza ML, Bernardinelli L, Caione P, et al: An Italian epidemiological multicentre study of nocturnal enuresis. *Br J Urol* 81:86-89, 1998.
22. Janet J: Les troubles psychopathiques de la miction: Essai de psychophysiologie normale et pathologique. *Diss Paris* 1890.
23. Frary LG: Enuresis: A genetic study. *Arch Pediatr Adolesc Med* 49:557-578, 1935.
24. Hallgren B: Enuresis: A clinical and genetic study. *Acta Psychiatr Neurol Scand* 32:1-159, 1957.
25. Bakwin H: Enuresis in children. *J Pediatr* 58:806-819, 1961.
26. Bakwin H: Enuresis in twins. *Arch Pediatr Adolesc Med* 121:222-225, 1971.
27. Robson WLM, Leung AKC, Brant R: The Genetic influence in primary nocturnal enuresis. *Nocturnal Enuresis* 2:4-6, 1992.
28. Eiberg H, Berendt I, Mohr J: Assignment of dominant inherited nocturnal enuresis (ENUR1) to chromosome 13q. *Nat Genet* 10:354-356, 1995.
29. Hollmann E, Von Gontard A, Eiberg H, et al: Molecular genetic, clinical and psychiatric associations in nocturnal enuresis. *Br J Urol* 81:37-39, 1998.
30. Arnell H, Hjälmås M, Jägervall M, et al: The genetics of primary nocturnal enuresis: Inheritance and suggestion of a second major gene on chromosome 12q. *J Med Genet* 34:360-365, 1997.
31. Von Gontard A, Hollmann E, Eiberg H, et al: Clinical enuresis phenotypes in familial nocturnal enuresis. *Scand J Urol Nephrol* 31:11-16, 1997.
32. Moffatt MEK: Nocturnal enuresis: Psychologic implications of treatment and nontreatment. *J Pediatr* 114:697-704, 1989.
33. Friman PC, Handwerk ML, Swearer SM, et al: Do children with primary nocturnal enuresis have clinically significant behavior problems? *Arch Pediatr Adolesc Med* 152:537-539, 1998.
34. De Graaf MJM: 40 years of being treated for nocturnal enuresis. *Lancet* 340:957-958, 1992.
35. Anonymous: Urology at the sharp end. *BMJ* 309:1378-1379, 1994.
36. Morison MJ: Parents' and young people's attitudes towards bedwetting and their influence on behaviour, including readiness to engage in and persist with treatment. *Br J Urol* 81:56-66, 1998.
37. Van Tijen NM, Messer AP, Namdar Z: Perceived stress of nocturnal enuresis in childhood. *Br J Urol* 81:98-99, 1998.
38. Haque M, Ellerstein NS, Gundy JH, et al: Parental perceptions of enuresis: A collaborative study. *Arch Pediatr Adolesc Med* 135:809-811, 1981.
39. Warzak WJ: Psychosocial implications of nocturnal enuresis. *Clin Pediatr* 38-40, 1993.
40. Hägglöf B, Andrén O, Bergström E, et al: Self-esteem before and after treatment in children with nocturnal enuresis and urinary incontinence. *Scand J Urol Nephrol* 31:79-82, 1997.
41. Brazelton TB: A child-oriented approach to toilet training. *Pediatrics* 29:121-128, 1962.

42. Hjälmås K: Urodynamics in normal infants and children. *Scand J Urol Nephrol* 114:20-27, 1988.
43. Robson WLM, Leung AKC: Developmental delay as a cause of enuresis. *J Urol* 159:1338-1339, 1998.
44. Mikkelsen EJ, Rapoport JL, Nee L, et al: Childhood enuresis. *Arch Gen Psychiatry* 37:1139-1144, 1980.
45. Nevéus T, Läckgren G, Stenberg A, et al: Sleep and night-time behaviour of enuretics and non-enuretics. *Br J Urol* 81:67-71, 1998.
46. Kawauchi A, Imada N, Tanaka Y, et al: Changes in the structure of sleep spindles and delta waves on electroencephalography in patients with nocturnal enuresis. *Br J Urol* 81:72-75, 1998.
47. Wolfish NM: Sleeping patterns and their effects on the etiology and treatment of nocturnal enuresis. *Nocturnal Enuresis* 5:4-5, 1996.
48. Page ME, Akaoka H, Aston-Jones G, et al: Bladder distension activates noradrenergic locus coeruleus neurones by an excitatory amino acid mechanism. *Neuroscience* 51:555-563, 1992.
49. Di Michele S, Sillén U, Engel J, et al: Desmopressin and vasopressin increase locomotor activity in the rat *via* a central mechanism: Implications for nocturnal enuresis. *J Urol* 156:1164-1168, 1996.
50. Yeung CK, Godley ML, Ho CKW, et al: Some new insights into bladder function in infancy. *Br J Urol* 76:235-240, 1995.
51. Carroll JL, Loughlin GM: Diagnostic criteria for obstructive sleep apnea syndrome in children. *Pediatr Pulmonol* 14:71-74, 1992.
52. Steers WD, Suratt PM: Sleep apnoea as a cause of daytime and nocturnal enuresis. *Lancet* 349:1604, 1997.
53. Richardson MA, Seid AB, Cotton RT, et al: Evaluation of tonsils and adenoids in sleep apnea syndrome. *Laryngoscope* 90:1106-1110, 1980.
54. Simmons FB, Guilleminault C, Dement WC, et al: Surgical management of airway obstructions during sleep. *Laryngoscope* 87:326-338, 1977.
55. Weider DJ, Sateia MJ, West RP: Nocturnal enuresis in children with upper airway obstruction. *Otolaryngol Head Neck Surg* 105:427-432, 1991.
56. Nowak KC, Weider DJ: Pediatric nocturnal enuresis secondary to airway obstruction from cleft palate repair. *Clin Pediatr* 37:653-658, 1998.
57. Friedell A: A reversal of the normal concentration of the urine in children having enuresis. *Arch Pediatr Adolesc Med* 33:717-721, 1927.
58. Poulton EM: Relative nocturnal polyuria as a factor in enuresis. *Lancet* 2:906-907, 1952.
59. Vulliamy D: The day and night output of urine in enuresis. *Arch Dis Child* 31:439-443, 1956.
60. Kawauchi A, Watanabe H, Miyoshi K: Early morning urine osmolality in nonenuretic and enuretic children. *Pediatr Nephrol* 10:696-698, 1996.
61. Vande Walle J, Hoebeke P, Van Laecke E, et al: Persistent enuresis caused by nocturnal polyuria is a maturation defect of the nyctihemeral rhythm of diuresis. *Br J Urol* 81:40-45, 1998.
62. Nørgaard JP, Pedersen EB, Djurhuus JC: Diurnal anti-diuretic-hormone levels in enuretics. *J Urol* 134:1029-1031, 1985.

63. Rittig S, Knudsen UB, Nørgaard JP, et al: Abnormal diurnal rhythm of plasma vasopressin and urinary output in patients with enuresis. *Am J Physiol* 256:F664-F671, 1989.
64. George CPL, Messerli FH, Genest J, et al: Diurnal variation of plasma vasopressin in man. *J Clin Endocrinol Metab* 41:332-338, 1975.
65. Steffens J, Netzer M, Isenberg E, et al: Vasopressin deficiency in primary nocturnal enuresis results of a controlled prospective study. *Eur Urol* 24:366-370, 1993.
66. Eggert P, Kühn B: Antidiuretic hormone regulation in patients with primary nocturnal enuresis. *Arch Dis Child* 73:508-511, 1995.
67. Rittig S, Knudsen UB, Nørgaard JP, et al: The diurnal rhythm of plasma atrial natriuretic peptide in children with nocturnal enuresis. *Scand J Clin Lab Invest* 51:209, 1991.
68. Vurgun N, Yiditodlu MR, Ýþcan A, et al: Hypernatriuria and kaliuresis in enuretic children and the diurnal variation. *J Urol* 159:1333-1337, 1998.
69. Watanabe H: Sleep patterns in children with nocturnal enuresis. *Scand J Urol Nephrol* 173:55-57, 1995.
70. Ohne T: The increase in c-Fos expression in vasopressin- and oxytocin-immunoreactive neurons in the paraventricular and supraoptic nucleus of the hypothalamus following urinary retention. *J Kyoto Pref Univ Med* 104:393-403, 1995.
71. Schaumburg HL, Hunsballe JM, Rittig S, et al: The effect of the full bladder on vasopressin secretion in healthy young adults. *Scand J Urol Nephrol* 31:20-30, 1997.
72. Akinyanju O, Agbato O, Ogunmekan AO, et al: Enuresis in sickle cell disease: I. Prevalence studies. *J Trop Pediatr* 35:24-26, 1989.
73. Readett DRJ, Morris JS, Serjeant GR: Nocturnal enuresis in sickle cell haemoglobinopathies. *Arch Dis Child* 65:290-293, 1990.
74. Figueroa TE, Benaim E, Griggs ST, et al: Enuresis in sickle cell disease. *J Urol* 153:1987-1989, 1995.
75. Medel R, Dieguez S, Brindo M, et al: Monosymptomatic primary enuresis: Differences between patients responding or not responding to oral desmopressin. *Br J Urol* 81:46-49, 1998.
76. Medel R, Ruarte AC, Castera R, et al: Primary enuresis: A urodynamic evaluation. *Br J Urol* 81:50-52, 1998.
77. Nørgaard JP: Urodynamics in enuretics: I. Reservoir function. *Neurourol Urodyn* 8:199-211, 1989.
78. Watanabe H, Azuma Y: A proposal for a classification system of enuresis based on overnight simultaneous monitoring of electroencephalography and cystometry. *Sleep* 12:257-264, 1989.
79. Blok C, Coolsaet BLRA, Mansour M, et al: Dynamics of the ureterovesical junction: Interaction between diuresis and detrusor instability at the ureterovesical junction in pigs. *J Urol* 136:1123, 1986.
80. Kirk J, Rasmussen PV, Rittig S, et al: Provoked enuresis-like episodes in healthy children 7 to 12 years old. *J Urol* 156:210-213, 1996.

81. Mattsson S, Lindström S: Diuresis and voiding pattern in healthy schoolchildren. *Br J Urol* 76:783-789, 1995.
82. Bloom DA, Park JM, Koo HP: Comments on pediatric elimination dysfunctions: The Whorf hypothesis, the elimination interview, the guarding reflex and nocturnal enuresis. *Eur Urol* 33:20-24, 1998.
83. Park JM, Bloom DA, McGuire EJ: The guarding reflex revisited. *Br J Urol* 80:940-945, 1997.
84. Schacter M: Considerations generales sur l' enuresis nocturne infantile. *J De Med de Paris* 52:619-621, 1932.
85. Şener F, Hasanoğlu E, Söylemezoğlu O: Desmopressin versus indomethacin treatment in primary nocturnal enuresis and the role of prostaglandins. *Urology* 52:878-881, 1998.
86. Robson WLM: Diurnal enuresis. *Pediatr Rev* 18:407-412, 1997.
87. Van Gool JD, de Jonge GA: Urge syndrome and urge incontinence. *Arch Dis Child* 64:1629-1634, 1989.
88. Fernandes E, Vernier R, Gonzalez R: The unstable bladder in children. *J Pediatr* 118:831-837, 1991.
89. Robson WLM, Jackson HP, Blackhurst D, et al: Enuresis in children with attention hyperactivity deficit disorder. *Southern Med J* 90:503-505, 1997.
90. Bachelard M, Sillén U, Hansson S, et al: Urodynamic pattern in infants with urinary tract infection. *J Urol* 160:522-526, 1998.
91. Robson WML, Leung AKC: Extraordinary urinary frequency syndrome. *Urology* 42:321-324, 1993.
92. Loening-Baucke V: Urinary incontinence and urinary tract infection and their resolution with treatment of chronic constipation of childhood. *Pediatrics* 100:228-232, 1997.
93. Dohil R, Roberts E, Verrier J, et al: Constipation and reversible urinary tract abnormalities. *Arch Dis Child* 70:56-57, 1994.
94. O'Regan S, Yazbeck S, Schick E: Constipation, bladder instability, urinary tract infection syndrome. *Clin Nephrol* 23:152-154, 1985.
95. Fernandes E, Reinburg Y, Vernier R, et al: Neurogenic bladder dysfunction in children: Review of pathophysiology and current management. *J Pediatr* 124:1-7, 1994.
96. Soler D, Borzyskowski M: Lower urinary tract dysfunction in children with central nervous system tumours. *Arch Dis Child* 79:344-347, 1998.
97. Reid CJD, Borzyskowski M: Lower urinary tract dysfunction in cerebral palsy. *Arch Dis Child* 68:739-742, 1993.
98. Bloom DA, Faerber G, Bomalaski MD: Urinary incontinence in girls' evaluation, treatment, and its place in the standard model of voiding dysfunctions in children. *Urol Clin North Am* 22:521-538, 1995.
99. Boemers TM, van Gool JD, DeJong TPVM, et al: Urodynamic evaluation of children with the caudal regression syndrome (caudal dysplasia sequence). *J Urol* 151:1038-1040, 1994.
100. Misra D, Mushtaq I, Drake DP, et al: Associated urologic anomalies in low imperforate anus are capable of causing significant morbidity: A 15-year experience. *Urology* 48:281-283, 1996.

101. Barkai L, Szabó L: Urinary bladder dysfunction in diabetic children with and without subclinical cardiovascular autonomic neuropathy. *Eur J Pediatr* 152:190-192, 1993.
102. Mattsson SH: Voiding frequency, volumes and intervals in healthy schoolchildren. *Scand J Urol Nephrol* 28:1-11, 1994.
103. Segura CG: Urine flow in childhood: a study of flow chart parameters based on 1,361 uroflowmetry tests. *J Urol* 157:1426-1428, 1997.
104. Holmdahl G, Hanson E, Hanson M, et al: Four-hour voiding observation in healthy infants. *J Urol* 156:1809-1812, 1996.
105. Robson WLM: Enuresis treatment in the US. *Scand J Urol Nephrol* 33:56-60, 1999.
106. Ferber R: *Solve Your Child's Sleep Problems.* New York, Simon & Schuster, 1985.
107. Forsythe WI, Butler RJ: Fifty years of enuretic alarms. *Arch Dis Child* 64:879-885, 1989.
108. Moffatt MEK, Harlos S, Kirshen AJ, et al: Desmopressin acetate and nocturnal enuresis: How much do we know? *Pediatrics* 92:420-425, 1993.
109. Bonde HV, Andersen JP, Rosenkilde P: Nocturnal enuresis: Change of nocturnal voiding pattern during alarm treatment. *Scand J Urol Nephrol* 28:349-352, 1994.
110. Oredsson AF, Jørgensen TM: Changes in nocturnal bladder capacity during treatment with the bell and pad for monosymptomatic nocturnal enuresis. *J Urol* 160:166-169, 1998.
111. Robson WLM, Leung AKE: Intranasal desmopressin (DDAVP) in the treatment of nocturnal enuresis: A review of efficacy studies. *Today's Therapeutic Trends* 2:35-42, 1993.
112. Aladjem M, Wohl R, Boichis H, et al: Desmopressin in nocturnal enuresis. *Arch Dis Child* 57:137-140, 1982.
113. Miller K, Goldberg S, Arkin B: Nocturnal enuresis: Experience with long-term use of intranasally administered desmopressin. *J Pediatr* 114:723-726, 1989.
114. Tuvemo T: DDAVP in childhood nocturnal enuresis. *Acta Paediatr Scand* 67:753-755, 1978.
115. Ramsden PD, Hindmarsh JR, Price DA, et al: DDAVP for adult enuresis: A preliminary report. *Br J Urol* 54:256-258, 1982.
116. Key DW, Bloom DA, Sanvordenker J: Low-dose DDAVP in nocturnal enuresis. *Clin Pediatr* 31:299-301, 1992.
117. Fjellestad-Paulsen A, Wille S, Harris AS: Comparison of intranasal and oral desmopressin for nocturnal enuresis. *Arch Dis Child* 62:674-677, 1987.
118. Harris AS, Nilsson IM, Wagner ZG, et al: Intranasal administration of peptides: Nasal deposition, biological response, and absorption of desmopressin. *J Pharm Sci* 75:1085-1088, 1986.
119. Skoog SJ, Stokes A, Turner KL: Oral desmopressin: A randomized double-blind placebo controlled study of effectiveness in children with primary nocturnal enuresis. *J Urol* 158:1035-1040, 1997.

120. Hogg RJ, Husmann D: The role of family history in predicting response to desmopressin in nocturnal enuresis. *J Urol* 150:444-445, 1993.
121. Hjälmås K, Hanson E, Hellström AL, et al: Long-term treatment with desmopressin in children with primary monosymptomatic nocturnal enuresis: An open multicentre study. *Br J Urol* 82:704-709, 1998.
122. Dimson SB: DDAVP and urine osmolality in refractory enuresis. *Arch Dis Child* 61:1104-1107, 1986.
123. Butler R, Holland P, Devitt H, et al: The effectiveness of desmopressin in the treatment of childhood nocturnal enuresis: Predicting response using pretreatment variables. *Br J Urol* 81:29-36, 1998.
124. Post EM, Richman RA, Blackett PR, et al: Desmopressin response of enuretic children. *Arch Pediatr Adolesc Med* 137:962-963, 1983.
125. Rushton HG, Belman AB, Zaontz MR, et al: The influence of small functional bladder capacity and other predictors on the response to desmopressin in the management of monosymptomatic nocturnal enuresis. *J Urol* 156:651-655, 1996.
126. Birkásová M, Birkás O, Flynn MJ, et al: Desmopressin in the management of nocturnal enuresis in children: A double-blind study. *Pediatrics* 62:970-974, 1978.
127. Evans JHC, Meadow SR: Desmopressin for bed wetting: Length of treatment, vasopressin secretion, and response. *Arch Dis Child* 67:184-188, 1992.
128. Rittig S, Schaumburg H, Schmidt F, et al: Characteristics of nocturnal enuresis based on home recordings of urine output and desmopressin response. *Pediatrics* 102:876, 1998.
129. Eller DA, Homsy YL, Austin PF, et al: Spot urine osmolality, age and bladder capacity as predictors of response to desmopressin in nocturnal enuresis. *Scand J Urol Nephrol* 31:41-45, 1997.
130. Rushton HG, Belman AB, Zaontz M, et al: Response to desmopressin as a function of urine osmolality in the treatment of monosymptomatic nocturnal enuresis: A double-blind prospective study. *J Urol* 154:749-753, 1995.
131. Chiozza ML, Plebani M, Scaccianoce C, et al: Evaluation of antidiuretic hormone before and after long-term treatment with desmopressin in a group of enuretic children. *Br J Urol* 81:53-55, 1998.
132. Läckgren G, Lilja B, Nevèus T, et al: Desmopressin in the treatment of severe nocturnal enuresis in adolescents: A 7-year follow-up study. *Br J Urol* 81:17-23, 1998.
133. Robson WLM, Leung AKC: Long-term effectiveness of desmopressin in the treatment of nocturnal enuresis. *Today's Therapeutic Trends* 11:135-141, 1993.
134. Horowitz M, Combs AJ, Gerdes D: Desmopressin for nocturnal incontinence in the spina bifida population. *J Urol* 158:2267-2268, 1997.
135. Robson WLM, Leung AKC: Side effects associated with DDAVP treatment of nocturnal enuresis. *J Singapore Paediatr Soc* 36:81-84, 1994.
136. Robson WLM, Leung AKC: Side effects and complications of treatment with desmopressin for enuresis. *J Natl Med Assoc* 86:775-778, 1994.

137. Robson WLM, Nørgaard JP, Leung AKC: Hyponatremia in patients with nocturnal enuresis treated with DDAVP. *Eur J Pediatr* 155:959-962, 1996.
138. Sukhai RN, Mol J, Harris AS: Combined therapy of enuresis alarm and desmopressin in the treatment of nocturnal enuresis. *Eur J Pediatr* 148:465-467, 1989.
139. Bradbury M: Combination therapy for nocturnal enuresis with desmopressin and an alarm device. *Scand J Urol Nephrol* 31:61-63, 1997.
140. Cendron M, Klauber G: Combination therapy in the treatment of persistent nocturnal enuresis. *Br J Urol* 81:26-28, 1998.
141. Hellström AL, Hjälmås K, Jodal U: Rehabilitation of the dysfunctional bladder in children: Method and 3-year follow-up. *J Urol* 138:847-849, 1987.
142. Wennergren H, Öberg B: Pelvic floor exercises for children: A method of treating dysfunctional voiding. *Br J Urol* 76:9-15, 1995.
143. Chai TC: New insights into the clinical value of oxybutynin. *J Urol* 160:644, 1998.
144. Forsythe WI, Redmond A: Enuresis and spontaneous cure rate: Study of 1129 enuretics. *Arch Dis Child* 49:259-263, 1974.
145. Hellström A, Hanson E, Hansson S, et al: Micturition habits and incontinence at age 17: Reinvestigation of a cohort studied at age 7. *Br J Urol* 76:231-234, 1995.
146. Malone PS, Wheeler RA, Williams JE: Continence in patients with spina bifida: Long term results. *Arch Dis Child* 70:107-110, 1994.

CHAPTER 15

Advances in Pediatric Pharmacology, Therapeutics, and Toxicology

Cheston M. Berlin, Jr, MD
University Professor of Pediatrics, Department of Pediatrics, and Professor of Pharmacology, The Milton S. Hershey Medical Center, The Pennsylvania State University College of Medicine, Hershey

ABSTRACT

This chapter reviews published studies in the field of pediatric therapeutics between July 1998 and July 2000. The most important area discussed in the first part of the chapter concerns the significant advances made in the labeling of drugs for children in the United States. Dr Harry Shirkey coined the term "therapeutic orphan" in 1968 to describe the state of children who were not being considered in either drug development or in drug clinical trials. This explains why about 80% of drugs listed in each edition of the *Physicians' Desk Reference* do not have labeling for the pediatric age group, especially children younger than 12 years. The recent legislative, regulatory, and pharmaceutical company activities to change this situation are summarized. These changes are current and promise to make significant contributions to the availability of drugs with adequate pediatric indications to the practicing physician.

Another important change in recent years has been the appreciation of the importance of placebo-controlled clinical trials for psychotropic medications in children. Trials with one of the selective serotonin reuptake inhibitors, as well as further studies involving the appropriate dosing and preparation of stimulant drugs for attention-deficit/hyperactivity disorder (ADHD), are also discussed. Several new areas that promise significant knowledge in therapeutics are in the treatment of osteoporosis (a neglected condition in pediatrics), arthritis (a condition for which drugs are used to treat the disease rather than the symptoms), and acquisition of data concerning transplacental transfer of human immunodeficiency virus (HIV) and use of multiple anti-HIV drugs for treatment of this virus in the pediatric population.

The past 4 years have been extremely exciting for pediatric drug therapy. The Food and Drug Administration Modernization Act (FDAMA) in 1997 and the FDA Final Rule in 1998 put emphasis on legislation and regulatory initiatives to promote pediatric drug development. FDAMA gave an incentive to the pharmaceutical industry to develop pediatric labeling of marketed drugs by providing a 6-month patent extension (exclusivity provision). As of September 1, 2000, the FDA has issued written requests to drug firms to conduct pediatric studies of 171 different drugs.[1] These studies would be for drugs already on the market. An excellent review of the entire subject of pediatric drug development was published recently.[2] The FDA Final Rule, which became effective as of December 2000, requires pediatric studies for many already approved drugs that might possess pediatric indications. As of February 2001, the FDA has extended exclusivity status to 27 drugs including ranitidine, ibuprofen, midazolam, fluvoxamine, and gabapentin.[1]

Other organizations have been instrumental in supporting this increased activity in drug development in children. The Committee on Drugs of the American Academy of Pediatrics has actively promoted initiatives in pediatric pharmacology since the submission to the FDA of the first edition of *Guidelines in Drug Testing in Children* in 1974 (revised in 1982 and 1998) (Box 1).

The Pediatric Panel of the United States Pharmacopeia (USP) has also been active in this area by reviewing and publishing monographs in the USPDI (Drug Information) that present pediatric data (indications, dosing, side effects, drug interactions) when such data are in the literature, even if lacking on the official

BOX 1.

American Academy of Pediatrics: Advocacy for Pediatric Drug Development

---

1974 – General Guidelines (submitted to FDA)
1977 – Ethical Guidelines for Pediatric Drug Studies
1979, 1998 – Lists of drugs needing pediatric labeling
1982 – Update of General Guidelines
1995 – Update of Ethical Guidelines
1998 – Update of General Guidelines

label. A recent initiative of the Pediatric Panel has been the issuing of guidelines for the education of children and adolescents in prescription and nonprescription drug usage.[3,4]

The pharmaceutical industry has responded through PhRMA (Pharmaceutical Research and Manufacturers of America) by collating and publishing efforts by the industry to study drugs in children for a wide variety of pediatric indications.[5]

The establishment of the Pediatric Pharmacology Research Units (PPRUs) by the Division of Maternal and Child Health, National Institutes of Child Health, National Institutes of Health, has resulted in firm scientific studies of selected drugs to provide data for pediatric labeling as well as investigation of basic science concepts. Seven units in academic medical centers were established in 1993, and the PPRUs were expanded to 13 units in 1998.[6] All of the above initiatives will continue to provide an increased number of drugs and indications for their use in the pediatric population.

This chapter reviews reports in the fields of pediatric pharmacology, therapeutics, and toxicology that were published between July 1998 and July 2000, with some earlier citations when appropriate.

DRUG ADMINISTRATION AND METABOLISM

Appropriate emphasis is now being paid to getting a drug to the pediatric patient. This must be an area of the highest priority. The caregivers of children seen for asthma exacerbations at 2 university pediatric emergency clinics were asked about their knowledge of using albuterol for their child. Each caregiver had stated that their child was receiving albuterol. Of 41 caregivers queried, 63% stated they were out of medication, 17% stated an incorrect dose, 44% stated an incorrect dosing frequency, and 24% stated an incorrect duration of use.[7] Previous reports have documented difficulties with drug dosage and duration, but this study reports a disturbing statistic—nearly two thirds of caregivers were out of medication for a chronic condition, and this contributed to an emergency department visit. It is hoped that efforts such as the education initiatives of the USP, as discussed above, will improve this situation.

Different routes of administration continue to be explored, especially for rapid onset of drug action. Status epilepticus needs rapid treatment; oral therapy is not possible except by transbuccal absorption. Midazolam (2 mg) squirted around the buccal mucosa stopped seizures of 75% of patients (40 episodes in 14 patients).[8]

The median time to seizure cessation was 6 minutes. The comparison treatment was 10 mg of rectal diazepam; this treatment stopped 59% of seizures (39 episodes in 14 patients), with a median time of cessation of 8 minutes. Even though the comparison was not between the same drug, buccal administration might be more reliably administered by the nonprofessional caregiver.

Rectal administration has been studied for multiple doses of acetaminophen for pain in neonates.[9] A dose of 20 mg/kg was used with unpredictable serum concentrations (most serum concentrations < 10 mg/L). The maximal serum concentrations after the first dose was 3.36 ± 2.11 mg/L. A correlation between adequate analgesia and serum concentration of acetaminophen has not yet been made in pediatric patients. Pain scores in this study were based on facial expressions of discomfort ranging from 0 (no pain) to 5 (obvious pain). Pain scores of 0 to 1 were associated with serum concentrations above 2.6 mg/L. The rectal route for analgesia may not be effective for young infants, hence the interest in buccal absorption as discussed above.

Adverse drug reactions (ADRs) have been the subject of major news stories in 1999-2000 and are a problem in both children and adults. A survey in Italy of 29 pediatric practices, including 24,000 children, showed that the overall incidence of ADRs for children aged 14 years and younger was 15 ADRs per 1000 children. The highest incidence of ADRs (34 per 1000) occurred in children aged 1 year and younger.[10] This overall incidence is 4 times greater than that reported to the Italian Ministry of Health. This study confirms that ADRs are underreported. In the United States, the USP has developed a reporting system (Med-MARX) that may provide a more accurate picture of the incidence of ADRs.

TREATMENT OF SYMPTOMS

One of the most common reasons for administering drugs to children is to treat the symptoms of an illness. The drugs used are usually over-the-counter (OTC) agents. Although widely used by and recommended for children, few controlled trials exist for many of these agents.

DIARRHEA

A study of 258 children (ages 2-11 years) with acute nonspecific diarrhea (all but 10 patients with negative bacterial cultures) in 12 sites in Mexico and the United States compared loperamide with placebo in a randomized controlled trial.[11] Children aged 2 to 5 years received (over a 48-hour period) an initial dose of 1 mg of loperamide, and children aged 6 to 11 years received 2 mg. After each subsequent unformed stool, each patient received 1 mg of drug or placebo to a daily maximum of 3 mg in children 2 to 5 years of age, 4 mg in children aged 6 to 8 years, and 6 mg in children aged 9 to 11 years. Children of all ages who received active drug had a statistically shorter time to last unformed stool and also a fewer number of unformed stools. Adverse events were not significantly increased with loperamide. Parents felt that the patients receiving loperamide did better symptomatically. Although nonspecific gastroenteritis is a limited, usually nonthreatening illness in children, loperamide may have a place in its therapy, particularly for families that may not be at home.

FEVER

We live in a fever-phobic country. Acetaminophen and ibuprofen are widely used as antipyretic agents for children. A common practice is alternating these 2 drugs in a febrile patient.[12] No data support this strategy, although 50% of practitioners advise their patients to do so. This practice is not new. The author recalls that alternating use of acetaminophen and aspirin was common 25 to 30 years ago. Alternating antipyretics may lead to incorrect dosing, especially of acetaminophen, with potentially serious adverse effects. The mechanism of action of these 2 antipyretics is the same; proper dosing (15 mg/kg per dose of acetaminophen or 10 mg/kg per dose of ibuprofen) of either drug with appropriate environmental strategies for fever control will be effective in nearly all cases.[13,14] Lessening the concern of the parents for fever in children is difficult; emphasis of correct dosing of a single antipyretic agent is appropriate.

SEDATION AND ANESTHESIA

In patients with cancer who were undergoing access of a central venous port, intranasal administration of midazolam (0.2 mg/kg by spray) decreased anxiety and discomfort as evaluated by parents and nurses, but patients (those older than 7 years) reported only decreased anxiety.[15] Two problems limit interpretation of this study; midazolam can produce amnesia, and there was an 8% dropout rate because of discomfort from the nasal administration of both the drug and placebo (both give a burning sensation). Some patients received as many as 10 puffs (0.1 mL). It would be interesting to repeat this study with buccal administration. Either route has the potential for rapid onset, and each is relatively noninvasive.

Analysis of adverse events occurring during sedation identifies that a higher proportion of these events are associated with cardiac arrests, inadequate resuscitation, and death/permanent neurologic sequelae when sedation is performed in non–hospital-based locations.[16] The authors of this study stress the need to use pulse oximetry for monitoring in a hospital setting (successful outcome) compared with nonhospital setting (where 4 of 5 patients had adverse outcomes).

An excellent review of sedation and anesthesia for children including dosages and drug choices depending on the procedure has been published by Krauss and Green.[17] An interesting part of this review is the discussion of ketamine, a safe and effective agent for significant outpatient procedures. It has a wide margin of safety. The well-known side effect of hallucinations during recovery described in adults is rarely seen in children.

IBUPROFEN

Ibuprofen is a widely used drug for antipyresis, inflammation, and analgesia. Concern that its widespread use, especially since becoming available OTC in 1995, might lead to an association with Reye syndrome (as did aspirin) seems eliminated with the data published by the manufacturer, McNeil Consumer Healthcare.[18] OTC pediatric sales have gone from none in 1989 to more than 1 billion 50-mg dosage units, with a continued decline in the number of reported cases of Reye syndrome up to 1997.

PREGNANCY

MEBENDAZOLE

Mebendazole is an anti-helminthic drug useful in treating hookworm infection. Hookworm is especially prevalent in developing countries, and the World Health Organization (WHO) estimates that 44 million pregnant women may be infected.[19] Hookworm infection may lead to iron deficiency anemia from intestinal blood loss. Mebendazole use during pregnancy was studied in 7087 women in Sri Lanka.[19] Women were interviewed after giving birth. Nearly 75% had taken mebendazole at least once during pregnancy. In the group of mothers taking mebendazole, 1.8% (97 of 5275) of infants had major congenital anomalies compared with 1.5% in the control group (26 of 1737) (odds ratio, 1.24; 95% CI, 0.80-1.91). No singular defect was observed in the mebendazole group. The incidence of stillbirths and perinatal deaths was significantly lower in the mebendazole group (1.9% vs 3.3%; odds ratio, 0.40-0.77). This difference was also seen for low birth weights (<1500 g) (1.1%

TABLE 1.
Psychotropic Drug Treatment During Pregnancy

Illness	Drug Therapy
Schizophrenia	Antipsychotic agents (haloperidol, phenothiazines)
Major depression	Tricyclic antidepressants*
Bipolar disorder	Lithium* and/or antipsychotic agent
Panic disorder	Fluoxetine
Obsessive-compulsive disorder	Fluoxetine

*Need therapeutic drug monitoring.

vs 2.3%). Even considering the issues associated with retrospective studies, mebendazole appears safe for use during pregnancy and may lead to a more favorable outcome for the infant.

DIETHYLSTILBESTROL

The follow-up of the status of women who were exposed to diethylstilbestrol (DES) during pregnancy continues.[20] Except for the increased risk of clear cell carcinoma, previously well described, there was no increased incidence of any other cancer in woman exposed to DES in fetal life (n = 3674) compared with unexposed women (n = 1220). The average age of these women is 38 years; continued follow-up will have to occur.

PSYCHOTROPIC AGENTS

The pharmacologic treatment of significant mental illness during pregnancy has always been a challenge. A major problem with assessing the risk to the infant has been the lack of long-term follow-up. Such follow-up is necessary to assess potential neurobehavioral effects throughout childhood. The Committee on Drugs of the American Academy of Pediatrics has published a statement on this issue that reviews existing data.[21] The guidelines for maternal therapy suggested in this statement for each of the significant psychiatric illnesses during pregnancy are listed in Table 1.

Long-term studies of neurodevelopment are much needed for the offspring of such pregnancies. These studies are also needed when mothers take these drugs during lactation.

NEONATOLOGY

Cisapride was a drug widely used for gastroesophageal reflux (GER) in infants and children. It was especially used in premature infants because GER may have adverse effects on swallowing (and hence nutrition) and respirations. Cisapride has potential cardiac toxicity; this appears to be related to serum concentration.[22] Its metabolism is mediated by the cytochrome system (P450 3A4 enzymes). Drugs that inhibit the cytochrome system (macrolide antibiotics, ketoconazole, fluconazole) will increase serum concentrations and may cause cardiac arrhythmias.[23] The degree of risk has been very controversial, but enough concern was raised for the company and the FDA to issue a safety warning in 1998. In 2000, the company announced it was withdrawing cisapride from the US market. This drug is an example of a potentially useful agent that rapidly gained widespread use perhaps without sufficient effort at monitoring and reporting adverse events.[24] The experience with cisapride also illustrates why the newborn infant remains a therapeutic orphan.

Apnea of prematurity may affect as many as 90% of premature infants with a birth weight of less than 1000 g. Management consists of environmental alterations such as positioning, ambient temperature, oxygen, stimulation, ventilation (intubation, positive airway pressure, or both) and use of the methylxanthines, theophylline or caffeine. Bhatia[25] has published a very useful review of the treatment of apnea of prematurity. The pharmacologic treatment of apnea of prematurity is not new, theophylline use being introduced in 1973.[25] The metabolite of theophylline is caffeine, and its use began shortly after that of theophylline. Caffeine has a much longer half-life than does theophylline (100 vs 30 hours) and has more stable plasma concentrations (therapeutic concentrations, 5-20 mg/L). The toxicity of caffeine is less than that of theophylline and is rarely seen at therapeutic plasma concentrations. Dosage is 10 mg/kg initially, then 2.5 mg/kg daily with therapeutic drug monitoring. What is new about the use of caffeine is that until 1999, no commercial preparation was available. For more than 20 years, each institution prepared its own supply from caffeine citrate and in-house sterilization. This made outpatient use very difficult, especially for those families living far from a neonatal/pediatric center. Erenberg et al[26] published a double-blind, placebo-controlled study of the efficacy of caffeine citrate. The drug was made available commercially in 1999 (Cafcit, Roxane).

LACTATION

SELECTIVE SEROTONIN REUPTAKE INHIBITORS

Perhaps the most common question asked pediatricians about drugs and lactation concerns antidepressants, especially selective serotonin reuptake inhibitors (SSRIs). Postpartum depression is common, and the SSRIs have received much attention because of their efficacy and safety (monitoring of serum concentrations not required). Stowe et al[27] studied 16 mother-infant pairs during maternal therapy with the SSRI paroxetine. The maternal dosage was 10 to 50 mg/d. The ages of the infants ranged from 4 to 55 weeks. Paroxetine appeared in all milk samples; the average concentration was 42 ng/mL. For most milk samples, the concentration of drug increased during a nursing period. The amount in milk increased with the maternal dose; milk concentrations at a maternal dose of 50 mg/d were about 100 ng/mL compared with about 20 ng/mL at 10 mg/d. Maternal serum concentrations ranged from 15 ng/mL to 164 ng/mL (2 mothers were below detection of 2 ng/mL). The serum concentrations of all 16 infants were below the detection concentrations. It would be comforting to know whether "below detection" meant no drug was delivered to the infant. There was no follow-up, including neurobehavioral testing of the infants. We may not possess sensitive-enough testing instruments to detect any neurodevelopmental effects on the central nervous system of infants exposed to psychoactive agents in utero or through lactation.

A retrospective study examined the weight gain of infants whose mothers took fluoxetine during pregnancy and lactation. The control group took fluoxetine only during pregnancy.[28] The maternal dosage during nursing varied from 20 to 40 mg/d, with 80% of mothers taking 20 mg/d. Infants exposed to fluoxetine gained an average of 392 g less between 2 weeks and 6 months of age than did infants not exposed to fluoxetine. The authors properly acknowledged that lack of objective data of drug concentration in either milk or infant plasma limits interpretation of this study. Perhaps mothers requiring postnatal fluoxetine might have more difficulties with feeding infants; a study of a group of mothers receiving fluoxetine and bottle feeding may answer this question.

METHADONE

Although the statement by the Committee on Drugs of the American Academy of Pediatrics on drug transfer in milk says that mothers receiving more than 20 mg/d of methadone should not breast-feed, data to support this seem to be missing.[29] McCarthy and Posey[30] studied 14 samples of milk from mothers receiving 25 to 180 mg/d of methadone. Methadone concentrations in milk ranged from 27 to 260 ng/mL (mean, 95 ng/mL), so that ingestion of 1 L of milk would contribute only about 100 μg of methadone. No adverse effects on the infants were seen. Breast-feeding should be permitted in women receiving methadone.

ANTIBIOTIC THERAPY

OVERPRESCRIBING OF ANTIBIOTICS AND OTITIS MEDIA

Overprescribing of antibiotics in children remains a problem and may be contributing to the emergence of relative or complete drug resistance by important bacteria. A large study of more than 47,000 children aged 3 to 72 months in 2 managed health care organizations (Boston and Seattle) investigated antibiotic use.[31] In these 2 cities, the average rates of antibiotic prescribing for children aged 3 to 36 months were 3.2 and 2.1 prescriptions per child per year, respectively. Thirty-five percent (Boston) and 23% (Seattle) of children received 4 or more prescriptions in 1 year. The older children (36-72 months) in Boston and Seattle received 2.0 and 1.5 prescriptions per child per year, respectively. More than half (56%) of prescriptions for antibiotics in the younger children (aged 3-36 months) and 40% for the group aged 36 to 72 months were for otitis media. Between 10% and 14% of prescriptions were for upper respiratory tract infections. The most significant finding was that 30% to 32% of prescriptions were for "unassigned" or "other" conditions. The latter did not include sinusitis and urinary tract infection. These categories almost certainly indicate overprescribing.

Otitis media may not always need to be treated with antibiotics. Assessment of the infant's or child's ear drum is a difficult diagnostic maneuver; one is always hopeful of finding a reason for fever in a young child. Many of the studies of results of not using antibiotics in children with otitis media have come from Europe. A study of 240 children investigated placebo or amoxicillin, 40 mg/kg per day, in a randomized, double-blind trial.[32] Clinical evaluations occurred at 4 and 11 days (tabulation of symptoms and clinical examination) and again at 6 weeks after therapy (symptoms, clinical examination, and tympanometry). The results are shown in Table 2. Findings on clinical examination were no different at day 4 and at 6 weeks. This study should provoke considerable debate concerning antibiotic treatment of otitis media. In the absence of a purulent drum, canal discharge, or both, many clinicians are withholding antibiotics.

The concern about drug-resistant organisms prompted the Communicable Disease Center in Atlanta, Georgia, to convene a Drug-Resistant *Streptococcus pneumoniae* (DRSP) Therapeutic Working Group.[33] The deliberations suggested a treatment scheme for DRSP of (1) high-dose amoxicillin (80-90 mg/kg per day) as the drug of choice for therapeutic failure, or (2) amoxicillin-clavulanate, (3) cefuroxime axetil, or (4) intramuscular ceftriaxone. This

TABLE 2.
Otitis Media Treated With Amoxicillin or Placebo

	Amoxicillin	Placebo
Symptoms at day 4	59%	72%
Median duration of fever	2 days	3 days
Analgesic use	2.3 doses	4.1 doses
Median duration of pain/crying	8 days	9 days

(Data from Damoiseaux R, van Balen F, Hoes A, et al: Primary care based randomized double blind trial of amoxicillin versus placebo for acute otitis media in children aged under 2 years. *BMJ* 320:350-354, 2000.)

report has received widespread interest, but many do not realize that these recommendations are for cases with DRSP and not for all cases of acute otitis media. Tympanocentesis is seldom done in the clinical setting. High-dose amoxicillin is not well tolerated by some children. Amoxicillin-clavulanate may be associated with a significant incidence of gastrointestinal complaints, and cefuroxime axetil is expensive.

Intramuscular ceftriaxone requires 3 daily consecutive injections (in our pediatric clinic the cost is $80 per injection). One hopes that newer agents may prove more effective and less expensive than current drugs for DRSP. The interest in not prescribing antibiotics for initial treatment of mild to moderate cases of otitis media is understandable.

STREPTOCOCCAL PHARYNGITIS

Compliance with a 10-day course of penicillin V administered 3 or 4 times a day has always been a challenge for the physician, patient, and parent. Amoxicillin, 750 mg, given once per day for 10 days (n = 79) is as effective as 250 mg of penicillin V administered 3 times daily for 10 days (n = 73).[34] The patients studied were between 3 and 18 years of age, and all cases were culture proven. At 4 to 6 days, 11% of amoxicillin-treated children were still culture positive as were 16% of children receiving penicillin V. At 14 to 21 days, the percentage of positive cultures was 5% and 4%, respectively.

RASHES WITH ANTIBIOTIC THERAPY

The child who develops a rash during and shortly after antibiotic therapy presents a challenge. Is the rash caused by the infection disease, a drug allergy, or neither? Huang and Borum[35] studied 86 children (aged 6 years and younger) referred to an allergy clinic to determine if the skin rash indicated a drug allergy. All had an upper respiratory tract infection. Eighty-five percent had an erythematous rash, 15% had urticaria, and 50% reported a rash with 2 or more different antibiotics. All rashes developed between 3 and 5 days of antibiotic therapy. The color photographs in the report are excellent and illustrate some extensive rashes. Scratch tests and intradermal tests against the antibiotic were negative in all but 1 of the 86 patients. The positive test was in a patient treated with sulfisoxazole-erythromycin. Penicillin radioallergosorbent (RAST) testing was negative in all patients tested. When well, all patients received an oral challenge with the offending drug; no adverse reactions occurred. In subsequent infections, 8 of 62 patients receiving a dye-free version of the antibiotic developed a mild rash managed with antihistamine therapy; these patients finished the antibiotic course. A group of 12 patients received an intravenous form of an antibiotic to which they previously had a reaction (10 cephalosporin and 2 penicillin); none had an adverse reaction. It is reassuring that rashes seldom indicate a drug allergy. The authors suggest an approach that includes skin and RAST testing for the suspected antibiotics and a careful oral challenge. This testing is best done by an allergist.

HIV INFECTION

Chemotherapy of HIV infection is changing so rapidly that published reviews are hard pressed to keep up with advances. In 1998, it was demonstrated that even abbreviated courses of zidovudine (AZT) decreased the incidence of transplacental transfer of HIV infection.[36] This study from New York State was able to distinguish infants whose mothers had received varying lengths of treatment with zidovudine. If the drug was given throughout pregnancy, the rate of infection was 6.1%; if given during birth, 10%; if given to the infant within the first 48 hours of life, 9.3%; and if given on day 3 or later, 18.4%. In untreated pregnancies and infants, the rate of HIV transfer was 26.6%. Follow-up was at 6 months of age. In a more recent study from Uganda, the effectiveness of zidovudine given to the mother during labor (600 mg first dose, 300 mg every 3 hours until delivery) and to the infant for 1 week after birth (4 mg/kg twice a day), was compared with that of nevirapine, given as a single dose (200 mg) to the mother during labor and as a single dose (2 mg/kg) to the infant after birth.[37] Nevirapine was more effective than zidovu-

TABLE 3.
Effect of Treatment on HIV Transmission

Age of Infant	% of Infants Infected	
	Zidovudine	Nevirapine
Birth	10.4	8.2
6-8 weeks	21.3	11.9
14-16 weeks	25.1	13.1

(Data from Guay L, Musoke P, Fleming T, et al: Intrapartum and neonatal single-dose nevirapine compared with zidovudine for prevention of mother-to-child transmission of HIV-1 in Kampala, Uganda: HIVNET 012 randomised trial. *Lancet* 354:795-802, 1999.)

dine at 6 to 8 weeks and at 14 to 16 weeks' post partum (Table 3). Long-term follow-up will be necessary. This study was done in a breast-feeding population. We await the results of studies with double- or triple-drug therapy for short courses. Developing countries may have to use these relatively inexpensive short courses until an effective vaccine is developed. It is gratifying to learn that prenatal and neonatal exposure to zidovudine does not cause any adverse effects in HIV-infected children followed up for as long as 5½ years.[38]

The treatment of children with HIV infection is also rapidly changing. The first drugs to be used in HIV-positive children were nucleoside analogues such as zidovudine and lamivudine.

Recently, protease inhibitors such as ritonavir have been used. A recent study included nucleoside inhibitors (zidovudine and lamivudine) only compared with these same 2 nucleoside inhibitors plus ritonavir. Another arm of the study used stavudine plus ritonavir.[39] The patients assigned to the 2 arms containing ritonavir had significantly greater lowering of plasma HIV viral load as measured by HIV-1 RNA. At least 50% of the patients assigned to the 2 arms containing ritonavir had undetectable plasma HIV-1 RNA levels compared with 12% of the patients assigned to the study arm containing only the 2 nucleoside inhibitors. However, enthusiasm must be tempered by the high incidence of side effects (21% severe, 72% moderate or worse) and discontinuation of drugs by study week 48 (62% in the nucleoside group and 28% and 35% in the 2 groups containing ritonavir). Also CD4 cell counts remained unchanged for patients in all 3 study arms. Combination drug therapy for HIV infection will continue to be developed until an effective regimen with minimal toxicity is found. Data showing reduction in mortality with double combination therapy (since 1993) and triple combination therapy (since 1996) in 106 Italian pediatric centers have been published.[40]

NEUROLOGY

SEIZURES

Although phenobarbital has been displaced as the initial single agent for childhood epilepsy, it is still used during pregnancy (preferred to phenytoin), during the neonatal period, and to prevent febrile seizures. A group of children with febrile seizures treated with phenobarbital demonstrated a decrease of 7 IQ points after 2 years compared with placebo. This group difference decreased to 4.3 IQ points after 6 months off therapy.[41] The same group was studied 3 to 5 years later after they had started school.[42] The difference in IQ between groups remained. The group previously treated with phenobarbital had a 3.71 point difference on Stanford-Binet IQ ($P = .09$, not significant), and an 8 point difference on the Wide Range Achievement Test (WRAT-R) ($P = .007$, significant). However, only 64% of the original patients could be studied. These studies support the negative effect on neurodevelopment of early phenobarbital treatment. Its use, especially in the neonatal period, should be reexamined. Follow-up studies of the newer anticonvulsants should be undertaken.

Both phenobarbital and phenytoin are equally but disappointingly effective in controlling neonatal seizures.[43] Only 43% of infants receiving phenobarbital and 45% of those receiving phenytoin had their seizures controlled. It is surprising that in the year 2000, there are no adequate studies of effective anticonvulsants in neonates. The neonate is a special category of the therapeutic orphan.

ANTIEPILEPTIC AGENTS AND BONE MINERAL DENSITY

Even short-term therapy (6 months to 3 years) with the anticonvulsants valproate and carbamazepine may result in an 8% decrease in bone mineral density (BMD) in children aged 6 to 12 years (mostly girls), compared with children not treated.[44] Boys as well as girls had elevated serum alkaline phosphatase levels, but only the girls had a significant decrease in BMD. The study had small numbers; therefore, it is premature to recommend increased calcium or vitamin D intake beyond that recommended by the American Academy of Pediatrics.[45] The difference between boys and girls may be explained by increased physical activity in the boys. Increased physical activity is associated with hip bone density in teenagers.[46] Physical activity on a daily basis may be a more important prognostic indication for BMD than is calcium intake.[46]

USE OF PSYCHOACTIVE MEDICATIONS IN CHILDREN

Drugs have been used extensively in children for the treatment of psychiatric conditions, including behavioral and learning problems, despite the fact that the first few adequate studies have only been done very recently. A very large study of the incidence of prescribing psychoactive mediations in children aged 2 to 4 years has been published.[47] The populations surveyed were 2 state Medicaid programs and one health maintenance organization. The total number of children involved was more than 250,000. The 3 classes of pyschoactive drugs prescribed were stimulants, antidepressants, and neuroleptics. Specific drugs tabulated were methylphenidate (MPH) and clonidine. Table 4 illustrates the increased use of these drugs between 1991 and 1995. Two interesting observations can be made. There has been a substantial increase (3-fold for MPH, 28-fold for clonidine) in the prescribing of these medications to a preschool population. For stimulants especially, it is intriguing to speculate as to how a diagnosis of attention deficit disorder (ADD) or attention-deficit/hyperactivity disorder (ADHD) in these young children was made. Likewise, the doubling of the use of antidepressants implies increased diagnosis of depression in an age group that may include preverbal children. The findings of this report vividly demonstrate the need for controlled studies of these medications in all pediatric age groups.

TABLE 4.
Use of Psychotropic Drugs in Children Aged 2 to 4 Years

	Prevalence (per 1000 Children)	
	1991	**1995**
Stimulants	4.1	12.3
Methylphenidate	3.7	11.1
Clonidine	0.1	2.3
Antidepressants	1.4	3.2
Neuroleptics	0.7	0.9

(Data from Zito J, Safer D, dosReis S, et al: Trends in the prescribing of psychotropic medications to preschoolers. *JAMA* 283:1025-1030, 2000.)

ADHD: STIMULANT THERAPY

The American Academy of Pediatrics has published a clinical practice guideline for ADHD.[48] This guideline emphasizes that criteria from the *Diagnostic and Statistical Manual of Mental Disorders, Fourth Edition* (DSM-IV) be applied to each child before this diagnosis is made. Therefore, information must be gathered from the patient, parents, and school personnel for proper evaluation. Drug therapy should only be undertaken after a thorough assessment with indicated tools of evaluation, including checklists and academic achievement tests. Approximately 10% of school-age children exhibit some elements of ADHD, but all do not require medication. Between 1990 and 1995, utilization data from the National Ambulatory Medical Care Survey showed that there was a 2- to 3-fold increase in the rate of office visits for the diagnosis of ADHD and a 3-fold increase in the prescribing of a stimulant drug.[49] Approximately 3% of office visits of children aged 5 through 18 years are for ADHD.

Adderall is a stimulant containing 2 salts of amphetamine (asparate and sulfate) and 2 salts of dextroamphetamine (saccharate and sulfate) in equal proportion. Adderall given once in the morning is equivalent (milligram for milligram) to twice-a-day dosing with MPH.[50] The highest dosage of MPH tested was 15 mg given twice a day. Both drugs were more effective than placebo. This comparison needs to be extended to higher doses. A second study, which used equivalent milligram dosages of Adderall and MPH, also showed day-long efficacy of a single morning dose of Adderall.[51] This study included a small group (n = 21) of children in an intensive 8-week summer behavior modification program. The omission of the lunchtime dose at school is certainly most desirable from a compliance standpoint and to avoid labeling a student as having a learning/behavioral problem. It is important to emphasize the potential positive benefits of behavioral intervention techniques in the management of AHDH and comorbid conditions such as oppositional defiant behavior.[52]

The issue of whether stimulant medication causes tics is a controversial one. Law and Schachar[53] studied 90 children with ADHD with and without tics. In a year-long study in which patients received placebo (n = 18) or MPH (n = 72), 19.6% of the patients (without prior tics) receiving MPH developed clinically significant tics versus 16.7% of those receiving placebo. In both groups, 33% who had preceding tics showed an increase in frequency of tics. The mean dosage of MPH used was 0.5 mg/kg twice a day, a significant dose. This dose, coupled with the long duration of a year of observation, supports the careful use of MPH in patients with tics. In a small group of 19 patients receiving an average of 0.3 mg/kg of MPH per dose or 0.6 mg/kg per day, an abrupt switch to placebo (2-week observation periods) and back again did not cause an increase in tics.[54]

OBSESSIVE COMPULSIVE DISORDER

Double-blind, randomized, placebo-controlled studies of pediatric neuropsychiatric disorders are rare. These disorders are of great importance for pediatric therapeutics. A multicenter (n = 12) trial of 107 children aged 6 to 12 years and 80 adolescents aged 13 to 17 years with obsessive compulsive disorder (OCD) was performed.[55] The patients were randomly assigned to receive sertraline (a selective serotonin reuptake inhibitor) or placebo for 12 weeks. The maximum dosage of sertraline used was 200 mg/d. All patients receiving sertraline improved by measurement of all 3 evaluation scales: Children's Yale-Brown Obsessive Compulsive Scale, National Institute of Mental Health Global Obsessive Compulsive Scale, and National Institute of Mental Health Clinical Global Impression Improvement Scale. Significant improvement did not occur until 4 to 6 weeks after starting drug therapy. The recommendation is that treatment of OCD begin with 50 mg/d of sertraline, followed by an upwards titration of the dosage at 6 to 8 weeks if no clinical response has occurred. Sertraline is well tolerated. The only statistically significant side effect was insomnia; 37% of patients receiving sertraline had insomnia compared with 13% of placebo patients. Other side effects observed were nausea (17% vs 7%), agitation (13% vs 2%), and tremor (7% vs 0%). One hopes that there will be more such trials involving psychotropic medications in children.

ASTHMA

Asthma has become the most prevalent chronic illness in pediatrics. In spite of expanded drug therapy, asthma is a frequent diagnosis for emergency department visits. The addition of nebulized ipratropium to the treatment regimen that asthmatic patients receive in the emergency department will significantly decrease the rate of hospitalizations for these patients.[56] In children with severe asthma (peak expiratory flow below 50% of the predicted value), the addition of ipratropium to nebulized albuterol and oral corticosteroid decreased the need for hospital admissions from 52.6% to 37.5%.

In a similar study conducted in the emergency department, children receiving ipratropium (a control group received nebulized saline) along with albuterol and oral corticosteroid for the first 3 nebulization treatments, had a slightly shorter treatment time (185 vs 215 minutes) and required fewer total albuterol doses (3 vs 4).[57] Admission rates were similar (18% vs 22%).

In a nonemergency outpatient setting, children with mild to moderate exacerbations of asthma (clinical asthma score utilizing wheezing and cough) responded equally well to either dexamethasone (a single intramuscular dose of 1.7 mg/kg) or a 5-day course of oral prednisone (2 mg/kg for 5 days).[58] The groups were small, with 15 patients receiving dexamethasone and 17 receiving prednisone. The use of a single dose of intramuscular dexamethasone removes the problem of compliance. In this study, 7 of 17 children receiving oral prednisone failed to receive 30% to 75% of the prescribed number of doses.

It is imperative that children with a chronic disease tightly adhere to all aspects of therapy. The study by Winkelstein et al[59] reminds us that much needs to be done in educating both children and their families about drug therapy. In a study of 30 families containing a school-age child with asthma, 93% of the children were taking inhaled asthma medication without adult supervision, but only 7% knew how to use a metered dose inhaler (MDI). Sixty percent of parents thought their child's MDI use was "excellent." It is not surprising that control of asthma was poor in this group; 77% had an emergency department visit and 27% required hospitalization within the previous 6 months. Seventy-three percent had a mean of 3 symptom-days per week, and 83% had a mean of 2.8 symptom-nights per week. In more than 50% of patients, the parents' reports of the drugs prescribed did not agree with the physicians' prescriptions for inhaled β-agonists, steroids, and cromolyn. Much needs to be done to better educate our pediatric population about prescribed medications.

ARTHRITIS

The pharmacology of arthritis is moving from treatment of symptoms to modifying the course of the disease. In addition to relatively small molecular weight drugs (eg, ibuprofen, methotrexate), large biological molecules are being used. Etanercept is a genetically engineered protein that blocks the action of tumor necrosis factor (TNF). TNF is a cytokine thought to play a major role in the pathogenesis of juvenile rheumatoid arthritis (JRA). It is elevated in the serum and present in the synovial fluid of patients with JRA. Etanercept is thought to act by binding TNF and preventing its biological inflammatory activity. In an open-label study of 69 patients (aged 4-17 years), 74% had clinical improvement after etanercept therapy.[60] These patients had active disease in spite of therapy with nonsteroidal anti-inflammatory agents and methotrexate. In a double-blind part of the study, 81% of patients receiving placebo had a flare of their disease compared with 28% of patients receiving etanercept. Adverse events were not different between the 2 groups. The use of large molecular agents will continue to proliferate as increasing knowledge of the precise molecular basis of many diseases is identified.

OSTEOPOROSIS

Osteoporosis has received little attention in pediatrics. A group of compounds known as bisphosphonates may provide the most exciting possibility of strengthening bone structure. Bisphosphonates work by inhibiting osteoclastic bone resorption.[61] The spectrum of diseases that may cause bone loss in children is lengthy. The most prevalent ones are steroid-induced osteoporosis, arthritis, and disease states such as paraplegia and neuromuscular conditions. The review by Srivastava and Alon[61] gives an excellent discussion of bone formation and remodeling and discusses the possible role for the bisphosphonates. Current studies will provide important information on their pharmacology, including adverse effects. This field is developing rapidly.

EYE DRUGS

Ocular pharmacology for the general pediatrician is usually limited to antibiotic preparations for conjunctivitis. The list of available antibiotics has been expanded in recent years with the addition of fluoroquinolones (ciprofloxacin, ofloxacin). These provide broad-spectrum coverage, but trimethoprim-polymixin has equal coverage and is less expensive.[62] Recently, a number of medications to treat allergic conjunctivitis have become available. These are divided into 3 groups: antihistamine and mast cell stabilizers (olopatadine), nonsteroidal anti-inflammatory agents (ketorolac), and antihistamine/vasoconstrictor combinations (nahazoline-antazoline). Cost may be the major difference between these drugs. A physician should acquire experience with one or two of these agents and become knowledgeable about the frequency of dosing and side effects. Other drugs used in the eye should be in the province of the ophthalmologist with experience in pediatric eye problems. The review by Wallace and Steinkuller[62] also emphasizes the possible systemic side effects from absorption of drugs placed in the eye.

SMOKING

Nicotine patches are safe to use in adolescents, but unfortunately they do not work.[63] After 6 weeks of nicotine patch use (15 mg per 16 hours), only 11% of 101 patients had biochemically proven abstinence from cigarettes. This percentage decreased to 5% at 6 months follow-up. No behavioral modification was used in this study. Prevention is the best therapy for cigarette smoking.

TOXICOLOGY

A recent excellent review of the management of toxic ingestions by children emphasizes the following principles:[64]

- Early treatment; this will allow gastric-emptying procedures.
- Induction of emesis by ipecac has become controversial; lavage of the patient if performed early (within 1 hour of ingestion) may be effective.
- The use of activated charcoal has received much attention. It is difficult for most children to drink the volume needed, so a nasogastric tube may be necessary.
- Whole bowel irrigation with a polyethylene glycol/electrolyte such as is used for bowel preparation is also being used. Irrigation may be especially indicated for substances that are poorly absorbed by charcoal.

ACETAMINOPHEN

Acetaminophen liver damage was studied in children aged 1 to 17 years.[65] The experience in 2 large children's hospitals (Kansas City, Mo and Seattle, Wash) comprised 322 children; intentional overdose was diagnosed in 140 (43%) of these children, accidental ingestion in 172 (53%), and therapeutic overdosage in 10 (3%). Liver damage occurred in 27 patients (8%); 17.9% in the intentional group but only 0.6% in the unintentional group. The therapeutic error group had a 10% incidence of liver damage. Liver damage was especially associated with patients who were initially seen more than 24 hours after ingestion. Therapeutic poisoning with acetaminophen is of concern because of the widespread use of this antipyretic, multiple and confusing product formulations containing different concentrations of acetaminophen, and inaccurate measurements of liquid formulations.[14] Kearns et al[66] published a useful review for pediatricians, emphasizing a "high-risk profile": administration of doses of acetaminophen that exceed 90 mg/kg per day to a sick child for more than 24 hours. This profile may be compounded by the simultaneous administration of cough and cold preparations that may also contain acetaminophen (not prominently labeled).

ENVIRONMENTAL CHEMICAL EXPOSURE (POLYCHLORINATED BIPHENYLS, METHYLMERCURY, LEAD)

There is much interest in potential adverse effects of environmental chemicals both during pregnancy and in early childhood. A Dutch study examined the growth (height, weight, head circumference) of 207 children at birth, 10 days of age, and at 3, 7, 18, and 42 months of age.[67] The children were further grouped according to cord and maternal plasma concentration of polychlorinated biphenyls (PCBs). Exposure to higher levels of PCBs resulted in a 165-g decrease in birth weight compared with that of infants with a low level of PCBs. Interestingly, small decreases in growth rate were seen in bottle-fed infants, but not in breast-fed infants, up until 3 months of age. Presumably, if a decrease in growth rate is caused by increased body burdens of PCBs, the breast-fed infants should show slower growth than the bottle-fed infants because of continued exposure through the mother's milk. There was no negative effect on growth in either breast-fed or bottle-fed infants from 3 to 42 months of age. Much more data are needed to determine the effect of environmental chemical exposure of any degree on children's short- and long-term growth and especially neurodevelopment.

In the Seychelles Islands, the effect of prenatal and postnatal methylmercury exposure on neurodevelopment was studied in 711 mother-child pairs.[68] The population of these islands depends on significant quantities of fish for daily food, and hence it is estimated that methylmercury levels in these children may be 10 to 20 times higher than those present in American children. Mercury exposure was determined by maternal and child hair samples. No serum samples (n = 49) had detectable levels of PCBs. With the use of 6 neurodevelopment scales, the authors found no effect on neurodevelopment at 66 months (5.5 years) of age.

There seems to be no end to studies conducted to examine the treatment of lead exposure. In a small group of children (n = 39) with elevated blood lead concentrations (30-45 μg/dL), 20 received environmental cleanup and placebo, and 19 received environmental cleanup and 2,3-dimercaptosuccinic acid (DMSA).[69] The double-blind study attempted to control for the characteristic DMSA odor (rotten eggs) by use of placebo bottles that previously were filled with DMSA capsules and then emptied and filled with placebo capsules. After 1 month, the blood lead levels were 33.2

μg/dL for the placebo group and 27.4 μg/dL for the DMSA group (P = .16). But at the 6-month follow-up visit, the levels were 25.1 μg/dL for the placebo group and 28.8 μg/dL for the DMSA group. This small study suggests that oral chelation therapy with DMSA may offer no benefit over environmental cleanup.

ETHYLENE GLYCOL POISONING

Ethylene glycol is commonly found in antifreeze, and injestion by children can occur. The toxicity of ethylene glycol affects the kidney and brain and is mediated by the metabolites glycoaldehyde, glycolic acid, glyoxylic acid, and oxalic acid. The formation of these metabolites is catalyzed by the enzyme alcohol dehydrogenase. A very promising treatment of this poisoning is the inhibition of this enzyme by 4-methylpyrazole (fomepizole).[70] Nineteen adults aged 19 to 73 years were studied. One patient died; the 18 patients who survived all needed hemodialysis in addition to treatment with fomepizole. All 10 patients who initially had normal renal function had no deterioration. The 9 patients who initially had elevated serum creatinine levels had a decrease in their creatinine levels during therapy. The serum metabolites of ethylene glycol also decreased during therapy. Few adverse reactions to fomeprizole occurred. Although no children were in this study, fomepizole should be considered for use in the treatment of this serious poisoning.

REFERENCES

1. Food and Drug Administration: Pediatric page. http://www.fda.gov/cder/pediatric/wrstats.htm, 2000.
2. Blumer J, ed: The therapeutic orphan: 30 years later. *Pediatrics* 104:581S-645S, 1999.
3. Bush PJ, Ozias JM, Walson PD, et al: Ten guiding principles for teaching children and adolescents about medicines. *Clin Ther* 21:1280-1284, 1999.
4. Menacker F, Aramburuzabala P, Minian N, et al: Children and medicines: What they want to know and how they want to learn. *J Soc Adm Pharm* 16:38-52, 1999.
5. Pharmaceutical Research and Manufacturers of America: *New Medicines in Development for Children 2000.* Washington, DC: Pharma, 2000.
6. Kearns G: The paediatric pharmacology research unit network: Proof of concept. *Paediatr Perinat Drug Ther* 3:9-14, 1999.
7. Simon H: Caregiver knowledge and delivery of a commonly prescribed medication (albuterol) for children. *Arch Pediatr Adolesc Med* 153:615-618, 1999.

8. Scott R, Besag F, Neville BGR: Buccal midazolam and rectal diazepam for treatment of prolonged seizures in childhood and adolescence: A randomized trial. *Lancet* 353:623-626, 1999.
9. van Lingen RA, Deinum HT, Qual CME, et al: Multiple- dose pharmacokinetics of rectally administered acetaminophen in term infants. *Clin Pharmacol Ther* 66:509-515, 1999.
10. Menniti-Ippolito F, Raschetti R, Da Cas R, et al: Active monitoring of adverse drug reactions in children. *Lancet* 355:1613-1614, 2000.
11. Kaplan MA, Prior MJ, McKonly KI, et al: A multicenter randomized controlled trial of a liquid loperamide product versus placebo in the treatment of acute diarrhea in children. *Clin Pediatr* 38:579-591, 1999.
12. Mayoral CE, Marino RV, Rosenfeld W, et al: Alternating antipyretics: Is this an alternative? *Pediatrics* 105:1009-1012, 2000.
13. Berlin CM: Fever in children: A practical approach to management. *Contemp Pediatr* 13:1S-8S, 1996.
14. Berlin CM: Acetaminophen and ibuprofen: Instructing parents on dosing. *Contemp Pediatr* 16:4S-11S, 1999.
15. Ljungman G, Kreuger A, Andreasson S, et al: Midazolam nasal spray reduces procedural anxiety in children. *Pediatrics* 105:73-78, 2000.
16. Coté C, Notterman D, Karl H, et al: Adverse sedation events in pediatrics: A critical incident analysis of contributing factors. *Pediatrics* 105:805-814, 2000.
17. Krause B, Green SM: Sedation and analgesia for procedures in children. *N Engl J Med* 342:938-945, 2000.
18. Prior M, Nelson E, Temple A: Pediatric ibuprofen use increases while incidence of Reye's syndrome continues to decline. *Clin Pediatr* 39:245-247, 2000.
19. de Silva NR, Sirisena JLGJ, Gunasekera DPS, et al: Effect of mebendazole therapy during pregnancy on birth outcome. *Lancet* 353:1145-1149, 1999.
20. Hatch EE, Palmer JR, Titus-Ernstoff L, et. al: Cancer risk in women exposed to diethylstilbesterol in utero. *JAMA* 280:630-634, 1998.
21. Committee on Drugs, American Academy of Pediatrics: Use of psychoactive medication during pregnancy and possible effects on the fetus and newborn. *Pediatrics* 105:880-887, 2000.
22. Khongphatthanayothin A, Lane J, Thomas D: Effects of cisapride on QT interval in children. *J Pediatr* 133:51-56, 1998.
23. van Haarst A, Gerben A, van't Klooster A, et al: The influence of cisapride and clarithromycin on QT intervals in healthy volunteers. *Clin Pharm Ther* 64:542-546, 1998.
24. Ward R, Lemons J, Molteni R: Cisapride: A survey of the frequency of use and adverse events in premature newborns. *Pediatrics* 103:469-472, 1999.
25. Bhatia J: Current options in the management of apnea of prematurity. *Clin Pediatr* 39:327-336, 2000.

26. Erenberg A, Leff R, Wynne B, et al: Results of the first double-blind placebo (PL)-controlled study of caffeine citrate (CC) for the treatment of apnea of prematurity (AOP). *Pediatrics* 102:756-757, 1998.
27. Stowe Z, Cohen LS, Hostetter A, et al: Paroxetine in human breast milk and nursing infants. *Am J Psychiatry* 157:185-189, 2000.
28. Chambers C, Anderson P, Thomas R, et al: Weight gain in infants breastfed by mothers who take fluoxetine. *Pediatrics* 104:e61, 1999.
29. Committee on Drugs, American Academy of Pediatrics: The transfer of drugs and other chemicals into human milk. *Pediatrics* 93:137-150, 1994.
30. McCarthy J, Posey BL: Methadone levels in human milk. *J Hum Lact* 16:115-120, 2000.
31. Finkelstein J, Metlay J, David R, et al: Antimicrobial use in defined populations of infants and young children. *Arch Pediatr Adolesc Med* 154:395-400, 2000.
32. Damoiseaux R, van Balen F, Hoes A, et al: Primary care based randomized double blind trial of amoxicillin versus placebo for acute otitis media in children aged under 2 years. *BMJ* 320:350-354, 2000.
33. Dowell S, Butler J, Giebink G, et al: Acute otitis media: Management and surveillance in an era of pneumococcal resistance: A report from the Drug-Resistant *Streptococcus pneumoniae* Therapeutic Working Group. *Pediatr Infect Dis J* 18:1-12, 1999.
34. Feder HM, Gerber MA, Randolph MF, et al: Once-daily therapy for streptococcal pharyngitis with amoxicillin. *Pediatrics* 103:47-51, 1999.
35. Huang S-W, Borum PR: Study of skin rashes after antibiotic use in young children. *Clin Pediatr* 37:601-608, 1998.
36. Wade NA, Birkhead GS, Warren BL, et al: Abbreviated regimens of zidovudine prophylaxis and perinatal transmission of the human immunodeficiency virus. *N Engl J Med* 339:1409-1414, 1998.
37. Guay L, Musoke P, Fleming T, et al: Intrapartum and neonatal single-dose nevirapine compared with zidovudine for prevention of mother-to-child transmission of HIV-1 in Kampala, Uganda: HIVNET 012 randomised trial. *Lancet* 354:795-802, 1999.
38. Culnane M, Fowler M, Lee SS, et al: Lack of long-term effects of in utero exposure to zidovudine among uninfected children born to HIV-infected women. *JAMA* 281:151-157, 1999.
39. Nachman S, Stanley K, Yogev R, et al: Nucleoside analogs plus ritonavir in stable antiretroviral therapy-experienced HIV-infected children. *JAMA* 283:492-498, 2000.
40. de Martino M, Tovo P-A, Balducci M, et al: Reduction in mortality with availability of antiretroviral therapy for children with perinatal HIV-1 infection. *JAMA* 284:190-197, 2000.
41. Farwell J, Lee Y, Hirtz D, et al: Phenobarbital for febrile seizures: Effects on intelligence and on seizure recurrence. *N Engl J Med* 322:364-369, 1990.
42. Sulzbacher S, Farwell JR, Temkin N, et al: Late cognitive effects of early treatment with phenobarbital. *Clin Pediatr* 38:387-394, 1999.

43. Painter MJ, Scher MS, Stein AD, et al: Phenobarbital compared with phenytoin for the treatment of neonatal seizures. *N Engl J Med* 341:485-489, 1999.
44. Kafali G, Erselcan T, Tanzer F: Effect of antiepileptic drugs on bone mineral density in children between ages 6 and 12 years. *Clin Pediatr* 38:93-98, 1999.
45. Committee on Nutrition, American Academy of Pediatrics: Calcium requirements of infants, children, and adolescents. *Pediatrics* 104:1152-1157, 1999.
46. Lloyd T, Chinchilli V, Johnson-Rollings N, et al: Adult female hip bone density reflects teenage sports-exercise patterns but not teenage calcium intake. *Pediatrics* 106:40-44, 2000.
47. Zito J, Safer D, dosReis S, et al: Trends in the prescribing of psychotrophic medications to preschoolers. *JAMA* 283:1025-1030, 2000.
48. Committee on Quality Improvement, Subcommittee on Attention-Deficit/Hyperactivity Disorder, American Academy of Pediatrics: Clinical practice guideline: Diagnosis and evaluation of the child with attention-deficit/hyperactivity disorder. *Pediatrics* 105:1158-1170, 2000.
49. Robison LL, Sclar DA, Skaer TL, et al: National trends in the prevalence of attention-deficit/hyperactivity disorder and the prescribing of methylphenidate among school-age children: 1990-1995. *Clin Pediatr* 38:209-217, 1999.
50. Manos M, Short E, Findling RL: Differential effectiveness of methylphenidate and Adderall in school-age youths with attention deficit/hyperactivity disorder. *J Am Acad Child Adolesc Psychiatry* 38:813-819, 1999.
51. Pelham W, Gnagy E, Chronis AM, et al: A comparison of morning-only and morning/late afternoon Adderall to morning-only, twice-daily, and three times-daily methylphenidate in children with attention-deficit hyperactivity disorder. *Pediatrics* 104:1300-1311, 1999.
52. Kolko D, Bukstein O, Barron J: Methylphenidate and behavior modification in children with ADHD and comorbid ODD or CD: Main and incremental effects across settings. *J Am Acad Child Adolesc Psychiatry* 38:578-586, 1999.
53. Law SF, Schachar RJ: Do typical clinical doses of methylphenidate cause tics in children treated for attention-deficit hyperactivity disorder? *J Am Acad Child Adolesc Psychiatry* 38:944-951, 1999.
54. Nolan EF, Gadow KD, Sprafkin J: Stimulant medication withdrawal during long-term therapy in children with comorbid attention-deficit hyperactivity disorder and chronic multiple tic disorder. *Pediatrics* 103:730-737, 1999.
55. March JS, Biederman J, Wolkow R, et al: Sertraline in children and adolescents with obsessive-compulsive disorder. *JAMA* 280:1752-1756, 1998.
56. Qureshi F, Pedtian J, Davis P, et al: Effect of nebulized ipratropium on the hospitalization rates of children with asthma. *N Engl J Med* 339:1030-1035, 1998.

57. Zorc JJ, Pusic M, Ogbern CJ, et al: Ipratropium bromide added to asthma treatment in the pediatric emergency department. *Pediatrics* 103:748-752, 1999.
58. Gries DM, Moffitt DR, Pulos E, et al: A single dose of intramuscularly administered dexamethasone acetate is as effective as oral prednisone to treat asthma exacerbations in young children. *J Pediatr* 136:298-303, 2000.
59. Winkelstein M, Huss K, Butz A, et al: Factors associated with medication self-administration in children with asthma. *Clin Pediatr* 39:337-345, 2000.
60. Lovell D, Giannini E, Reiff A, et al: Etanercept in children with polyarticular juvenile rheumatoid arthritis. *N Engl J Med* 342:763-769, 2000.
61. Srivastava T, Alon US: Bisphosphonates: From grandparents to grandchildren. *Clin Pediatr* 38:687-702, 1999.
62. Wallace DK, Steinkuller PG: Ocular medications in children. *Clin Pediatr* 37:645-652, 1998.
63. Hurt R, Croghan G, Beede S, et al: Nicotine patch therapy in 101 adolescent smokers. *Arch Pediatr Adolesc Med* 154:31-37, 2000.
64. Shannon M: Ingestion of toxic substances by children. *N Engl J Med* 342:186-191, 2000.
65. Alander SW, Dowd D, Bratton SL, et al: Pediatric acetaminophen overdose. *Arch Pediatr Adolesc Med* 154:346-350, 2000.
66. Kearns G, Leeder J, Wasserman G: Acetaminophen intoxication during treatment: What you don't know can hurt you. *Clin Pediatr* 39:133-144, 2000.
67. Patandin S, Koopman-Esseboom C, De Ridder MAJ, et al: Effects of environmental exposure to polychlorinated biphenyls and dioxins on birth size and growth in Dutch children. *Pediatr Res* 44:538-545, 1998.
68. Davidson PW, Myers GJ, Cox C, et al: Effects of prenatal and postnatal methylmercury exposure from fish consumption on neurodevelopment: Outcomes at 66 months of age in the Seychelles Child Development Study. *JAMA* 280:701-707, 1998.
69. O'Connor M, Rich D: Children with moderately elevated lead levels: Is chelation with DMSA helpful? *Clin Pediatr* 38:325-331, 1999.
70. Brent J, McMartin K, Phillips S, et al: Fomepizole for the treatment of ethylene glycol poisoning. *N Engl J Med* 340:832-838, 1999.

Index

B

C

D

F

G

H

I

J

K

L

M

O

P

Q

R

S

T

U

Z

Order your *Advances* today! Simply complete and detach this card and drop it in the mail to receive the latest information in your field.

Information and insights you won't find anywhere else—straight from the experts!

YES! Please start my subscription to the ***Advances*** checked below with the current volume according to the terms described below.* I understand that I will have 30 days to examine each annual edition.

Please Print:

Name ______________________

Address ______________________

City ______________ State ________ ZIP ________

Method of Payment

❑ Check (payable to **Mosby**; add the applicable sales tax for your area)

❑ VISA ❑ MasterCard ❑ AmEx ❑ Bill me

Card number ______________ Exp. date ________

Signature ______________________

❑ **Advances in Anesthesia**
$93.00 (Avail. December)

❑ **Advances in Cardiac Surgery**
$97.00 (Avail. January)

❑ **Advances in Dermatology**
$95.00 (Avail. November)

❑ **Advances in Internal Medicine**
$89.00 (Avail. December)

❑ **Advances in Nephrology**
$96.00 (Avail. October)

❑ **Advances in Otolaryngology—Head and Neck Surgery**
$99.00 (Avail. July)

❑ **Advances in Pediatrics**
$89.00 (Avail. July)

❑ **Advances in Surgery**
$85.00 (Avail. October)

❑ **Advances in Vascular Surgery**
$95.00 (Avail. October)

**Your Advances service guarantee:*

When you subscribe to an ***Advances***, you will receive notice of future annual volumes about two months before publication. To receive the new edition, you need do nothing—we'll send you the new volume as soon as it is available. (Applicable sales tax is added to each shipment.) If you want to discontinue, the advance notice allows you time to notify us of your decision. If you are not completely satisfied, you have 30 days to return any ***Advances***.

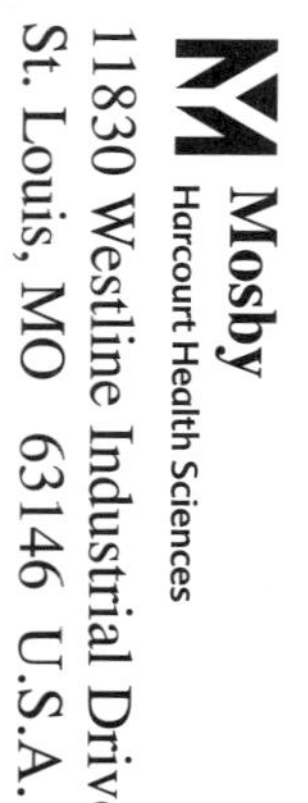

BUSINESS REPLY MAIL

FIRST-CLASS MAIL PERMIT NO 7135 ORLANDO FL

POSTAGE WILL BE PAID BY ADDRESSEE

PERIODICALS ORDER FULFILLMENT DEPT
MOSBY
HARCOURT HEALTH SCIENCES
6277 SEA HARBOR DR
ORLANDO FL 32821-9852

VISIT OUR HOME PAGE!

www.mosby.com/periodicals